Every Family in the Land

Understanding prejudice and discrimination against people with mental illness

REVISED EDITION

Edited by

Arthur H Crisp

MD, DSc, FRCP, FRCP(Ed), FRCPsych

Emeritus Professor of Psychological Medicine, University of London;
Chairman, Changing Minds Campaign, Royal College of Psychiatrists

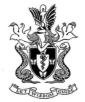

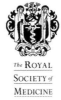

The ROYAL
SOCIETY of
MEDICINE

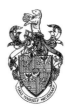

British Library Cataloguing in Publication Data
A catalogue record for this book is available from the British Library

ISBN 1-85315-573-X

Distribution in Europe and Rest of World:
Marston Book Services Ltd, PO Box 269, Abingdon, Oxon OX14 4YN, UK
Tel: +44 (0)1235 465500   Fax +44 (0)1235 465555

Distribution in the USA and Canada:
Royal Society of Medicine Press Ltd, c/o Jamco Distribution Inc, 1401 Lakeway Drive,
Lewisville, TX 75057, USA
Tel: +1 800 538 1287   Fax: +1 972 353 1303
E-mail: jamco@majors.com

Cover photograph: Pine carving 'The Arrangement' by Arthur Crisp. Photograph by Toby Crisp (www.tobycrisp.co.uk)

Phototypeset by Phoenix Photosetting, Chatham, Kent
Printed and bound in Great Britain by Goodmanbaylis, Worcester

Contents

Contributors

Ian Ainsworth-Smith, MA
Chaplain, St George's Hospital, London and Honorary Canon, Southwark Cathedral, London, UK

V Y Allison-Bolger, MB, ChB, MRCPsych
Consultant Psychiatrist, Cumbria, UK

Anon
Members, Action on Addiction, UK

Janey Antoniou, MSc
Service user, UK

Tom Arie, CBE, FFPHM, FRCPsych, FRCP
Professor Emeritus of Health Care of the Elderly, Nottingham University, UK

Simon Armson, MSc, FRSA
Chief Executive, The Samaritans, London, UK

Susan Bailey, MB, ChB, FRCPsych
Consultant Adolescent Forensic Psychiatrist, Manchester; Chairman, Children's Working Party, Changing Minds Campaign, Royal College of Psychiatrists, London, UK

Annie Bartlett, MA, MPhil, MB, BChir, MRCPsych
Senior Lecturer and Consultant in Forensic Psychiatry, St George's Hospital Medical School, London, UK

Anthony W Bateman, MA, MB, BS, FRCPsych
Consultant Psychiatrist in Psychotherapy, Halliwick Psychotherapy Unit, St Ann's Hospital, London, UK

Robert Bluglass, CBE, MD, FRCP, FRCPsych
Emeritus Professor of Forensic Psychiatry, University of Birmingham, UK

Nicky Bryant, BSc
Development Director, Downing College, Cambridge; formerly Chief Executive, Eating Disorders Association, Norwich, UK

Tom Burns, MD, DSc, FRCPsych
Professor of Social Psychiatry, University of Oxford, UK

Peter Byrne, MA, MB, MRCPsych
Senior Lecturer and Consultant Psychiatrist, University College London; Chairman, Media Working Party, Changing Minds Campaign, Royal College of Psychiatrists, London, UK

Marco Chiesa, MD, MRCPsych
Cassel Hospital, London, UK

Anthony Clare, MD, FRCPI, FRCPsych
Professor of Psychiatry, University of Dublin, Eire

Jeremy Coid, MD, FRCPsych
Professor of Forensic Psychiatry, University of London, UK

Christopher Cordess, MA, MB, ChB, FRCP, FRCPsych
Honorary Professor of Forensic Psychiatry, University of Sheffield, UK

John Cox, DM, FRCP(Ed), FRCPsych
Professor of Psychiatry, Keele University; former President (1999–2002), Royal College of Psychiatrists, London, UK

Arthur Crisp, MD, DSc, FRCP, FRCP(Ed), FRCPsych
Chairman, Changing Minds Campaign, Royal College of Psychiatrists, London; President 1999–2000, Section of Psychiatry, Royal Society of Medicine; Emeritus Professor of Psychological Medicine, University of London, UK

Sidney Crown, MRCS, LRCP, PhD, FRCP, FRCPsych
Consulting Psychotherapist, Royal London Hospital, London, UK

Carla Drahorad, MA
Cassel Hospital, London, UK

Mary Eminson, MA, MB, ChB, MRCPsych
Consultant Child Psychiatrist, Lancashire, UK

Dylan Evans, PhD
Department of Philosophy, King's College London, UK

Clive Evers, MBE, BA
Director of Information and Education, Alzheimer's Society, London, UK

Philip Fennell, PhD
Reader in European and Medical Law, Cardiff Law School, Cardiff, UK

Peter Fenwick, MB, BChir, FRCPsych
Senior Lecturer, Institute of Psychiatry, London, UK (retired)

Simon Fleminger, MA, MB, MChir, PhD, MRCPsych
Consultant Neuropsychiatrist, Maudsley Hospital, London, UK

Michael Gelder, DM, FRCP, FRCPsych
Emeritus Professor of Psychiatry, University of Oxford; Chairman, Research Advisory Committee, Changing Minds Campaign, Royal College of Psychiatrists, London, UK

Paul Gilbert, BA, MSc, PhD, DipClinPsychol, FBPsS
Professor of Clinical Psychology, University of Derby, UK

Nicholas Glozier, MA, MSc, MRCPsych
Consultant Psychiatrist, Institute of Psychiatry, University of London, London, UK

Sir David Goldberg, DM, FRCP, FRCP(Ed), FRCPsych
Emeritus Professor of Psychiatry, Institute of Psychiatry, University of London, UK

John Gunn, MD, FRCPsych
Emeritus Professor of Forensic Psychiatry, Institute of Psychiatry, University of London, UK

Anna Harrison-Hall, MA
North Devon Hospital, Barnstaple, UK

Deborah Hart, BA, AIMPR
Head, Department of External Affairs, Royal College of Psychiatrists, London, UK

Oscar Hill, FRCP, FRCPsych
Consultant Psychiatrist (retired)

Sheila Hollins, MB, BS, FRCPsych, MRCPCH
Professor of Psychiatry of Disability, University of London, UK

Jeremy Holmes, MA, MD, FRCPsych
Consultant Psychiatrist and Psychotherapist, North Devon Hospital, Barnstaple, UK

Patricia Hughes, MSc, MB, ChB, DObstRCOG, FRCPsych
Psychoanalyst and Senior Lecturer/Consultant in Psychotherapy, St George's Hospital Medical School, London, UK

Hugo Jacobs
Service user, UK

Richard Jameson
Trustee, Community Activities Project, Ealing, London, UK

Kay Redfield Jamison, PhD
Professor of Psychiatry, Johns Hopkins School of Medicine, Baltimore, USA

Andrew Johns, MB, BS, BSc, FRCPsych
Consultant Forensic Psychiatrist and Honorary Senior Lecturer, Denis Hill Medium Secure Unit, South London and Maudsley NHS Trust, London, UK

John Kellett, MA, MB, BChir, FRCP, FRCPsych
Senior Lecturer in Psychiatry of Old Age, St George's Hospital Medical School, London, UK (retired)

Robert E Kendell, CBE, MB, BChir, FRCP, FRCP(Ed), FRCPsych
Former President (1996–1999), Royal College of Psychiatrists, London, UK and Chief Medical Officer for Scotland (deceased)

Julian Leff, MD, FRCPsych, FFPHM
Emeritus Professor of Social and Cultural Psychiatry, Institute of Psychiatry, University of London, UK

Rosemary Lethem, MA, MB, BChir, PhD, MRCPsych
Consultant Psychiatrist, Sheffield, UK

Nicky Lidbetter, BSc
Honorary Assistant Director, National Phobics Society; Non-executive Director, Manchester Mental Health Partnership, UK

Roland Littlewood, MB, DPhil, FRCPsych
Professor of Anthropology and Psychiatry, University of London, UK

Sally Mitchison, BA, MB, BS, MRCPsych
Consultant Psychiatrist, Sunderland, Tyne and Wear, UK

Charles Montgomery, MB, BS, MRCPsych
Wonford House Hospital, Exeter, UK

Parimala Moodley, MB, ChB, FRCPsych
Consultant Psychiatrist, South West London and St George's Mental Health NHS Trust, UK

John F Morgan, MA, MB, BChir, MRCPsych
Senior Lecturer, Department of Psychiatry, St George's Hospital Medical School, University of London, UK

Julia Neuberger, MA
Rabbi; Chief Executive, King's Fund, London, UK

Susan Noakes, BSc
Formerly Acting Executive Director, Depression Alliance, UK

Kingsley Norton, MD, FRCPsych
Senior Lecturer in Forensic Psychiatry, St George's Hospital Medical School, London; Consultant Psychiatrist, Henderson Hospital, Sutton, UK

Anton Obholzer, MB, ChB, FRCPsych
Consultant Psychiatrist, Tavistock Clinic, London, UK

Mawlana Sikander Khan Pathan
Liaison Officer/Muslim Chaplain, Balham Mosque and Tooting Islamic Centre, London, UK

Jill Peay, BSc, PhD
Barrister at Law, Reader in Law, London School of Economics and Political Science, UK

Rachel Perkins, BA, MPhil, PhD, FBPsS
Consultant Clinical Psychologist and Clinical Director, Rehabilitation and Continuing Care Service, South West London and St George's Mental Health NHS Trust, UK

Brice Pitt, MD, FRCP, FRCPsych
Professor Emeritus, Psychiatry of Old Age, University of London; Chairman, Road Show Working Party, Changing Minds Campaign, Royal College of Psychiatrists, London, UK

Barbara Pointon, BMus
Family carer, member of local committee of the Alzheimer's Society; formerly Principal Lecturer in Music, Homerton College, Cambridge, UK

Roy Porter, BA, PhD
Professor of the History of Medicine, The Wellcome Trust, London, UK (deceased)

Felix Post, MD, FRCP, FRCPsych
Formerly Emeritus Physician, Bethlem and Maudsley NHS Trust, London, UK
(deceased)

Andrew Powell, MA, MB, BChir, MRCP, FRCPsych
Consultant Psychotherapist, Oxford; Chair, Spirituality and Psychiatry Special
Interest Group, Royal College of Psychiatrists, London, UK (retired)

Cliff Prior, BA
Chief Executive, Rethink, London, UK

Claire Rayner, OBE
Journalist, UK

Gerald FM Russell, MD, FRCP, FRCP(Ed), FRCPsych (Hon)
Emeritus Professor of Psychiatry, University of London, UK

Mark Salter, MB, BS, MRCPsych
Consultant Psychiatrist, Homerton Hospital, London, UK

Norman Sartorius, MD
Chairman, World Psychiatric Association, Geneva, Switzerland

Duncan Selbie, MSc, MHSM, DipHSM
Chief Executive, South East London Strategic Health Authority, UK

Rosemary Shelley, BSc
Trustee, Eating Disorders Association, UK

Michael Shooter, MA, MB, BChir, FRCPsych
President, Royal College of Psychiatrists, London, UK

Andrew Steptoe, BSc, DPhil, DSc, FBPsS
Professor of Psychology, University College London, UK

Anthony Storr, MB, BChir, FRCP, FRCPsych
Formerly Honorary Consultant Psychotherapist, Oxford, UK (deceased)

George Szmukler, MD, FRCPsych, FRANZCP
Consultant Psychiatrist and Medical Director, South London and Maudsley NHS
Trust, UK

David Taylor, BSc
Helpline volunteer, National Phobics Society, UK

David Tidmarsh, MD, FRCPsych
Consultant Psychiatrist, Broadmoor Hospital, UK (retired)

Philip Timms, MRCS, LRCP, MRCPsych
Senior Lecturer in Community Psychiatry, Guy's, King's and St Thomas's School of
Medicine, London, UK

David Trotman, PhD
Formerly Chief Executive, Action on Addiction, UK

André Tylee, MD, FRCGP, MRCPsych (Hon)
GP, Surrey, UK

Fiona Warren, MA
Robert Baxter Research Fellow, St George's Hospital Medical School, London, UK

Peter D White, MD, BSc, FRCP, FRCPsych
Senior Lecturer, St Bartholomew's Hospital, London, UK

Ruth White, MA, MPhil, MRCPsych
Senior Lecturer and Honorary Consultant, Worcester Royal Infirmary, UK

Melba Wilson, BA, MSc
Chair, Wandsworth Primary Care Trust; formerly Policy Director, Mind, London, UK

Lewis Wolpert, CBE, DIC, PhD, FRS
Professor of Biology as Applied to Medicine, University College London, UK

Preface

Perspectives on stigmatisation, distancing and discrimination

Arthur Crisp

It has been my privilege to bring together in this publication contributions addressing the frequent stigmatisation of and discrimination against people with mental disorders and related mental health problems. Its origins lie in the related five-year long national campaign to reduce such stigmatisation mounted by the Royal College of Psychiatrists in the UK and Eire and launched in October 1998, and in the opportunity offered by the 1999–2000 academic programme of the Royal Society of Medicine's Section of Psychiatry, also here in the UK. The contents include texts delivered and discussed within this series of one-day conferences, plus subsequent complementary contributions. This book is a revised and updated print version of an earlier electronic publication (Crisp 2001: www.stigma.org/everyfamily).

Since the time of Goffman's seminal tome with a sociological perspective on the subject, it has often been politicised. In particular, psychiatry and psychiatrists have sometimes been castigated for worsening stigmatisation through the generation of diagnostic labels. Moreover, the caring face of medicine in respect of those who suffer mental illnesses has less often been acknowledged than the custodial roles thrust upon it by society. But doctors must also accept this responsibility for generating a new set of labels that have rapidly usurped previous ones used throughout recorded history to provide discriminatory identification; and moreover recognise that diagnostic labelling, like the stigmatising process itself, seeks potentially negative generic characteristics at the expense of individuality.

For doctors, the diagnostic process is the cornerstone of practice, hopefully not personally driven by negative so much as altruistic intent. It aspires to be a scientific method whereby, once labelled, the natural course of any presenting disorder can best be predicted, along with the impact of further interventions, including treatments. It is psychiatry's obligation, in developing such classifications, to justify this process as sufficiently often valuable for the sufferer – also, properly, to acknowledge that, as with many other illnesses, it is not always helpful and not often exclusively so. From this position it is my hope that the following text will shed some light on fundamental aspects of our seemingly intractable need to stigmatise people labelled as mentally ill, and to discriminate socially against them.

The campaign itself is entitled "Changing Minds: Every Family in the Land". The subtitle is intended to convey the widespread and common nature of many mental illnesses and mental health problems. The slogan "One in Four" has also crept into the campaign, for example as the title of a two-minute trailer film that has been shown in many UK cinemas, again to convey the lifetime risk of experiencing such a level of distress. It reminds us that mental illnesses are ubiquitous, very different one from another, and relate to the vast reservoir of people with "concealed" mental illnesses rather than just the minority of us in whom they are "visible", for example presenting with severe or chronic behavioural disabilities. Such a high risk can generate its own fears and defensive reactions. The sooner that effective preventive approaches and better psychological, social and physical treatments arise, especially those that also empower the individual, the sooner will this fear be muted.

This book has certain other features. Unashamedly – but also hopefully – humbly "medical" in its core approach, primarily it addresses half a dozen mental illness categories and those who suffer with them. These diagnostic categories and labels are respectively *anxiety disorders*, *depression* and its ramifications, *schizophrenia*, *dementia*, *eating disorders* and *excessive use of drugs and alcohol*. It is clear from the campaign's national survey of public perceptions of people with these illnesses that they attract some generic stigmatisation but also several negative perceptions that vary with the diagnostic label. We need to consider not the stigmatisation but the stigmatisations of people with one or other of this range of illnesses.

First, though, in Part 1, Roy Porter gives us a historian's scholarly perspective of the largely enduring nature of stigmatisations of people with mental illnesses. Does this constitutional tendency imply biological origins, at least for some of the mechanisms underlying the processes? Roland Littlewood shows us that there are also important culture-bound elements.

Part 2 reveals stigmatisation as experienced in the present day by those with mental illnesses, or who have suffered them in the past; also the experience of their families, carers and those in related health care professions. Two professional health carers are amongst those describing the impact of their mental illness and of others' attitudes to them. Some other contributors, who have described their illness and its stigmatising consequences most graphically, have felt the need to use pseudonyms or to remain totally anonymous, such is the potential threat of this end of the spectrum of stigmatisations. Public attitudes like these frequently reinforce the afflicted person's self-doubt and shame. Self-disclosure and related availability of help from others become more remote possibilities. Finally, in this part, we key into the experiences and views of expert professionals involved in a variety of social settings. These include the very special problems that dual and multiple stigmatisations can bring, stemming from clustering such as dual diagnosis or from an illness coupled with ethnic minority status. David Goldberg concludes with a timely "Whither psychiatry?" contribution.

Part 3 is dedicated to knowledge and theories concerning the biological, social and psychological origins of the human propensity to stigmatise others. Why do we have this exaggerated tendency to regard some others negatively? What behaviours do they exhibit that trigger these reactions in us? If we are to tackle such crude and damaging responses in order to protect both the mentally ill and ourselves, then we need to understand ourselves better than our natures and our present upbringings readily permit.

Part 4 addresses all seven mental disorders. Authors have been charged with exploring the extent to which knowledge, notions or theories concerning the causes of these illnesses, as distinct from their expression, contribute to our negative perceptions of people experiencing them. Does an exclusive belief in heredity sometimes bring absolution from personal responsibility or, contrariwise, indictment based on a notion of immutable taint. Mental illnesses, so often identified as part and parcel of the sufferer him- or herself, can be a major challenge to the need to believe in free will and choice, which is a core ingredient of mankind's existence in many cultures.

Part 5 attempts to address the vexed question of "personality disorder", perhaps the most controversial of all current medical diagnostic labels, and potentially one of the most stigmatising. Often defined by attributes such as persistent antisocial behaviour or social inadequacy, it bears the same uncomfortable relationship to psychiatric illness as does another constitutional condition – obesity – to physical illnesses. Are they in fact "illnesses"? By definition constitutional in nature, both conditions are identified as risk factors for "other" illnesses, and invoke strong professional and social needs for intervention. In this part, authors attempt to make sense of this matter and, importantly, examine the potential for enlightened understanding and help that might justify application of the medical diagnostic process to this particular arena.

When personality disorder is discussed, the Law cannot be far behind, and Part 6 is devoted to it. At its worst the Law ensures that the solutions to related social problems are reduced to their under-resourced behavioural manipulation by others (e.g. psychiatrists), who also then become damaged by stigmatisation. Ideally the Law provides a vehicle for sensitive and enlightened intervention that best serves the interests of all concerned. Whereas these days other groups of disadvantaged disabled people fight vigorously for their rights, this is much less often the case with the mentally ill. In this context it will be important to discover how the new human rights legislation in the UK may strengthen the capacity of people with mental illness to defend themselves with or without external advocacy.

Suffering has long been linked to the peaks of human creativity and nobility of spirit. Aristotle saw it as invariably so. It is also an idea that underwrites Christianity and other religions. In Puritan times depression was seen as the proper condition for mankind. Experiencing and acknowledging it did not block the creative outpourings of either Milton or Bunyan. Burton, floundering in a chronic melancholy state, was able, insightfully, to compose and have published his *Anatomy of Melancholy*. Can the mental suffering associated with mental illnesses and vulnerability to them ever breed the kind of creativity that mankind values so highly? Is it a prerequisite? Severe mental illness can lead to a barren existence, but how often is it true that, as Schultz, creator over decades of the immortal *Peanuts* cartoon strip, is alleged to have said: "All is a product of anxiety and melancholy"? Was Tchaikowsky's alleged and tortured suppression of his homosexuality the essential driving force to his creativity? Is Elgar's cello concerto a product of his grief at the destruction of an era? Was Byron's periodic anorexia nervosa essential to his poetic productivity? Was Proust's obsessive/compulsive disorder the basis of his monumental texts? In Part 7 we are priviliged to sit in on excellent discourses on this matter. Relatedly, eight colour plates carry reproductions of paintings produced by artists, some of them professional, which also reflect poignantly their states of mind.

Spirituality not only can enable us to accept suffering but can also breed compassion and love. The churches today are sometimes to the fore in befriending people who briefly or otherwise develop mental illnesses. Religions can provide compassionate teaching, guidelines and rules of conduct that find their expressions within such befriending and caring approaches to those with mental illness. The origins of befriending – biological, religious and secular – are central to our further understanding of attitudes to people with mental illnesses. Part 8 is the product of inviting representatives of three religious groups in the UK to explore these matters.

Since the spirit of this publication is to analyse and understand as much as possible in order to do something about the stigmatisation of the mentally ill, Part 9 is devoted to proposals to reduce it and its related social discrimination. Since lack of empathy with the mentally ill is a strident statement by those allegedly mentally well, the advice that we stop and listen is timely, as is the pioneering project to discriminate positively in favour of the mentally ill within the workplace. Also timely is the need to improve legislation to protect those disabled by mental illnesses. Is it possible to practise medicine given a propensity for mental illness? Two authors show us that it can be done and how it can be done. Doctors are no more immune to mental illnesses than others, and with one in four of us vulnerable, nor should they expect to be. Reference is also made here to other concurrent campaigns to tackle stigmatisation. The publication concludes with outlines of the current Royal College of Psychiatrists' Campaign and its toolkit (www.changingminds.co.uk) and a final chapter addressing possible origins of our need to label others, often negatively, when a mental illness is the affliction.

Finally, the overall text is bracketed between contributions – Foreword and Epilogue – by two successive presidents of the Royal College of Psychiatrists.

As a "medical" signature to this piece, may I remind us that experiences, translated into memory and its development, are contingent on the latter's biology. This includes the chemical changes associated with learning and unlearning that are available to harness new information and discard harmful memories. Whilst this may be a slow process, it may also be long-lasting.

Arthur H Crisp

Acknowledgements

First and foremost, I am deeply grateful to the authors. Some of them contributed to the original Royal Society of Medicine's Section of Psychiatry academic programme, 1999-2000, which was inspired by the Changing Minds Campaign of the Royal College of Psychiatrists. The complex assemblage of those initial authors owes a great deal to the crucial help given to me at the time by Mrs Liz Cowan, the campaign administrator. My very grateful thanks go to her. The programme and this book have also received a seal of approval from the College campaign and the College itself. The Editor values this greatly and is most appreciative.

More than anyone else, Mrs Heather Humphrey has subsequently helped me to develop the book. This has involved engaging many more authors to flesh out and add to the book's themes. Above all it has involved a sustained effort of communication with all the authors, coupled with many hours of careful copyediting and liaison with publishers. I am deeply grateful to her and also to her husband, Dr Michael Humphrey, who expertly and freely proofread every chapter.

Initially the book was published in electronic form, both on its own website (www.stigma.org/everyfamily) and as a CD-ROM. This was funded jointly by the Sir Robert Mond Memorial Trust (I am deeply grateful for the encouragement and sustained support of Richard Hornsby, Chief Executive), and the Section of Psychiatry of the Royal Society of Medicine. At this stage the RSM also formally approved and endorsed the book.

Now, through the generosity of Partnerships in Care (PiC), we are also able to publish this revised and updated print version. I am deeply grateful to Peter Farrier, Managing Director of PiC, for this support. In this electronic age many of us still hanker after bound books that we can pick up and carry round and read anywhere. The colour plates are an addition, funded again through the generosity of the RSM's Section of Psychiatry. They depict paintings and sculptures held in the Bethlem Museum and have been generously made available through the professional guidance, energy and goodwill of the Chief Archivist, Patricia Allderidge. Alison Campbell, Managing Editor, and her assistants at RSM Press have been tremendous in their enthusiasm and professional approach.

The good things about this book are due to the input of those people I have referred to above. Any deficiencies are down to the Editor. We all hope that readers will find this work useful and informative.

AHC

This publication has been sponsored by Partnerships in Care
www.partnershipsincare.co.uk

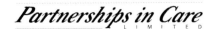

Provider of specialist mental health services

Foreword

Why stigma matters

Robert E Kendell

The stigma of mental illness is in many ways both the most important handicap people with mental disorders have to face and the most important challenge confronting contemporary psychiatric services. It is the stigma, and the feelings of guilt and shame, or the defensive denial, that go with it, that makes people with psychiatric symptoms reluctant to seek treatment, or even to accept that their symptoms exist and might be a manifestation of mental disorder.

Anyone who has suffered from a mental illness is liable to be discriminated against, even if they have made a full recovery. Once the label has been pinned to them it is harder for them to obtain employment commensurate with their skills, to marry anyone who is not similarly afflicted themselves, to obtain a mortgage, to emigrate or even to obtain holiday insurance. As a result, their self-esteem and self-assurance are undermined. Stigma also contributes to the persistent underfunding of services for the mentally ill. When there is intense competition for resources, as there frequently is, any new funds tend to go to services for the kinds of patients the public regard as most deserving: children with life-threatening diseases, perhaps, or people with cancer or heart disease, but not the mentally ill. And when there is a financial crisis – an oft-recurring situation in the NHS – ministers and managers quickly learn that the easiest budget to cut, because it is the least likely to provoke a public outcry, is the mental health budget (Bottomley 1998).

The causes of this stigmatisation are complex and largely derived from deeply rooted cultural attitudes to madness, and assumptions about the nature of mental illness. The behaviour of people identified by their fellows as mad, or by psychiatrists as psychotic, is often bizarre and unpredictable, and occasionally violent. They may be preoccupied with absurd beliefs and imaginary voices, and express emotions quite inappropriate to their circumstances. More fundamentally, their responses to ordinary social cues and expectations are strange and unnerving, and as a result their friends, neighbours and relatives can no longer identify with them, or understand why they behave as they do. This loss of the ability to identify or empathise is crucial in setting the scene for stigmatisation, and it is made worse by the anxiety that madness provokes. Our concept of ourselves as rational beings guided by reason and intelligence is crucial to our self-confidence and self-esteem; and encountering a fellow human being who has lost their reason and whose behaviour is no longer rational is profoundly disturbing, because it implies that the same might happen to us. That is why the mentally ill are mocked as well as feared, for mockery reduces the implied threat they pose. It is also why we are so keen to establish a clear gulf between the mentally ill and normal people like ourselves. The idea that mental health and psychosis might merge into one another is disturbing and unwelcome because it draws attention to the possibility of a transition from the former to the latter. In most cultures, including our own, madness is regarded as lifelong and incurable, despite the occurrence of prolonged periods of quite normal behaviour. It is also regarded as hereditary, although other less dramatic mental disorders, like depressions and anxiety states, are commonly attributed to lack of willpower or weakness of character.

Psychiatrists try to insist that there is no fundamental difference between mental illness and physical illness, that the boundary between them is arbitrary and that the distinction between them is based on long-discredited philosophical assumptions about the relationship between mind and matter. Unfortunately this cuts no ice, either with laymen or even with other doctors. Cultural assumptions about the nature of mental illness are too deeply rooted to be susceptible to rational arguments. Only vivid personal experiences incompatible with the stereotype are adequate to bring about change.

Even so, the stigma is almost certainly reducing, but decade by decade rather than year by year. People who are, or have been, mentally ill are currently stigmatised less in Western Europe and North America than in most other parts of the world, and less now than they were a generation ago. This is partly in response to the availability of demonstrably effective treatments that have greatly improved the outlook for several types of illness. It is also in response to increasing awareness of the ubiquity and diversity of mental illness. All stigmatised minorities, whether they be homosexuals, cowards or the mentally ill, are stigmatised in part because they are assumed to be small, clearly defined minorities. Once it becomes apparent that the stigmatised behaviour or minority is actually quite common, and often merges insensibly into what we regard as normality, it becomes much harder to regard such people as fundamentally different. This is one of many reasons why the World Health Organization's demonstration that in Europe depressive illness ranks with ischaemic heart disease and cerebrovascular disease as one of the three leading contributors to the overall burden of disease is so welcome (Murray and Lopez 1997).

As the stigma declines people slowly become more willing to admit to themselves, to their friends and relatives and to the wider public that they are, or have been, mentally ill. People are more willing now than they were even a decade ago to admit to having had a depressive illness, or to having an adolescent daughter with anorexia nervosa or a parent with dementia. Ronald Reagan and his family were able to say publicly that he was suffering from Alzheimer's disease. Twenty years earlier Harold Wilson and his family were not. Schizophrenia, though, is usually still veiled in the euphemism, "mental health problems", and contemporary politicians appear to regard it as more electorally damaging to reveal their history of mental illness than their homosexuality. The insistence of many people suffering from chronic debilitating fatigue that, whatever the medical profession may say, they are suffering from a genuine "organic" illness – ME or myalgic encephalomyelitis – is another telling illustration of the stigma still associated with mental illness and the lengths to which people will go to avoid any suggestion that their symptoms might be psychogenic.

It was against this background that the Royal College of Psychiatrists launched its Changing Minds Campaign in October 1998 and, a year later, that the Royal Society of Medicine's Section of Psychiatry arranged a series of five multidisciplinary conferences on the theme of reducing the stigmatisation of mental disorders. The College's campaign is running for five years and, as with its earlier Defeat Depression Campaign, the attitudes of a representative sample of the general adult population were assessed beforehand to establish a baseline against which to measure subsequent change. Six different types of mental illness will be targeted in the course of the campaign – schizophrenia, dementia, depressions, anxiety states, alcohol and drug dependence, and eating disorders – and simple factual information about each is being widely disseminated in leaflet form. The ubiquity of these and other mental disorders is also emphasised by the campaign's central slogan: "Every Family in the Land". The College realises, though, that factual information alone, however skilfully it is worded and however widely it is promulgated, can never combat stigma effectively on its own.

The various target audiences, from schoolchildren to the general public to the medical profession itself, will need to be involved emotionally as well as intellectually if entrenched attitudes are to change. To this end, much time and energy are being devoted to the preparation of videotapes, of a brief film to be shown alongside the advertisements in cinemas throughout the land, and to ways of confronting the medical profession – including psychiatrists themselves – with its own use of stigmatising, derogatory terms to refer to patients with various kinds of mental illness.

No one expects the stigmatisation of mental illness to have ceased to be a significant problem by the time the campaign ends in the autumn of 2003, but if the College and the other organisations working alongside it can perceptibly speed up the slow waning of stigmatisation and discrimination, it will have achieved something of real importance.

References

Bottomley V (1998) Letter to *The Times* (London), Monday 16 February.

Murray CJL & Lopez AD (1997) Global mortality, disability and the contribution of risk factors: Global Burden of Disease Study. *Lancet* **349**: 1436–42.

Dedication

This book is dedicated to all those who have experienced stigmatisations as a result of their mental illnesses; and to the aims of the Royal College of Psychiatrists' anti-stigma campaign, 1998–2003.

Part 1

The history of stigmatisation of the mentally ill

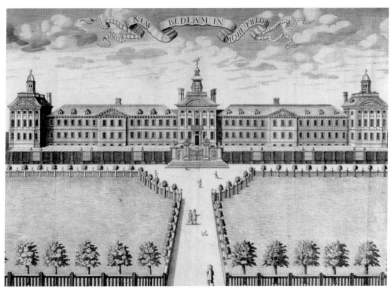

Bethlem Hospital at Moorfields

1

Is mental illness inevitably stigmatising?

Roy Porter

If stigma is, in Goffman's definition, "the situation of the individual who is disqualified from full social acceptance", historically speaking the mentally ill have borne the brunt of stigma more than most other disadvantaged groups. This chapter attempts to show how many subsidiary processes have contributed to this deplorable outcome; including institutionalisation, diagnostic specificity, visualisation and legal penalisation. At the same time it points out that the attribution of mental illness has served, at some times, as a *destigmatising device*, to obviate what were perceived as worse taints, notably, back in the sixteenth and seventeenth centuries, possession by the Devil.

In more recent times two main circumstances have contributed to lessening the stigmatising functions of mental illness. On the one hand, the complaint in question can be ascribed to a somatic (rather than a spiritual or psychological) source, as with the diagnosis of a neurological origin. On the other hand, the malady can be argued to be an affliction of a superior set of people. Somatisation and gentrification combined in the eighteenth century in the case of 'the English malady' and in the nineteenth in neurasthenia.

Thirty years ago, Ida Macalpine and Richard Hunter declared that mad King George had never been mad at all. Rather, the third Hanoverian had been suffering from variegate porphyria, an inherited metabolic condition. Proclaiming the significance of these findings, the mother-and-son psychiatric pair made much of the notion that the monarch had at long last been rescued from what Macalpine called the 'taint' of madness – he had, thank goodness, been suffering all the time from a relatively clean, respectable organic disease. Mental disorder has commonly attracted aspersions of disgrace (Macalpine and Hunter 1969). How interesting then, that, in the twentieth century, psychiatrists – of all people! – can still be heard calling it a 'taint'!

Modern thinking about stigma is indebted, above all, to the work of Erving Goffman, who defined it as "the situation of the individual who is disqualified from full social acceptance" and thus explained its roots:

> *"The Greeks, who were apparently strong on visual aids, originated the term stigma to refer to bodily signs designed to expose something unusual and bad about the moral status of the signifier. The signs were cut or burnt into the body and advertised that the bearer was a slave, a criminal, or a traitor – a blemished person, ritually polluted, to be avoided, especially in public places.*
>
> *Later, in Christian times, two layers of metaphor were added to the term: the first referred to bodily signs of holy grace that took the form of eruptive blossoms on the skin; the second, a medical allusion to this religious allusion, referred to bodily signs of physical disorder. Today the term is widely used in something like the original literal sense, but is applied more to the disgrace itself than to the bodily evidence of it. Furthermore, shifts have occurred in the kinds of disgrace that arouse concern."*
>
> (Goffman 1970)

Goffman taught us to think of stigma not as a natural mark of inferiority but as a product of social labelling. Stigmatising involves projecting onto an individual or group judgments about what is inferior, repugnant, or disgraceful. It translates disgust into the disgusting, apprehensions of danger into the dangerous. It is thus the creation of spoiled identity; first it singles out difference, next calls it inferiority, and finally blames those who are different for their otherness.

Some, for instance the American scholar Sander Gilman, see this demonising process operating primarily in psychological and anthropological ways, regarding it as an almost inescapable consequence of the human tendency to order the world by way of demarcating selfhood and otherness – Black and White, Insiders and Outsiders, Natives and Foreigners, Gay and Straight, Pure and Polluted, and so forth. In such books as *Difference and Pathology* and *Disease and Representation*, Gilman has drawn attention to our deep-seated, indeed unconscious need to construct such "them-and-us" schemes, in which our fragile sense of self-identity is reinforced through the pathologization of pariahs. To set the sick apart sustains the fantasy that we are whole (Gilman 1985, 1988). Disease may thus constitute a powerful classificatory tool, and medicine has contributed its fair whack to the stigmatising enterprise. Amongst the many groups scapegoated and anathematised by this "them and us" cognitive apartheid, those branded insane have, of course, been prominent.

How stigmatising has worked in the case of insanity has attracted widespread attention. Michel Foucault for instance argued that the mad became more decisively discriminated against from late medieval times because they filled the gap in the exclusionary imagination left by lepers, those unclean creatures, officially treated as socially dead nonpersons, who were then beginning to disappear from Europe (Foucault 1961). Thomas Szasz, who has highlighted the sinister elision between the noun "invalid" and the adjective "invalid", notably maintained that the stigmatising of the mad was the successor to the hunting of the witch. Madness thus was a witch-hunting charge pinned upon "deviants", both to enhance social control through victim-blaming, and also to further psychiatric empire-building (Szasz 1970, 1972).

One stigma will work to reinforce another. The blot of mental illness has been variously deepened by the taints of ugliness, blackness, homosexuality or femaleness (the stigmatisation of the madwoman is a topic too vast to be addressed here, and so I shall say no more about it) (Showalter 1986; Gilman 1989). Tarring with the same brush and guilt by association have been common. Psychiatrists often complain that their own specialty is itself, by association, tainted with the stigma of mental illness - they are, you might say, hoist on their own petard.

I shall not, however, in this brief account even begin to venture anything like a potted history of the stigmatisation of the mentally ill from the palaeolithic to the present, a task both grandiose and sterile (Fabrega 1990, 1991a,b). Rather, I wish to single out a few areas for discussion, each intended to illuminate the question posed in my title: is mental illness inevitably stigmatising?

And I shall begin with a counter-example designed to show that, *pace* Szasz, the category of mental illness has occasionally worked to the opposite effect. Consider witchcraft. Throughout the early modern period, the witch was perhaps the supreme stigma-carrier, for she would quite literally bear on her body the *stigmata diaboli* – blemishes, warts, moles or birthmarks, often to be found in "secret places", for instance the armpit or the genitals. In *maleficium* accusations, much hinged upon interpretation of those *stigmata* (which, in heinous cases, might be invisible) (Sharpe 1996; Thomas 1971).

To sustain a witchcraft charge in court, certain standard behavioural and physical manifestations normally had to be proven via formal forensic procedures. Expert witnesses were heard, amongst them physicians. There is no reason to assume that physicians entertained a greater scepticism towards the reality of witchcraft and diabolism than other accredited experts: their testimony was often positive and ended in convictions. But familiarity with the vagaries of the diseased organism, and the opportunity to contest authority with the clergy, often led doctors to insist that supposed signs of possession – convulsions, anaesthesias, tics, swoonings, trances, and so forth – were the work not of Satan but of sickness. Ambroise Paré and Johannes Wier, eminent sixteenth-century practitioners, published treatises showing how natural malaises like melancholia would precipitate these manifestations. In one well-documented case, the physical origin of witchcraft symptoms was eloquently argued by the English physician, Edward Jorden, a contemporary of Shakespeare (MacDonald 1991).

With three other doctors, Jorden was summoned to testify in the case of Elizabeth Jackson, arraigned on a charge of bewitching the 14-year-old Mary Glover. This girl had begun to suffer from "fittes . . . . so fearfull, that all that were about her, supposed that she would dye"; she had become speechless and occasionally blind; her left side was anaesthetised and paralysed. Classic symptoms: but was it sorcery or sickness? Glover had initially been treated by leading physicians from the College. When she failed to respond to their treatment, they pronounced, perhaps predictably, that there was something "beyond naturall" in it. Jorden demurred, however, finding for disease.

He defended his disease theory of Glover's condition in a book whose title highlighted his claims: *A Briefe Discourse of a Disease Called the Suffocation of the Mother. Written uppon occasion which hath beene of late taken thereby, to suspect possession of an evill spirit, or some such like supernaturall power. Wherein is declared that divers strange actions and passions of the body of man, which in the common opinion are imputed to the Divill, have their true naturall causes, and do accompany this disease* (1603). Jorden named Glover's condition the "suffocation of the mother" [i.e., matrix or womb], or simply the "mother", those phrases being interchangeable in seventeenth-century parlance with "hysteria". Such symptoms as the oesophagian ball, constrictions, respiratory and digestive blockages, and panic feelings of suffocation, all pointed to a uterine pathology. In this Jorden drew heavily upon ancient authority, giving some airing to the notion, found in Hippocrates, of the wandering womb. Above all, relying on Galen, he argued that uterine irregularities – menstrual blockage, amenorrhoea, the retention of putrescent "seed", and assorted other "obstructions" – generated "vapours" which wafted through the body, inducing physical disorders in the extremities, the abdomen, and even the brain – something made possible by the sympathetic interactivity of the entire organic system. A power of "sympathy" linked the womb to the head, the seat of the imagination; to the senses, which determined feelings; and finally to the "animal soul", which governed motion – thereby producing the paroxysms, twitches, palsies, convulsive dancing, stretching, yawning, etc., so often misattributed to possession, yet properly explained by "the suffocation of the mother". Jorden's overwhelming concern was to establish a *natural* explanation.

The upshot of a medical intervention like Jorden's, if successful, might be twofold. On the positive side, it could exonerate a woman from being a diabolical accomplice, and her very life might thus be spared. On the negative, medical exposure might then draw to her the charge of being guilty of "imposture" – being a fake witch. The result might thus be both destigmatisation and restigmatisation.

Or take a further and parallel instance in which the mental illness diagnosis erased a stigma: suicide (MacDonald and Murphy 1990). Throughout Christendom "self-murder" had been both sin and crime, an offence against God and King. Since Tudor times juries had routinely returned verdicts of *felo de se* (wilful self-murder), entailing severe posthumous punishments: the corpse was denied Christian burial, being interred at a crossroads, a stake through the heart; and the felon's property was forfeit to the Crown.

As in so many other theatres of life, the Restoration and then the Enlightenment brought a transformation. It soon become standard for coroners' courts, sometimes on the basis of medical opinion, to reach a *non compos mentis* verdict, whether or not there was any real history or independent sign of mental instability in the victim: was not suicide itself proof sufficient of derangement? This medicalisation or psychologisation of self-destruction sanctioned a regular Christian burial and put a stop to the escheat of the victim's possessions. The old vilification of the suicide might thus give way to sympathy. David Hume and others offered enlightened defences of suicide, and fashionable society meanwhile condoned the deed, holding death preferable to dishonour (Minois 1999; Sprott 1961). The psychiatrisation of witchcraft and suicide affords two instances of a much broader development in Western society: the formulation of the insanity defence (Smith 1981; Walker 1968). That is a plea whose desirability is not in itself uncontroversial. Szasz for one has contended that the stigma of being labelled "mad" may be far more damaging to someone's social standing than that of being "bad". Criminalisation is less degrading than psychiatrisation, and a psychiatric record may well be more scarring, more permanent, than a criminal. In taking his punishment the felon is at least credited with free will, and he thereby repays his debts to society. Nothing is more crippling, argues Szasz, than a victim culture (Szasz 1972, 1984).

The stigma attached to mental illness has commonly been all the more dire because it has been reinforced by formidable engines of exclusion: more were locked away in lunatic asylums than in gaols, and often for longer terms. Such institutionalisation makes stigma stick by rendering difference into legal status. In his influential *Madness and Civilization*, Foucault (1961) argued that the age of reason inaugurated a Europe-wide "great confinement". All social groups identifiable with "unreason" found themselves at risk of being locked away. And if paupers, the aged and ill, ne'er-do-wells, petty criminals, prostitutes and vagabonds formed the bulk of this body of 'unreason', symbolically their leaders were the lunatics.

Foucault's point was that this "great confinement" amounted to far more than mere physical sequestration: it represented a degradation of the status of the insane. Hitherto, by dint of peculiarity, madness had possessed a fascinating power, perhaps uttering deep if obscure truths: when insanity spoke, society had listened. Once institutionalised, however, madness was robbed of all such allure, dignity and truth. It was reduced from a positive – or, at least, powerful – state to an utterly negative condition ("unreason"). Shut up in madhouses, lunatics resembled wild animals caged in a zoo: it was easy to view them not as sick people but as beasts (Foucault 1961; Scull 1993).

If institutionalisation creates and reinforces spoiled identity, so does the related agency of nomenclature. The possession of technical languages enhances the professional power to stigmatise, and naming means blaming and shaming (Burke and Porter 1995). Psychiatric labelling generally serves to turn the transient into the permanent, the superficial into the essential, and the act into the type, all supposedly indexical of the person within. The gentleman who was "easy come, easy go" with his income became a case of moral insanity, the man who practised sodomy became the homosexual, the sexually active woman the nymphomaniac (Prichard 1835; Foucault 1979).

Such habits of thought spurred the emergence, towards 1900, of new biomedical theories that deemed insanity a hereditary taint. To generations of psychiatrists whose daily occupation lay in watching living death in asylum back-wards, sober realism pointed to such "degenerationist" beliefs: disorders were ingrained; they got worse over the generations. Degenerationist psychiatry successively staked greater territorial claims to the unearthing of mental disease where it had not been suspected before. Inordinate drinking became medicalized as alcoholism, and many erotic "perversions" were freeze-framed by psychopathology in and after Richard von Krafft-Ebing's pathbreaking *Psychopathia Sexualis* (1886). Abnormal children and women, "inverts" and other "perverts" were deemed mentally ill and often confined. Such conclusions expressed the fears of an elite anxious about the dangerous degeneracy of the rabble, who, many psychiatrists warned, were endangering civilization with mental imbecility at precisely the time when Social Darwinism was warning that only fit societies would survive (Nordau 1920; Chamberlin and Gilman 1985; Dowbiggin 1985).

Seeming bearers of an *imprimatur* of reality, labels mushroom. Requiring energetic revision every few years, today's *Diagnostic and Statistical Manual* reveals a proliferation of different, and often overlapping or incompatible terminologies, some disappearing and reappearing from edition to edition, in a patently unscientific manner (Kutchins and Kirk 1997). In a postal ballot held in 1974, the members of the American Psychiatric Association voted, by a rather slim margin, to delete homosexuality from its catalogue of mental disorders. That poll followed frenzied and sometimes violent lobbying; the Association's conventions had been stormed by Gay Lib activists, and a conference had been addressed by a cloaked and hooded "Dr Anonymous", who declared himself gay and proceeded to disclose that over 200 fellow members of the Association were also homosexual, thereby in effect threatening to "out" the closet gays.

This notorious affair so utterly smacks of pantomime – the nullification of a major psychiatric disorder by ballot – that it is tempting to assume it must have been a oneoff event, uniquely scandalous. But the whole history of the *Diagnostic and Statistical Manual* has been one of non-stop wheeling and dealing, the only difference being that the diagnostic horse-trading has usually taken place behind closed doors.

DSM started small – the first edition in 1952 was a bare hundred pages – but it just grew and grew. Issued in 1994, DSM-IV ran to 900 pages and 300 disorders. This is partly because, over the years, the act of diagnosis assumed greater practical consequence: a patient with an authorized DSM-coded diagnosis is one whose treatment can be billed to third-party insurers, Health Maintenance Organisations, or Federal bodies. And diagnostic terms have come and gone like summer fashions. In some cases the fate of a candidate diagnostic category has hung in the balance. Thus in drafts for the revised DSM-III, a new entity called "Masochistic Personality Disorder" was put up for membership. Sufferers were said to display personalities disposed to make people angry, and to forego pleasures in an abnormal manner. Rightly suspecting that the Committee identified this as a woman's complaint, feminist psychiatrists exposed the diagnosis as a none too subtle way of stigmatising the victims of abusive husbands and lovers, and they turned the tables by coming up with a mirror-image diagnosis for men: "Delusional Dominating Personality Disorder". The Committee – all male, with the exception of the chairman's wife! – found this riposte hard to stomach.

The verbal languages which enact stigmatisation have been paralleled and supplemented by visual codes (Kromm 1984; Gilman 1982; MacGregor 1989). Common wisdom has assumed that madness is as madness looks, and popular assumptions of this kind have been conventionalised by artists and writers. In satires, cartoons or on the stage, the insane have standardly been depicted as ferocious, resembling wild beasts, with dishevelled locks, straw in their hair, their clothes ragged and torn, or sometimes wearing barely a stitch. Further conventions have hammered such messages home. Just as the cuckold had his horns, so it was standard in the age of Erasmus to portray the fool as a figure with a stone in the forehead, the Stone of Folly: the character flaw was thus written all over the person. The court jester and the stage fool wore motley, caps and bells, and carried bladder and pinwheel, the carnivaleseque accoutrements of folly.

Artists and writers were then joined in this stereotyping process by psychiatry itself. From the Greeks onwards, medicine claimed to be able to identify madness, no less than other conditions, through the discerning gaze. Spasms, convulsions, fainting fits, paroxysms, prostration and paralyses were taken as indications of epileptic insanity, mania, melancholy and hysteria. Physical appearance, in particular the face, was equally revealing within that holistic system of medical humoralism which saw humours, complexions and temperaments, the inner and outer, as a continuum. The choleric person, who, in the extreme case, became maniacal, suffered from excess bile or choler; the melancholic was victim of surplus black bile or melancholy, and could be identified by swarthiness of skin, dark hair and eyes or "black looks" – note, as always, the stigmatising property of blackness.

Humoral identifications were supplemented by a further medical legacy from the Greeks: physiognomy, or the art and science of using facial features to tell character and, by extension, pathology. Physiognomists believed in the significance of both permanent, anatomical, features – the size and shape of chin, nose, brow, bonestructure, etc. – and more labile aspects: a disposition to scowl, frown or smile, patterns of muscular tension, attention, animation. Artists studied the physiognomical expression of emotional extremes – crazed grief, joy, anger, rage. Case-notes kept by asylum doctors paid close attention to facial features, and students combining artistic and anatomical interests, such as Charles Bell in early nineteenth-century Britain, made special studies of the physiognomy of the mad.

Indeed the drive to identify, classify and diagnose the insane by their appearance flourished as never before in the Victorian era. Why? Because all over Europe and North America they were being swept in their droves into lunatic asylums, providing unmatched opportunities for the study of appearances en masse, and thus for the tracing of behavioural quirks over long periods. The classic Mongoloid, or Down's Syndrome type, thus became an object of scientific visibility, knowledge and interest only in the 1870s, because it was only then that vast idiots' asylums (as they were called) were established, and such people were herded together for the first time in conspicuous contiguity (Zihni 1989).

If the monster asylum gave doctors opportunities and incentives to study the appearances of lunatics, the growth of textbooks and journals, and the development of cheaper engraving and lithographic processes, led to a huge expansion in the production, reproduction and diffusion of standardised images of the insane. The medico-scientific world thus imprinted upon the minds of all interested parties the authorised representations of the madman, through a stock repertoire of illustrated medical texts.

The coming of photography then lent the enterprise further impetus and authority, for was not the subjective eye and hand of the draughtsman thereby replaced by the objective, optical science of the camera? Such psychiatrists as Hugh Diamond, superintendent at the Surrey Asylum, aspired to create a complete photographic record of insanity, so as to perfect diagnostic taxonomies, and to mark improvements or deteriorations in individual cases (Gilman 1976).

This was an ambiguous enterprise, to say the least. For one thing, with the extremely long exposures required by early photography, the patients whose traits were to be perpetuated by silver nitrate were required to sit or stand stock still for a minute or more. Clearly, they must have been made to pose. The resulting pictures were thus not documentary snapshots but projections of the profiles filling the mind's eye of medical superintendents.

These dangers – of stigma being in the eye of the beholder – stick out like a sore thumb in the chequered career of Jean-Martin Charcot, chief of the Salpêtrière from the 1860s (Micale 1987; Charcot 1987, 1991; Didi-Huberman 1982; Goetz, Bonduelle and Gelfand 1995). Charcot viewed that huge Parisian institution as a "museum of living pathology", and it became synonymous with the displaying of hysterics, neuropaths and the insane.

Systematic observation provided the basis for the vast photograph collection which Charcot built up there. Using patients and patients' photos, he was committed to unremitting scrutiny of hysterical pathology – motor and sensory symptoms, bizarre visual abnormalities, tics, migraine, epileptiform seizures, somnambulism, hallucinations, word blindness, alexia, aphasia, and so forth. For him it was axiomatic that, it being a real disease, hysteria must be biologically universal: "l'Hystérie a toujours existé", he declared, "en tous lieux et en tous temps".

And the so-called Napoleon of the neuroses did indeed have some success in mapping hysteria onto the body. He was delighted to discover, for instance, hysterogenic points, zones of hyper-sensitivity which, when fingered, provoked an attack, analogous perhaps to the pressing of an electric light switch – the direct successors, we could hardly resist saying, to the *stigmata diaboli* of the old witch trials. Such a "discovery" confirmed his conviction of the reality of what he styled "latent hysteria".

Yet his early faith that the investigation of hysteria would systematically reveal demonstrable neurological substrates proved increasingly forlorn or premature. He claimed, nevertheless, at least to have established the series of stages of manifestations, from *petite hystérie* through *hystérie ordinaire* up to the *grande attaque d'hystéro-epileptique*.

Also talented as an artist, Charcot's protégé Anselm Richer sketched innumerable cases for the Salpêtrière's teaching collection. Between them they aimed to demonstrate that a reliable pictorial record survived of hysterics throughout the course of history. On the basis of an examination of religious paintings dating from medieval times onwards, their *Les Démoniques dans l'Art* contended that the mystics, demoniacs and saints portrayed therein had typically been hitherto undiagnosed hysterics (Charcot and Richer 1887). The volume concluded with a lengthy chapter, illustrated by Richer with the plates from his own study of hysteria, on "hysteria today". This identified all the impressions of hysteria from more than thirteen centuries as prefigurations of contemporary, scientific work on hysteria. The stigmas were permanent; they had merely been wrongly interpreted.

Ours is not the first generation to question stigmatisation or to seek to counter it. Historically, as already noted, one strategy has been to seek to discredit stigma by medicalisation: the party in question is not, after all, sinful or satanic but sick, and hence absolved of blame or responsibility. Within this broad medical paradigm, certain sorts of explanations have further been construed as less stigmatising than others. In the psychiatric domain, somatic diagnoses have typically been viewed as less demeaning, through assigning the malaise not to the will or personality but to the body (Shorter 1992, 1997).

An example. The "new philosophy" which became dominant from the seventeenth century represented the body as a machine, and eighteenth-century doctors popularised the colloquial disease label "nerves" and coined the word "neurosis" (Piñero 1983). Within this mechanical model of the organism, confused thoughts, feelings and behaviour were typically attributed to some or other defect of the sense organs and their attendant nervous networks. Low spirits were represented as a cross to be borne by those swanning around in High Society, those sensitive souls singled out for superiority. Such melancholy ladies and gentlemen were, it was argued, patently not fundamentally warped in the will but deserving of sympathy. The fashionable physician, George Cheyne, flattered them in his *The English Malady* by insisting that that condition was "as much a bodily Distemper as the Small-Pox or a Fever" (Cheyne 1733). He was thus not disposed to think in terms of primary mental disorder. Nevertheless, it taxed diplomacy, he stressed, assuming a patient's friendly disposition, to find the right tactful phrases when handling conditions of that type:

> *"nervous* Distempers especially, *are under some* Kind of *Disgrace and Imputation,* in the Opinion of the *Vulgar* and *Unlearned;* they pass among the Multitude, for a lower Degree of *Lunacy,* and the first Step towards a *distemper'd Brain;* and the best Construction is *Whim, Ill-Humour, Peevishness or Particularity;* and in the Sex, *Daintiness, Fantasticalness, or Coquetry."*

> (Cheyne 1733)

Such diagnostic ambivalence among the ignorant and prejudiced challenged bedside tact:

> *"Often when I have been consulted in a Case, before I was acquainted with the Character and Temper of the Patient, and found it to be what is commonly call'd Nervous, I have been in the utmost Difficulty, when desir'd to define or name the Distemper, for fear of affronting them or fixing a Reproach on a Family or person."*

> (Cheyne 1733)

His contemporary, Richard Blackmore, reported similar difficulties. "This Disease, called Vapours in Women, and the Spleen in Men, is what neither Sex are pleased to own", he emphasised:

> *"for a doctor cannot ordinarily make his Court worse, than by suggesting to such patients the true Nature and Name of their Distemper. ... One great Reason why these patients are unwilling their Disease should go by its right Name, is, I imagine, this, that the Spleen and Vapours are, by those that never felt their Symptoms, looked upon as an imaginary and fantastick sickness of the Brain, filled with odd and irregular Ideas... the persons who feel it are unwilling to own a Disease that will expose them to Dishonour and Reproach."*

> (Blackmore 1725)

Any imputations of shamming would properly be scotched, insisted Dr Nicholas Robinson, once it was made clear that such disorders were not "imaginary Whims and Fancies, but real Affections of the Mind, arising from the real, mechanical Affections of Matter and Motion"; for "neither the Fancy, nor Imagination, nor even Reason itself ... can feign a ... a Disease that has no Foundation in Nature" (Robinson 1729).

The somatising approach to troubled spirits and disordered emotions illustrated here had an important secondary consequence. Precisely because Cheyne and others would have no truck with the notion that such disturbances were primary diseases of the soul or mind, but were rather caused by defective nerves, those very disorders could assume a certain legitimacy, even an aura. It might, indeed, be considered a badge of distinction to be suffering from the English malady, because it was, by definition, a top people's disease, rather as, in earlier centuries melancholy had been the courtier's affliction. Somatisation thus allowed it to be presented as a malady more flattering than stigmatising. Gentrification has always been a choice strategy for alleviating stigma.

Another instance of these stigma-reducing processes – gentrification and recourse to somatic diagnosis – is offered by neurasthenia. Introduced around 1860, George Beard's new disease category may be seen as a classic attempt to re-assign mental symptoms – anxiety, despair, fretfulness, insomnia and nightmares, fatigue, etc. – to neurological causes. Also nominated as a top people's condition, neurasthenia was a diagnostic label popular for a generation or two with doctors and patients alike, before it lost credibility when it failed to authenticate its claimed neurological foundations (Oppenheim 1991; Rosenberg 1962; Wessely 1995; Lutz 1995).

At that point it became easy for hostile medical critics to trash it as a fantasy or to expose the so-called neurasthenic as a fraud, the ignominious demise of the diagnosis being transferred to taint the patients themselves. It was said that at the Johns Hopkins Hospital "the neurasthenic patient is treated by physicians ... with ridicule or a contemptuous summing up of his case in the phrase 'there is nothing the matter, he is only nervous' ". In the USA Smith Jelliffe described neurasthenics as "purely mental cases. Laziness, indifference, weakness of mind and supersensitiveness characterise them all. They are ... ill because of lack of moral courage". Even those sympathetic to neurasthenics could not avoid a note of irritation and condescension. Such patients were "the terror of the busy physician", according to Guthrie Rankin, "occupied by their symptoms beyond reason", traipsing from physician to physician where they "write down their sensations in long memoranda which they hasten to read and to explain". It all sounds like a dress-rehearsal for the stigmatising of ME sufferers today.

Regarding destigmatising strategies, let us return to homosexuality (Bullough 1979; Greenberg 1988). Challenging the demonising degenerationist sexology mentioned earlier, the twentieth century brought psychodynamic outlooks, notably Freud's reading of homosexuality as arrested development and later theories purporting to show how adolescents become gay through mother-fixation or absent fathers. Critics, however, argued that, while masquerading as "progressive", such views were in reality the expressions of anti-gay stigmatisation; the leading exponent of such opinions, Dr Charles Socarides, has been characterised as a rampant homophobe (LeVay 1996).

The English-born but US-based neuroanatomist Simon LeVay has in turn advanced the "born that way" case: like all other sexual orientation, homosexuality is, he claims, encoded into the brain. Experiments allegedly reveal that the size of a certain nucleus in the hypothalamus varies with sexual orientation – it is largest in heterosexual males, smaller in homosexual males and, as it happens, smallest of all in females.

Adducing other evidence too – experiments which showed that rats turned "gay" if their hormonal balance was altered – LeVay has proclaimed that the homosexuality question is at last being solved: being gay is neither a matter of choice nor a consequence of upbringing, but is inscribed into biological destiny. Sexual orientation lies in one's genes, brain or metabolism, embedded in one's very nature.

The idea that homosexuality is inborn has, of course, been voiced before, for Nazi eugenicists used comparable arguments to prove that gays, like Jews, gypsies and schizophrenics, were inherently and indelibly diseased or degenerate. Nevertheless, LeVay is convinced that scientific evidence for the "born that way" theory offers the best destigmatising strategy for the gay community. In a nation where many are convinced that to choose to be gay is to opt for evil, being born that way would logically remove the blame.

I have been discussing two key and often interlinked anti-stigma strategies: somatisation and gentrification. I shall close by mentioning one further circumstance in which mental disorder finds release from stigma: when it is perceived to confer prized powers. Sometimes madness has been viewed as a divine affliction, honoured as a revelation of holiness. Within Christianity, that faith founded upon the madness of the Cross, believers could hardly avoid seeing gleams of godliness in the simplicity of the idiot or the abnormal transports of mystics. Strands of Medieval, Reformation and Counter-Reformation theology held that Folly could be a medium for Divine utterance and bade it be heard.

Similarly mental illness avoids stigmatisation when it is viewed as creative (Jamison 1993; Becker 1978). From the Greeks onwards, it could be construed as a mark of distinction. Plato spoke of the 'divine fury' of the poet, and Aristotle was to paint the portrait of the melancholy genius (Simon 1978). Such views were fleshed out in the Renaissance by Ficino and other humanists; to dub a poet "mad" was to pay him a compliment. Michael Drayton thus praised Kit Marlowe:

"For that fine madness still he did retain,
Which rightly should possess a poet's brain."

In the early modern period, the melancholic was often regarded as gifted, special. And, at least in fiction and on the stage, melancholy malcontents like Prince Hamlet abounded. In our own day, addressing afflictions like Tourette's syndrome, Oliver Sacks has taught us to see not stigma but the special (Sacks 1981, 1985).

The true solution, of course, to the problem of psychiatric stigmatising would be the public acceptance, without shame, of mental disorder. But that would be crying for the moon.

References

Becker G (1978) *The Mad Genius Controversy.* London: Sage.

Blackmore Sir R (1725) *A Treatise of the Spleen and Vapours.* London: Pemberton.

Bullough V (1979) *Homosexuality: A History.* New York: American Library.

Burke P & Porter R (1995) (eds). *Languages and Jargons: Contributions to a Social History of Language.* Cambridge: Polity Press.

Chamberlin JE & Gilman SL (1985) (eds). *Degeneration: The Dark Side of Progress.* New York: Columbia University Press.

Charcot J-M (1987) *Charcot the Clinician: The Tuesday Lessons – Excerpts from Nine Case Presentations on General Neurology Delivered at the Salpêtrière Hospital in 1887–88* (translation and commentary by Goetz CG). New York: Raven Press.

Charcot J-M (1991) *Clinical Lectures on Diseases of the Nervous System* (ed. Harris R). London: Routledge.

Charcot J-M, Richer P (1887) *Les Démoniaques dans l'Art.* Paris: Delahaye and Lecrosnier.

Cheyne G (1733) *The English Malady; or, A Treatise of Nervous Diseases.* London: G Strahan.

Didi-Huberman G (1982) *Invention de l'Hystérie: Charcot et l'Iconographie Photographique de la Salpêtrière.* Paris: Editions Macula.

Dowbiggin I (1985) Degeneration and hereditarianism in French mental medicine 1840–1890: psychiatric theory as ideological adaptation. In: Bynum WF, Porter R & Shepherd M (eds). *The Anatomy of Madness*, Vol. 1. London: Tavistock: 188–232.

Fabrega Jnr F (1990) Psychiatric stigma in the classical and medieval period. *Comprehensive Psychiatry* **31**: 289–306.

Fabrega Jnr F (1991a) The culture and history of psychiatric stigma in early modern and modern western societies: a review of recent literature. *Comprehensive Psychiatry* **32**: 97–119.

Fabrega Jnr F (1991b) Psychiatric stigma in non-western societies. *Comprehensive Psychiatry* **32**: 534–51.

Foucault M (1961) *La Folie et la Déraison: Histoire de la Folie à l'Age Classique.* Paris: Librairie Plon. [Translated and abridged by Howard R as *Madness and Civilization: A History of Insanity in the Age of Reason.* New York: Random House, 1965/London: Tavistock, 1967.]

Foucault M (1979) *The History of Sexuality*, Vol. 1: *An Introduction* (translated by Hurley R). London: Allen Lane.

Gilman SL (1976) *The Face of Madness: Hugh W. Diamond and the Origin of Psychiatric Photography.* New York: Brunner-Mazel.

Gilman SL (1982) *Seeing the Insane: A Cultural History of Madness and Art in the Western World*. New York: Wiley, in association with Brunner-Mazel.

Gilman S (1985) *Difference and Pathology*. Ithaca: Cornell University Press.

Gilman S (1988) *Disease and Representation. From Madness to AIDS*. Ithaca: Cornell University Press.

Gilman S (1989) *Sexuality: An Illustrated History*. New York: Wiley.

Goetz CG, Bonduelle M & Gelfand T (1995) *Charcot. Constructing Neurology*. Oxford: Oxford University Press.

Goffman E (1970) *Stigma: Notes on the Management of Spoiled Identity*. Harmondsworth: Penguin: 9.

Greenberg DF (1988) *The Construction of Homosexuality*. Chicago: University of Chicago Press.

Jamison KR (1993) *Touched with Fire: Manic-Depressive Illness and the Artistic Temperament*. New York: Free Press.

Krafft-Ebing R von (1886) *Psychopathia Sexualis*. Stuttgart: Verlag von Ferdinand Enke.

Kromm J (1984) Studies in the iconography of madness, 1600–1900. PhD dissertation, Emory University.

Kutchins H & Kirk SA (1997) *Making Us Crazy: The Psychiatric Bible and the Creation of Mental Disorders*. New York: Free Press.

LeVay S (1996) *Queer Science. The Use and Abuse of Research into Homosexuality*. Cambridge, MA: The MIT Press.

Lutz T (1995) Neurasthenia and fatigue syndromes, social section. In: Berrios GE, Porter R (eds). *A History of Clinical Psychiatry. The Origin and History of Psychiatric Disorders*. London: Athlone: 533–44.

Macalpine I & Hunter R (1969) *George III and the Mad Business*. London: Allen Lane.

MacDonald M (1991) *Witchcraft and Hysteria in Elizabethan London. Edward Jorden and the Mary Glover Case*. London: Routledge.

MacDonald M & Murphy TR (1990) *Sleepless Souls: Suicide in Early Modern England*. Oxford: Clarendon Press.

MacGregor JM (1989) *The Discovery of the Art of the Insane*. Princeton: Princeton University Press.

Micale MS (1987) Diagnostic discriminations: Jean-Martin Charcot and the nineteenth-century idea of masculine hysterical neurosis. PhD dissertation, *Yale University*.

Minois G (1999) *History of Suicide: Voluntary Death in Western Culture*. Baltimore: Johns Hopkins University Press.

Nordau MS (1920) *Degeneration*. London: Heinemann.

Oppenheim J (1991) *"Shattered Nerves": Doctors, Patients and Depression in Victorian England*. Oxford: Oxford University Press.

Piñero JML (1983) *Historical Origins of the Concept of Neurosis* (translated by Berrios D). Cambridge: Cambridge University Press.

Prichard JC (1835) *A Treatise on Insanity and Other Disorders Affecting the Mind*. London: Sherwood, Gilbert and Piper.

Robinson R (1729) *A New System of the Spleen*. London: Bettesworth.

Rosenberg C (1962) The place of George M. Beard in nineteenth century psychiatry. *Bulletin of the History of Medicine* **36**: 245–59.

Sacks O (1981) *Migraine: Evolution of a Common Disorder*. London: Pan Books.

Sacks O (1985) *The Man Who Mistook His Wife for a Hat*. London: Duckworth.

Scull A (1993) *The Most Solitary of Afflictions: Madness and Society in Britain, 1700–1900*. New Haven: Yale University Press.

Sharpe J (1996) *Instruments of Darkness. Witchcraft in England 1550–1750*. London: Hamish Hamilton.

Shorter E (1992) *From Paralysis to Fatigue. A History of Psychosomatic Illness in the Modern Era*. New York: Free Press.

Shorter E (1997) *A History of Psychiatry*. New York: Free Press.

Showalter E (1986) *The Female Malady: Women, Madness, and English Culture, 1830–1980*. New York: Pantheon Press.

Simon B (1978) *Mind and Madness in Ancient Greece*. Ithaca: Cornell University Press.

Smith R (1981) *Trial by Medicine: Insanity and Responsibility in Victorian Trials*. Edinburgh: Edinburgh University Press.

Sprott SE (1961) *The English Debate on Suicide from Donne to Hume*. London: Open Court Publishing.

Szasz TS (1970) *The Manufacture of Madness*. New York: Dell.

Szasz TS (1972) *The Myth of Mental Illness: Foundations of a Theory of Personal Conduct*. London: Granada.

Szasz TS (1984) *The Therapeutic State: Psychiatry in the Mirror of Current Events*. Buffalo: Prometheus Books.

Thomas K (1971) *Religion and the Decline of Magic: Studies in Popular Beliefs in Sixteenth and Seventeenth-Century England*. London: Weidenfeld & Nicolson.

Walker N (1968) *Crime and Insanity in England*. Vol. i. *The Historical Perspective*. Edinburgh: Edinburgh University Press.

Wessely S (1995) Neurasthenia and fatigue syndromes. In: Berrios GE & Porter R (eds). *A History of Clinical Psychiatry. The Origin and History of Psychiatric Disorders*. London: Athlone, 509–32.

Zihni LS (1989) The history of the relationship between the concept and treatment of people with Down's Syndrome in Britain and America from 1866 to 1967. PhD dissertation, University College London.

2 Cultural and national aspects of stigmatisation

Roland Littlewood

We know little of how culture and nationality determine the popular stigmatisation of psychiatric illness. Nonetheless, "culture" in the widest sense seems to influence the invalidating or other response to illness (and indeed to its associated professionals and to relatives of those affected).

There is evidence that popular understanding of mental illness, and thus the social response, may determine the actual prognosis of severe mental illness, independently of any recourse to medical treatment. Indeed, it has now become generally accepted that schizophrenia has "a better prognosis" in the Third World (Cooper and Sartorius 1977). The smaller proportion of "poor outcome" patients, such as those found in the WHO International Pilot Study of Schizophrenia and the Determinants of Outcome Study, have been attributed to differences in the attribution of individual responsibility for illness (Warner 1994) and to different concepts of personal identity (Horwitz 1982). The value placed on the autonomous individual in industrialised, largely Western, cultures has been said to accentuate the social extrusion of a chronic psychiatric patient who assumes personal responsibility for the illness, and this then makes for a worse prognosis.

Warner (1994) has proposed that the course of schizophrenia is related to gender roles, to class and social identity, and to labour dynamics: more specifically that unemployment of the mentally ill in capitalist economies leads to a loss of selfesteem, status and independence; in developing societies, the mentally ill individual is supposedly extruded less because of a graduated accommodation of work to presumed ability (Cooper and Sartorius 1977). Some argue that non-industrialised societies are simply more cohesive, with clear social roles independent of personal choice, and which have categorisations of illness which attribute to the illness an external causation such as sorcery, thus removing responsibility from the individual patient and making for a better outcome (Waxler 1976). Nuclear (and thus Western) families are said to be less accepting of mental illness than are extended families. Cooper and Sartorius (1977) assume that in non-industrialised societies the environment for schizophrenic patients is "supportive and tolerant and [with] little risk of prolonged rejection, isolation, segregation and institutionalisation."

Horwitz (1982) makes a useful distinction between such *psychiatric* models – in which societies respond by extrusion to the independently existing symptoms of an underlying disease process, and hence the popular conceptualisations may be judged true or false – and the *t* or labelling model – in which the illness is itself understood as the individual responding to a culturally variable perception of minor deviance, both individual and others then shaping this deviance in the direction of a conventionally accepted disease category. Some sociological interpretations place particular emphasis on the social process of labelling in itself; others stress the way individuals make their identity through or against such ascriptions and extrusions.

Whatever the more general cultural and historical influences on local responses to psychiatric illness, it is at the level of individual conceptions of illness (or "deviance"), in its experience, recognition and immediate consequences, that we are likely to find a link between broader economic and cultural meanings and the immediate consequences of identified illness. There are, however, few direct crosscultural comparisons between local recognition of illness; these usually devise an ordinal scale of Western attitudinal measure such as "stigmatisation" and then use translated versions of the questionnaire with some assumption of comparability of meaning (Askenasy 1974). An exception is the cross-cultural study of Wig and his colleagues using vignettes in three developing countries (Wig et al. 1980).

Whilst the distinction between "conceptualisation of psychiatric illness" and "response to psychiatric illness" has some heuristic value, it of course begs the question of actual causation. Even at the pragmatic level of devising questionnaires and rating scales it is not easy to say whether the question is concerned with existing ideas about the "nature" of psychiatric illness itself or with strategic attitudes to identified psychiatrically ill individuals. Ethnographically the distinction may be relatively arbitrary but most studies tend to emphasise one or other position.

Anthropological accounts have concentrated on understandings of psychiatric illness (or analogous patterns) within the general field of local values and social structure. Using a broad framework of medical or cognitive anthropology they have examined the terminology, nosologies and logical structure of local ethnomedicines, how these relate to other key local cultural concepts, classifications of illness, gender, human action and the natural world, and what notions of the person, theodicy, moral choice and contingency they evoke. Such studies traditionally examine a well-known small-scale population; they are concerned not with cross-cultural comparison but with local meaning. Unlike health policy psychiatric studies they do not start from, say, schizophrenia as the given independent variable and then assess local understandings of it, but examine the whole broad field of commonsense concepts from which patterns which recall the psychiatrist's field of interest may emerge.

Before we can compare attitudes to mental illness cross-culturally, we first have to consider whether "mental illness" or an analogous category is recognised by a society. On the vexed question of "Are psychiatric illnesses universally recognised?", the consensus seems that something akin to chronic schizophrenia is recognised as a distinct and undesirable state, usually but not always aligned to a more general category recalling physical illness, and that it is characterised primarily by continued unintelligibility (Horwitz 1982). In both Trinidad and Boston (USA) relatives respond especially to altered appearance and inexplicable actions, and they rate these as the most disturbing (Littlewood 1988; Scheper-Hughes 1987). Patterns *recalling* (and in this type of study we cannot presume *identity with*) the medical concepts of acute psychosis, mental handicap, personality disorder or neurosis may, however, be understood in a variety of ways – as moral choices, anti-social behaviour, "physical" or "psychological" illnesses, or simply as points located on a spectrum of possible everyday action and experience.

The analytical schemata we apply to such local understandings may be quite diverse: "modern" or "traditional" ideas, "naturalistic" or "personalistic" aetiology, "instrumental" or "ultimate" causality, "indexical" or "referential" notions of the person, or simply a qualitative approach which avoids anything like an etic/emic dichotomy.

Townsend (1979) has argued from cross-cultural studies which included both psychiatrists and lay people that local commonsense conceptions in any society may shape the practical professional response more than explicit psychiatric theory. Using historical data, others have proposed that popular and professional categorisations alike are a function of wider changes in notions of moral order. Western notions of psychiatric illness, as determined by questionnaire interviews, seem relatively unstable over short periods of time (Murphy 1976), but it is difficult to identify the specific associated factors in public opinion, whether these are particular health education programmes, general shifts in conceptualising or empathising with deviant and unusual patterns, changing prognosis, or just an increasing familiarity with patients.

In certain East African societies in the 1960s, a "naturalistic" explanation went with expectations of a poor prognosis, an "ultrahuman" explanation with expectations of a better prognosis (Edgerton 1966). In Britain and Hawaii, also in the 1960s, the reverse held (Askenasy 1974). It is uncertain how much such local ethnomedical categories in themselves actually predict the observable community response. In rural Botswana madness is more likely to be seen as caused by sorcery than is epilepsy, and less likely to be seen as "contagious" (and hence presumably less likely to be seen as "physical"); yet Western biomedical treatment is more likely to be sought for schizophrenia than epilepsy (Ben-Tovim 1987). Nor does what people say they know, or do, necessarily mean that this is indeed what they do in actual situations. Thus, in India, China, Ireland and elsewhere, one can certainly find distinct oral and written traditions which place a "positive" value on insanity, but it is uncertain whether this results in a more general empathy with, or refusal to extrude, identified patients. Conversely, in Trinidad, a generally elicited rejecting notion of *madness* may be rather more benign in actual practice (Littlewood 1988). While in Hawaii, serious psychiatric illness is seen as the intelligible result of social factors, there is still considerable distrust of the patient: in England the reverse (Askenasy 1974). Concepts recalling the English word *insanity*, such as *pagol* (Bengali) or *pissu* (Sinhalese), may carry with them some notion of eccentric but meaningful value, but this may be no more than a common but "weak" connotation, akin to *bad* in Afro-American Englishes or crazy in British English. Such terms have to be considered in actual use: in one situation analogues of *insane* or *mad* may refer to subjective experience, in another to observed behaviour. It seems plausible that the subjective connotation is associated with less social extrusion in practice.

Unless named "universal" (etic, here psychiatric) categories are used in these studies, it is difficult to place immediate practical decision making in a standardised framework susceptible to cross-cultural study, and anthropology like other interpretative social sciences can be faulted for generalising from local accounts. To use even a vignette in cross-cultural studies of attitudes to psychiatric illness assumes, as does the "psychiatric model", that this description has some primacy that can be generalised across societies without too much loss of meaning. The assumption that such questions can be asked with comparable meaning across cultures has been criticised for isolating psychiatric and psychological patterns defined as separately existing entities, even those with a biological component, both in psychiatry and psychology. To generalise about local conceptions and responses in a similar way is even more doubtful – similar to drawing cross-cultural conclusions about "marriage" or "religious belief". This is not to argue that any attempt at a cross-cultural comparison is invalid; merely that the limitations of any such methodology have to be borne in mind: any question we *can* ask in different languages, in different societies and under different economic assumptions, will inevitably transform local meanings, social context and political process. Any comparative attempt will single out that which does appear to be translatable or transferable across cultures, and will thus emphasise the apparently universal over the diverse.

A common statement within the mental health professions is that ethnic minority groups in Britain are more likely to stigmatise mental illness than does the White European population, thus explaining later recourse to treatment and justifying higher rates of "sectioning" under the Mental Health Act. This has not actually been demonstrated and it remains uncertain why it might be so: perhaps competitive economic striving in a climate of limited opportunity is such that one has to maximise every single competitive personal advantage and cannot afford the luxury of empathy with those who are mentally ill? Or past experience with colonial and post-colonial mental hospitals before migration, to which only the more dangerous were admitted?

In a continuing study, Sushrut Jadhav and I, together with colleagues in India, Sri Lanka, Trinidad and elsewhere, have been collaborating on a relatively "culture-free" stigmatisation questionnaire derived in Bengali, Sinhalese and English which we have field-tested in Britain and these countries. Early results suggest that responses to questions such as "Would you be happy if your child's teacher was like this?", following a vignette using a lay description of schizophrenia, were actually least stigmatising in a slum area of Calcutta and most stigmatising in Port-of-Spain, Trinidad, White British responses being somewhere in between. To generalise about cross-cultural differences in stigmatisation however seems premature given the paucity of our current knowledge.

References

Askenasy AR (1974) *Attitudes Toward Mental Patients: A Study Across Cultures.* The Hague: Mouton.

Ben-Tovim DI (1987) *Development Psychiatry: Mental Health and Primary Health Care in Botswana.* London: Tavistock.

Cooper JE & Sartorius N (1977) Cultural and temporal variations in schizophrenia: a speculation on the importance of industrialisation. *British Journal of Psychiatry* **130**: 50–5.

Edgerton RB (1966) Conceptions of psychosis in four East African societies. *American Anthropologist* **66**: 408–425.

Horwitz AV (1982) *The Social Control of Mental Illness.* New York: Academic Press.

Littlewood R (1988) From vice to madness: the semantics of naturalistic and personalistic understandings in Trinidad local medicine. *Social Science and Medicine* **27**: 129–48.

Murphy HBM (1976) Review of Askenasy (1974). *Transcultural Psychiatric Research Review* **13**: 49–51.

Scheper-Hughes N (1987) "Mental" in "Southie": individual, family and community responses to psychosis in South Boston. *Culture, Medicine and Psychiatry* **11**: 53–78.

Townsend JM (1979) Stereotypes and mental illness: a comparison with ethnic stereotypes. *Culture, Medicine and Psychiatry* **3**: 205–30.

Warner R (1994) *Recovery from Schizophrenia: Psychiatry and Political Economy*, 2nd edn. New York: Routledge.

Waxler NE (1976) Social change and psychiatric illness in Ceylon: traditional and modern conceptions of disease and treatment. In: Lebra W (ed). *Culture-Bound Syndromes, Ethnopsychiatry and Alternative Therapies.* Honolulu: University Press of Hawaii.

Wig NN, Suleiman MA, Routledge R, Srinivsa Murthy R, Ladrido-Ignacio L, Ibrahim HHA & Harding TW (1980) Community reactions to mental disorders: a key informant study in three developing countries. *Acta Psychiatrica Scandinavica* **61**: 111–126.

Acknowledgement

This paper uses material previously published in *The Lancet* 1998; **352**: 1055–7.

Part 2

People's perceptions of the mentally "ill" and the experiences of users and carers

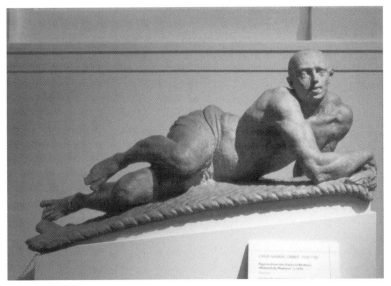

Caius Gabriel Cibber, *Melancholy*

3 The Royal College of Psychiatrists' survey of public opinions about mentally ill people

Michael Gelder

Introduction

It might be said that there is no need to carry out another survey of stigmatising opinions about people with mental illness. Everyday observation, the accounts of patients, and the results of surveys show that mental illness is a stigma. There are, however, several reasons for a further enquiry. First, there has been no recent study of a representative sample of the population of the UK and recent events, especially the development of community care, may have led to changes in opinions. Second, previous surveys have not differentiated between different kinds of mental disorder, for example Trute et al. (1989) asked about "someone who had been a patient in a psychiatric hospital", Jalali et al. (1978) asked about someone "hospitalized for mental illness", and the Scottish Association for Mental Health (1998) enquired about "people with mental health problems" – phrases that could include conditions ranging from schizophrenia to eating disorders. Third, the Royal College of Psychiatrists had decided to campaign against the stigmatisation of mentally ill people and it was desirable to measure opinions at the start of the campaign as a baseline against which its effects could be measured on a later occasion. A fuller account of the study is published elsewhere (Crisp et al. 2000).

How the survey was carried out

The investigation was carried out on behalf of the College by the Office of National Statistics as part of their regular surveys of national opinion, using their standard methodology. The questions in the survey were formulated after a search of the literature and from the results of a study of focus groups carried out for the College by Research Quorum.

The sample was drawn from a national sample of postal sectors stratified by region of Great Britain, and by the proportion of households renting from local authorities and with the head of household in social groups 1–5 and 13. Within each of the sectors chosen in this way, 30 addresses were selected randomly; if there was more than one household at the address, one was selected randomly. In each household one person aged 16 years or older was chosen randomly. Proxies were not taken if this person was not available. An advance letter was sent to each address giving a brief account of the survey, which contained questions about some general issues as well as about mental health.

Experienced interviewers asked questions about the composition of the household and variables related to demography and employment, before asking about opinions concerning psychiatric illness. Replies to the latter were recorded on 5-point scales ranging from complete agreement to complete disagreement with a statement read by the interviewer. This format was chosen because it had worked well in other surveys carried out by the Office of National Statistics. The interview began with a practice question, namely "Thinking about someone who has severe depression, I would like you to look at this card and tell me which point on the scale from 1–5 best describes a person with severe depression. Point 1 means that they are always thinking of themselves, point 5 means that they are always thinking of other people". When the interviewer was confident that the respondent understood the procedure, she went on to ask eight questions about severe depression. The questions were from a review of the literature combined with the results of focus groups. Respondents were asked whether patients with severe depression are dangerous to others, unpredictable, hard to talk to, feel different from the rest of us; are to blame for their illness, could pull themselves together, would not improve with treatment, and will never recover. The same questions were then asked about each of the disorders chosen for the anti-stigma campaign, namely schizophrenia, dementia, panic attacks, eating disorders, alcoholism, and drug addiction.

The results of the survey

Of the 2679 adults approached, 9% could not be contacted and 25% refused to be interviewed (at this stage respondents were unaware of the subject of the survey). These figures are within the range of negative responses to other ONS opinion surveys. When the main subject of the interview was revealed, only a further 3% refused to take part. As noted above, respondents who refused were not replaced. In the resulting sample 45% were male, 14% were single, and 95% were white. The last figure is representative of the population of the UK but the small number of non-white respondents does not allow evaluation of differences between these two groups within the population

In scoring the replies, a negative response is the sum of ratings 1 + 2. The figures in Table 1 are percentages of respondents endorsing ratings of 1 or 2. Table 1 shows that respondents did not have a single opinion about all the psychiatric disorders. Consider first the rows in Table 1.

Table 1. Percentage of respondents endorsing negative opinions about mental disorders. Percentages are rounded to the nearest whole number with 95% confidence limits in brackets

	Severe depression	Schizophrenia	Dementia	Panic attacks	Eating disorder	Alcohol addiction	Drug addiction
Dangerous	23 (21–25)	71 (69–74)	19 (17–21)	26 (23–28)	7 (5–8)	65 (62–68)	74 (71–79)
Unpredictable	56 (54–59)	77 (75–80)	53 (50–56)	50 (47–54)	29 (26–31)	71 (68–74)	78 (75–80)
Hard to talk to	62 (59–65)	58 (56–61)	60 (57–63)	33 (30–35)	38 (35–41)	59 (57–62)	62 (62–68)
Feel different	43 (40–45)	58 (55–61)	61 (57–64)	39 (37–42)	49 (46–52)	35 (33–38)	48 (45–51)
Self to blame	13 (11–15)	8 (6–9)	4 (3–5)	11 (10–13)	35 (32–38)	60 (57–63)	68 (65–70)
Pull self together	19 (16–21)	8 (7–9)	4 (3–5)	22 (20–24)	38 (35–41)	52 (49–56)	47 (44–50)
Not respond	16 (14–17)	15 (13–17)	56 (54–59)	14 (12–15)	9 (8–11)	11 (10–13)	12 (10–14)
Not recover	23 (21–26)	51 (48–54)	82 (80–85)	22 (20–24)	11 (10–13)	24 (22–28)	23 (21–26)

Dangerousness

There are clear differences between the percentages of respondents rating as dangerous, patients suffering from the various disorders. More than two thirds of people responded that patients with schizophrenia and people with drug addiction are dangerous to others. Almost as many held this opinion about people with alcoholism. Far fewer respondents rated as dangerous to others patients with severe depression, panic attacks and dementia. That only 7% rated people with eating disorders as dangerous provides a base rate for the other disorders.

Unpredictable

The percentages of people endorsing the opinion that patients are unpredictable follow a pattern similar to those for dangerousness, although the differences between disorders are less extreme. About three quarters of respondents thought that patients with schizophrenia and substance abuse are unpredictable, and half held the same opinion about patients with severe depression, dementia and panic attacks. Almost a third rated people with eating disorders as unpredictable.

Hard to talk to

About 60% of respondents held this opinion about patients with all disorders except panic attacks and eating disorders. For the latter, these opinions were held by 33% and 38% respectively.

Feel different from the way we all feel at times

People with alcoholism were rated as feeling different by the least number of respondents (put in another way, more respondents thought that they feel the way that everyone does at times). Around 60% of respondents endorsed the opinion that people with schizophrenia and dementia felt differently, and almost a half held this opinion about people with eating disorders and drug addiction.

Have only themselves to blame for their condition

This stigmatising opinion was held most frequently about drug addiction (67%) and alcohol addiction (60%). Few of the respondents attached similar blame to people with schizophrenia, severe depression, dementia or panic attacks, but a third thought this about people with eating disorders.

Could pull themselves together if they wanted to

The pattern of response is similar to that for blame though less extreme. About a half of respondents thought that this statement applied to people with alcohol and drug addictions, and almost as many to eating disorders. Few recorded this opinion about people with schizophrenia or dementia but, despite a recent national Defeat Depression Campaign, almost a fifth of respondents applied it to people with severe depression.

Would improve if given treatment

Most people recognised the possibility that, with the exception of dementia, patients with mental disorders would improve with treatment.

Will never recover fully

Most held this opinion about dementia and half held it about schizophrenia. Less than a quarter thought that the other disorders would not recover.

Table 2. Percentage of respondents of different ages endorsing the opinion that patients with mental disorders are dangerous to others. Percentages rounded to the nearest whole number; 95% confidence limits in brackets

	16–24 years (n=194)	25–64 years (n=1182)	65 and over (n=361)
Depression	28 (21–36)	21 (18–24)	26 (21–31)
Schizophrenia	83 (75–90)	75 (72–78)	54 (49–60)
Alcoholism	80 (73–87)	68 (65–71)	49 (42–54)
Drug dependence	86 (80–91)	75 (72–79)	63 (56–70)

The patients' perspective

By looking down the columns in Table 2 we can assess the likelihood that patients with the various disorders will meet people who hold each of the eight opinions.

Patients with schizophrenia will find that about three quarters of the people they meet think that they are or were dangerous and unpredictable, more than a half expect that it will be difficult to talk to them, and half think that they will never recover. However, few of the people they meet will think that they are to blame for their illness or able to pull themselves together, or that they will not respond to treatment. It could be said that people are fearful but not unsympathetic.

More than half the people encountered by patients with severe depression will think them unpredictable and hard to talk to, but only about a quarter fear that they could be dangerous. Few will think that they are to blame for their illness but almost a fifth will think that they could pull themselves together. Most will expect that they will improve with treatment and eventually recover.

Rather more than half the people encountered by patients with dementia will expect them to be unpredictable and hard to talk to. They also expect that they will not respond to treatment. Four in five expect that they will not recover. Almost everyone will be sympathetic, recognising that these patients are not to blame for their illness and cannot pull themselves together. Patients with panic attacks will meet fewer people with unfavourable opinions. However, half will think them unpredictable, a third expect that they will be hard to talk to, and a quarter will fear that they could be dangerous to others. A fifth will think that they could pull themselves together, and a similar proportion that they will not recover.

Patients with eating disorders will find that more than a third of the people they meet think them hard to talk to and lack sympathy, thinking that they are able to pull themselves together, and to blame for their condition. Most people will expect them to improve with treatment and to recover eventually.

People with alcohol addiction will encounter many people with unfavourable opinions. Almost two in three will fear that they could be dangerous and rather more will think that they are unpredictable. More than half will expect them to be hard to talk to, able to pull themselves together, and to blame for their condition. However, most will think that they would respond to treatment and will recover eventually.

People with drug addiction will meet even more people with stigmatising opinions. Three in every four will expect that they are dangerous to others, and unpredictable. Two in three expect them to be hard to talk to. The same proportion will think them to blame for their condition and about half will think them able to pull themselves together. Most expect that they would respond to treatment and will recover eventually.

The effects of knowing someone with a mental disorder, and of age

Respondents were divided into those who said that they knew someone with a mental disorder and those who did not (note that the question did not specify any particular type of mental disorder). Their responses to the questions about dangerousness and being hard to talk to were examined. Contrary to expectation, respondents who knew someone with a mental disorder were not more sympathetic. The sole exception was that slightly fewer people who knew someone with a mental disorder said that patients with severe depression are dangerous to others.

Respondents were divided into three age groups, 16–24 years, 25–64 years and over 65 years, and their responses about dangerousness were examined. Fewer of those in the last group endorsed unfavourable opinions about schizophrenia, alcoholism and drug addiction than did either of the other groups.

Conclusion

Stigmatising opinions are frequent in the community but the nature of these opinions differs according to the disorder. People with schizophrenia are stigmatised by opinions that they will be dangerous, unpredictable and hard to talk to. However most people recognise that they are not to blame for their condition. People with alcohol or drug addiction are even more stigmatised than those with schizophrenia: almost as many people expect them to be dangerous and unpredictable and more than half think them to blame for their condition. People with severe depression are rather less stigmatised in that few people expect them to be dangerous but more than half expect them to be unpredictable and hard to talk to. People with eating disorders are stigmatised the least of the seven conditions studied, but even so a third of the population think that they are to blame for their condition, and that it will be hard to talk to them.

The results indicate that a campaign to reduce stigma must take account of these differences between disorders, The opinion that is held about all the disorders is that it will be hard to talk to those who suffer from them. It is an opinion which isolates patients and prevents the public from gaining a greater understanding of the problems of the mentally ill.

References

Crisp AH, Gelder MG, Rix S, Meltzer HI & Rowlands OJ (2000). The stigmatisation of people with mental illness. *British Journal of Psychiatry* **177**: 4–7.

Jalali B, Jalali M & Turner F (1978) Attitudes to mental illness: its relation to contact and ethnocultural background. *Journal of Nervous and Mental Disease* **166**: 692–700.

Scottish Association for Mental Health (1998) *Attitudes to Mental Health*. Edinburgh: SAMH.

Trute B, Tefft B & Segall A (1989) Social rejection of the mentally ill: a replication study of public attitude. *Social Psychiatry and Psychiatric Epidemiology* **24**: 69–76.

4 Living with anxiety: Social phobia – my story

David Taylor

My name is David and until recently I was a heroin addict with some twenty years of addiction behind me. Now, I'm totally drug-free, teetotal and enjoy life in recovery. I am ever grateful to the National Phobics Society for all their warmth and support, and perhaps if I'd have known of their existence twenty years ago I wouldn't have turned to substance abuse in the first place. I can now openly admit without shame that the problems that toppled me into the pit of addiction were actually mental health problems: anxiety, depression and non-existent self-esteem. My story is quite disturbing really, what should have been a very bright future turned into a 20-year nightmare of shame, degradation and self-hatred. I graduated with a science degree at 20 years of age, and this is the story of how I went down from there instead of up.

Rationalising why such things happen is difficult because the reasons are complex and not always apparent. A traumatic childhood was my undoing. However public opinion and my own ignorance towards mental health issues were contributors in exacerbating my problems rather than being part of the solution. I know only too well about ignorance, insensitivity and the tendency to stigmatise and marginalise those who are already reeling in pain. Sadly the problem not only lies with the public; our institutions and our places of work would all benefit from having their awareness raised in areas of mental health and social responsibility.

Childhood and adolescence

My childhood was austere and insecure in many ways; I was an unwelcome arrival to an already struggling family unit with one parent an alcoholic and the other emotionally aloof. I still feel the tensions to this day: frequent outbursts of unpredictable rage from my father and a peculiar coldness from my mother. I must have been so confused and scared as a child – it's written all over my face in old photographs. In a family where one was equally likely to be blessed with a drunken sign of the cross or screamed at and physically abused for no apparent reason, defence strategies were all important to my survival.

I became hypervigilant early on, studying changes in facial expression and reading atmospheres for potential threat. I lived very much in my own head, choosing not to be seen and not heard. Primary school probably found me to be quiet and withdrawn, and maybe here support and intervention could have changed things but I doubt it. Here was a child, stigmatised by his parents, being further stigmatised because of an inability to relax and simply be himself socially. In spite of home life, I passed my eleven plus and went on to grammar school where many of my problems really came to fruition. Here I struggled to find my identity, an insecure working class lad amongst what seemed like a sea of middle class bright stars. The teaching regime was severe, thriving on humiliation rather than reward, on academic achievement rather than personal growth. I was trapped between home life and school life, with no real sense of security, no one to confide in, no one to soothe my adolescent fears. On my eleventh birthday I was beaten mercilessly by my father and my relationship with him was over. I was seething with anger and contempt for him. Around the age of twelve I learned he was dying with cancer of the liver and I had to live with my feelings in silence. My father was unaware that he was dying and my mother was unaware that I knew – I was told by a sister. My father eventually died when I was 15, a shadow of himself, a dead bag of bones in the front room. I was numb, unable to cry, filled with relief and guilt for feeling that way. I was on my own totally and looked to schoolwork as a distraction and a way out of the misery that I'd so far known. I took my O levels three weeks after my father's burial and put on a very brave face, passing all eight.

At 17 whilst studying for A levels, I experienced my first panic attack in full view of my classmates. Not only was I extremely embarrassed and frightened by the experience, I was confused about what was happening to me: was I cracking up at last? From that terrible day I lived in dread of further attacks, which usually came when I was placed on the spot in a trapped social setting. My social anxiety went through the roof, as did my self-blame. I began to question whether I was going insane and slipped into depression.

At this point in my life I could quite reasonably have been given support and advice about my emotional distress and in doing so I would not have internalised "there is something wrong with me". Instead of receiving empathy from teachers I was treated with ridicule and insensitivity, being singled out to sit in the front of the class, being hauled out to the blackboard, being forced to read out aloud in class; all situations which heightened my feelings of self-consciousness and shame. At the time it felt as though I was being punished for something I really could not help, I felt like a laughing stock.

Social anxiety and chemical crutches

At university I held things together but I began drinking quite heavily and experimented with amphetamines as a way of lifting me out of depression and social anxiety; without them I was introspective and anxious all the time. My ignorance and lack of insight was frightening – I should have sought professional help at this time but felt unable to talk about how I felt, choosing only to punish myself and beat myself up for the way I felt. I believed I was weak and strange perhaps. In my final year at university I was required to present a dissertation to the department and in absolute desperation actually inflicted an injury to my head to absent myself from this nightmare – my tutor was adamant that I give the lecture or fail my finals. Here again I felt stigmatised because of my weakness and the inability of others to grasp the depth of my anguish. Perhaps I should never have struggled so hard to better myself educationally but at the time I felt I was doing the right thing. My eventual graduation proved to be a total anticlimax because I didn't genuinely feel worthy of it. The rest is history really – an addictive cycle of shame, depression and anxiety that swallowed my career, my life and every ounce of my self-respect.

My first job ended in tears when it was discovered that I had been charged with the possession of a minute amount of amphetamine. This was a criminal offence I know, and my employers were not interested whatsoever in any plea of mitigation from me. I was consigned to the dole queue without a second thought.

By the time I was 23 I was addicted to opiates and by the time I was 27 I had a criminal record – an addict, no longer employable, not even a person in the eyes of some people. I was eventually imprisoned for a drug-related offence, and here my treatment can only be described as barbaric. Even in prison an addict is treated with contempt and disgust. I was detoxed in a strip cell – a cell with only a mattress, where all my clothing was removed. I was stapled into a nylon smock. The whole prison system beggars belief and I find it too painful to discuss even now.

How I survived such a long spell of addiction I don't know, such was my self-hatred and despair, I didn't care whether I died or not. At no time did I encounter the understanding, acceptance and compassion that is vital to a person's recovery; instead I was met with prejudice and a readiness to stereotype and isolate and criminalise.

To ask for compassion may be too idealistic a notion, but to ask for understanding certainly isn't. The only way that can be achieved is through education and destigmatising mental health issues so that sufferers don't hide in shame blocking their recovery. For me probably the most potent medicine was the understanding and fellowship of people who have actually been there and come out on the other side. Maybe the way forward lies in utilising the enormous amount of experience that lies with ex-sufferers and sufferers alike. In fact it should be our duty to raise awareness and change public and professional opinion.

5 Living with depression

Hugo Jacobs

Background

I suffer from appalling bouts of depression which result in me being hospitalised and given electro-convulsive therapy. Prior to being hospitalised during these bouts, I hibernate at home avoiding everybody. When I am well, I run my own business. I am the opposite to a depressed person, extrovert, energetic and wanting to get involved with everybody. The difference is terrifying and very visible to anybody who knows me.

Mental illness – a stigma?

To me mental illness is stigma ("stigma – *a distinguishing mark or characteristic of a bad or objectionable kind*", *Oxford English Dictionary*). Initially I refused to say that I suffered from "mental illness". That was something confined to real "loons" not me. Mental illness brings vivid pictures of "One Flew over the Cuckoo's Nest" – and carries a stigma which I was desperate to distance myself from. I did this by making my own mental illness something rather different … "The difficulty is that I create too much energy in my brain. If the excess energy does not get used up, then I do not sleep. If I don't sleep then after a period of about two weeks, I get physically exhausted and go downhill rapidly." This is somewhat different from saying, "I am a standard depressive".

In reflection, the reason I said this (and too an extent still do) is that the word depression carries so much stigma. Depression needs a different name. It is too overused and mostly associated with an indifferent day rather than a life threatening illness.

Nurturing the stigma – the unsaid

My experience is that people do not know how to react to friends/colleagues with mental illness. Do they ask how you are feeling ? Do they show sympathy ? Do they ask what the matter is ? NO. The usual reaction is to pretend that all is normal and nothing is said. However, as soon as I leave the room, I know it is.

Avoid it or tackle it head on?

I firmly believe that it is much easier to tackle the stigma of mental illness by being very open about it and using humour. "I've just been a patient in a lunatic asylum" usually breaks the ice. This directness creates an ease of dialogue, which provides a far better environment in which to discuss the subject. The relaxed head-on approach creates interest. People seem fascinated to establish what exactly does go on within a mental hospital. They want to know about the illness and it's devastating impact. It's as if they are having a conversation they ought not to have, so they want to get the most out of it.

It should be noted that in my experience the older generation is much less able to handle this approach than the younger. I have had my comments totally ignored on a number of occasions. Clearly, some of the older generation think that mental illness is a taboo subject and are uncomfortable when it is discussed.

6 Living with manic depression: Personal perspectives from a psychologist

Kay Redfield Jamison

It was difficult to make the decision to be public about having a severe psychiatric illness. I am a clinician with state licences that enable me to practise in the District of Columbia and California, and I have hospital privileges at the Johns Hopkins School of Medicine. I am a scientist who studies and writes about the illness I have, and I knew as a result of my disclosure that my work would be subject to a different kind of scrutiny. I am potentially liable to malpractice claims; I am a teacher of young doctors; and, like most people, I was brought up to be private about personal matters.

But privacy and reticence can kill. The problem with mental illness is that so many who have it – especially those in a position to change public attitudes, such as doctors, lawyers, politicians, and military officers – are reluctant to risk talking about mental illness, or seeking help for it. They are understandably frightened about professional and personal reprisals.

As a scientist and clinician, and most especially as a person, I was extremely reluctant to discuss having a psychotic form of manic-depressive illness. That it would be difficult to tell people, I assumed. That it would be less difficult than continuing to remain silent, I hoped.

I had studied and written about depression and manic depression for 20 years, was a full professor with clinical privileges at a major university teaching hospital, and had the unequivocal support of my husband, family, friends, and department chairman at Johns Hopkins. My illness had been under good control for many years. If I couldn't go public about it now, how could I hope that others might do so?

I decided, finally, to write a book about it. I also agreed to talk with a reporter from the *Washington Post* who was doing a story about my work. I hoped that by revealing my own experiences I could let others know what having such a devastating yet seldom discussed illness was like.

To say the least, manic depression had brought a certain level of emotional intensity into my life. It had also brought psychotic manias and suicidal depressions. From the time I was 16, my life had been an unpredictable, often terrifying, occasionally glorious storm of moods, thoughts, and behaviors. Yet despite this, thanks to excellent psychiatric care and highly effective medication, I'd managed to keep my illness hidden, except from a few friends and the physicians with whom I worked most closely. The thought of now telling my colleagues and patients filled me with horror. I assumed that once I had told them the truth, their perceptions of me would never again be the same.

I should have realised that the various responses from people would be complicated – and they were. There was much uncomfortable silence, and there were remarks that were witty, insensitive, generous, wonderful, or cruel. The responses, in short, were very human. A few days after the *Washington Post* story appeared, for instance, our gardener approached me outside of our house. Referring both to the article and to my rather manic tendency in the later summer months to order, with great enthusiasm, hundreds of vivid spring bulbs, he said, "Gosh, Dr Jamison. If I'd known that you had that kind of problem, I would have planted more subdued colours." It was a perfect comment, perfectly unexpected, and one that still makes me laugh whenever I think about it.

Telling my patients turned out to be not nearly as difficult as I imagined. Most of them were simply stunned. "You seem so normal," said one. "So Brooks Brotherish." Others were not so surprised. Two patients, fellow professors, expressed the hope that the academic community would become more aware of the extent of mental illness within its ranks. And both remarked, with a surprising degree of bitterness, more tolerant. Most asked me what medication I was on and wondered which side effects I had experienced. But I was interested to note, in every instance, how quickly our psychotherapy sessions reverted to their usual form and focus. My patients were eager to get on with the business of their lives.

I particularly dreaded going back to Johns Hopkins once the *Washington Post* article came out. The first day, I found myself slinking along the corridors of the hospital, identification badge flipped over so my name was hidden, trying to be inconspicuous. Ordinarily neither an anxious person nor a shy one, I was frightened beyond measure at the prospect of encountering the residents. When I walked into the seminar that I teach with a colleague, there was an unnerving silence, and I could feel the acute discomfort in the room. No one seemed to know what to say. Soon, however, everyone was lost in the topic at hand and the initial unease was gradually replaced with warmth and an unspoken support. The teaching rounds later that afternoon were likewise both distracting and, reassuringly, collegial. My self-consciousness began to fade, replaced by the more usual sense of pleasure I find in teaching and spending time at the hospital.

For the most part, it became easier still. The following week, the chief resident dropped by my office to congratulate me. It should not have had to have been a brave thing to do, she said, but it probably was. She told me she had distributed the *Post* article to all of the residents, several of whom suffered from mood disorders themselves. And, a few days later, I had a long discussion with another resident, who confessed that he had struggled with severe depression for years. In the weeks that followed, many other residents, interns, medical students, and faculty approached me to talk about their problems with depression and their concerns about the consequences of being open about their illnesses. For the first time I saw, concretely, that some good might come from my disclosure.

Several weeks later, I went to the annual meeting of the American Psychiatric Association in Miami. I knew that all news travels fast, and I was not eager to face people. To say the least. In fact, I didn't want to go at all, and nearly didn't.

Yet those colleagues who actually approached me were remarkably supportive. Most said they'd had absolutely no idea I had manic-depressive illness, and most thought my decision to be open about it was a good one. Many spontaneously hugged me and wished me well. A few, however, seemed terribly uncomfortable, averting their eyes and saying nothing. I found the silence chilling; it remains an ongoing, if increasingly less frequent source of discomfort to me. I have also become resigned to the fact that one never knows what other people truly think.

Then there was the sheer number of people who called to request clinical consultations, more than 50 in the first few days after the *Post* article. I heard from doctors, attorneys, students, scientists, teachers, and businessmen, almost all of whom described inordinate, and probably quite realistic, fears about repercussions in their work life if colleagues found out they suffered from mental illness. Some worried about being asked to leave medical school, others that their professional licences would be revoked. Many others – including several members of Congress – simply called or wrote to offer their support. I carried one remarkably kind and supportive letter around with me for weeks. Written by a senior US Senator, its generosity and fierce support saw me through many a dark hour when I was racked with self-doubts about my decision.

The response from the public was overwhelming with the publication in 1995 of my memoir, *An Unquiet Mind* (Jamison 1995). Within weeks, letters flooded in (more than 5,000 to date). Most of the writers shared their own or family members' experiences with depression and manic-depression. The level of despair and frustration was palpable. Hundreds sent manuscripts, poems, or artwork they had composed while manic, depressed or recovering from their illnesses. Some letters, however, were vicious, saying, for example, that because manic-depression was a genetic illness, it was a "blessing that I hadn't had children", that I'd "spared the world of yet another destructive psychotic". Other letters were themselves overtly psychotic – many astonishingly so – and yet others berated me for "abandoning my Christian faith", making it clear that madness and despair were precisely what I deserved. Others were simply anti-science, anti-medicine, anti-genetics, or anti-psychiatry – but often mean-spirited and highly personal, as well. Their cruelty hurt, as it was designed to do, and I occasionally found myself frightened or sobbing after reading a particularly vitriolic letter or diatribe.

But, all things considered, speaking out about my illness has had a freeing effect. I'm much more able to say what I feel now. And for every discomfort about the loss of privacy, for every fear of a personal or professional reprisal, there is also relief in the honesty. For the most part, people have been more understanding than I could have imagined. It is true that a few colleagues have – quite publicly – questioned my judgement for writing about my illness, and yet others have questioned my professional ethics for not having written earlier. One has no choice but to be somewhat philosophical.

The entire process has drawn my family more tightly together. We've begun talking about an illness that for far too long we ignored or skirted around. It's become a part of our casual conversation, a more natural part of our lives. A few months after my "coming out", for instance, my then 11-year-old niece wrote a school report about manic-depressive illness, expressing herself with a frankness and knowledge unimaginable to me at that age. "This report," she wrote, "tells the stories of my family's pains and triumphs. It tells of the sorrows caused by manic-depressive illness, which has sometimes torn my family apart. But this report also explains that even in the face of this often fatal disease, people can succeed."

My niece has already succeeded not only in being honest about her family, but also in making me very glad that I have finally been more honest about myself.

Reference

Jamison KR (1995) *An Unquiet Mind.* New York: Alfred A Knopf.

Comment on Chapter 6

Tom Burns

Professor Jamison's keynote presentation of her experience of manic depression and of deciding to acknowledge publicly her illness dramatically exemplified this process. Her presentation, like her book *An Unquiet Mind*, mixed intimately the scientific and the intensely personal. How had her revelation been received? With some prejudice but overwhelmingly with support and admiration. Colleagues usually, patients always, and politicians and opinion formers from quite unpredictable sources applauded her honesty.

Professor Jamison attributed much of this to her supportive departmental head. My experience of both colleagues and patients with senior mental health positions is that they are rarely stigmatised within the profession. Professor Jamison, by her vivid demonstration of extraordinary professional productivity and success alongside her illness, begins the essential process of dispelling the myth that the mentally ill cannot contribute, that they are doomed to dependency. It is this juxtaposition of illness and productivity that has the power to dilute the stigma. The authentic voice of experience as embodied in Professor Jamison far outweighs many heavy academic tomes in changing public opinion. High-profile individuals, who admit to the struggle they have with a mental illness despite their conspicuous success, will achieve infinitely more than well-meant and successfully managed public campaigns.

Discussion of Professor Jamison's contribution demonstrated how welcome her stand had been, although some mental health professionals with mental illnesses commented that their colleagues had not been that supportive. Not surprisingly nurses were found to be more so than doctors! Issues of managing diagnosis in a way that is sensitive to cultural variation were also raised.

The task of reducing stigma and discrimination for the mentally ill was well mapped out by this contribution. We were helped to recognise both the ubiquity of stigma and also its enormous variation across time and social groupings. Professor Jamison's brave and powerful story gives a clear way forward and a hope that much can be achieved. It remains vital, however, to recognise the role that discrimination plays in human behaviour. Only by acknowledging our own vulnerability to it and understanding it better can we achieve the goal of reducing its detrimental impact on the mentally ill. Externalising it and demonising it are not helpful. In the campaign to reduce stigma we should start by not stigmatising stigma.

7 A psychiatrist lives with bipolar affective disorder

Rosemary Lethem

Introduction

In 1999, I wrote "a selective autobiography", looking back on over thirty years' experience of recurrent affective disorder. Although I had had this in mind for some time, the trigger came from attending a meeting of the Stigma Campaign at the Royal College of Psychiatrists in May 1999. Subsequently I offered the script to the campaign and was invited to make this contribution.

I am a clinician in my forties, married, with three pre-teenage children. My illness started in my teens but for much of my adult life its significance was not realised, even though the number of episodes has reached well into double figures. It was not diagnosed as bipolar affective disorder (BAD) II until 1999. By then I had developed a rapid cycling disorder. I have experienced a number of incapacitating depressive episodes, but the highs have been mild.

Having a recurrent, poorly controlled mental illness is an ever present reality which has been the single most important influence, other than my family of origin, on the course of my life. It underlies the seemingly random sequence of studies and jobs in my teens and twenties and continues to challenge me on both personal and professional fronts.

Autobiography

I had a comfortable though geographically mobile childhood. The first hint of the struggles ahead came when I was 12 years old. The year before, my family had made yet another move and I had started the fifth of six schools. Mid-term, I was promoted to the year above and within a few weeks developed what I now recognise as a depressive illness with biological features, which persisted for months. It did not receive appropriate attention, nor stop me becoming top of the class, but the pattern was set for the rest of my teenage years, which were academically achieving but left me lonely and socially unskilled.

I enjoyed sixth form, but could not catch up on developmental tasks. To my enormous surprise, I got a place at Cambridge to read Natural Sciences and duly went up, aged 17, where I spent probably the unhappiest days of my life. Uncomprehendingly, I became severely depressed very rapidly. Six weeks into term I was briefly hospitalised, before spending the rest of the year at home, largely without treatment. (The intention had been that I should transfer to the equivalent student health service: I have recently learned that it did not then exist.) My salvation came through getting a job, during which I recovered and learnt some social skills. I returned the following academic year; so did the depression. Fortunately psychiatric follow-up had been pre-arranged and I got through my degree, extremely successfully in academic terms, with supportive psychotherapy throughout.

In my twenties things were healthier. No psychiatrists. I did a PhD, considered studying medicine, became a management trainee instead (which I loathed, partly due to being seriously depressed once again), and eventually qualified as a doctor in 1983. After house jobs I became an SHO in psychiatry, having discussed the idea with my Cambridge psychiatrist. The same pattern continued: I got depressed, soldiered on and passed exams at the first go.

In 1987, now married, I moved to London, after which my illness became much more severe. Twins arrived in 1987 and another baby (unscheduled) in 1989. I became depressed half way through both pregnancies. Other than briefly at university, medication was not prescribed until 1989. I responded to physical treatments but in retrospect antidepressants have precipitated mild hypomania and probably contributed to rapid cycling. I took them continuously from 1989 to 1999.

In 1990 I relapsed to the point where I could no longer force myself to function, culminating in a period of nearly six months in hospital. Once I was admitted I stopped speaking, eating and drinking, and had ECT, the first of four series of treatments to date. After discharge came the first of three periods at a day hospital. I took lithium for seven years, during which the severity of episodes attenuated. I have been on the receiving end of several psychological therapies, on which my view is that the presence or absence of non-specific, Rogerian qualities in the therapist outweighed theoretical considerations. I trained, part-time, as a senior registrar and was accredited in 1996. I am sure that the severity of my illness was not recognised and cannot recall any real discussion of its impact.

On moving to Sheffield, I hoped, naively, that I might have left all the turmoil behind, but from 1997 there has been a series of lows, mild highs and mixed episodes. I did not take sick leave until felled by a major depressive episode last autumn.

In 1999, thirty years on, I met my Cambridge psychiatrist. I asked if I had ever been high, to which the answer was clearly yes. It has been disconcerting to discover that evidence existed then for the bipolar nature of my illness. Writing my "autobiography" also demonstrated likely highs. Only my husband has suspected.

Consequences

The parts of my life story which I have chosen to include illustrate particular themes. The first is the effect of mental illness at various life stages.

The onset in my early teens had vast consequences. It moulded my character as well as directed the nature of life events. From puberty onwards I was unable to complete developmental tasks on time, with profound consequences. Thirty years on, I think I have managed to compensate to a considerable extent, so that I am one of the few who defies the statistics.

The experience of mental illness as a student was particularly frightening. I was naive, away from home for the first time and unaware that I was ill. Students with serious mental illness often will not seek help, in contrast to those with "stress" or personal problems, and the impact on their lives can be devastating. Follow-up may need to be assertive, and must ensure that a safety net is set up, particularly where enquiry has established evidence of earlier problems.

Mental illness interferes with the training of doctors. This is obvious during periods of frank illness, but I suspect frequently goes unrecognised. The way medical training is structured, with its series of unrelated jobs, frequent changes of location and lack of coherent supervision, mitigates against recognition, treatment and support. Sometimes there is active concealment, in my own case through ignorance and shame. The amount of time needed to rehabilitate, and the sheer disruption to career development and life in general, are often not recognised. There is great pressure, from within and without, to carry on. Personally, however, I probably got through to my consultant job because of, rather than despite, the system – although I nearly stopped myself at times. I have never regretted the decision to study medicine but with the benefit of hindsight would have chosen a different specialty.

A second theme concerns the consequences of not understanding fully until 1999 that I suffered from a poorly controlled mental illness rather than being personally inadequate. What difference would this have made? Episodes of illness would have been recognised and treated as such: I might have struggled less, but possibly achieved less too. However, it is destructive to believe that in some fundamental way one is "substandard". Over 15 years in psychiatry the awareness gradually dawned that I had suffered from some severe illness episodes and that as a person I was achieving and robust, but I have no doubt that it would have been preferable to have had this understanding from the start.

Thirdly, living with a severe, recurrent illness means facing vulnerability and uncertainty. My history to date, and the natural history of the illness, dictate that there will be future episodes. There are no treatment guidelines for people of my diagnosis and chronicity. I will remain on medication for the foreseeable future. What is my prognosis? I wouldn't choose to go on living the way I have had to, especially over the last 15 years, and do not share Professor Jamison's view, that, on balance, having BAD has been worth the experiences.

There have been significant consequences for my husband and children, but they do not fall within the scope of this chapter. There are consequences for the ability generally to work. The disruption caused by recurrent or poorly controlled illness should not be underestimated. It can lead to real or apparent underachievement as "soldiering on" and loss of continuity make it difficult to build up a successful career.

Working as a doctor raises the major issue of fitness to practice on health grounds. I and others have had to consider whether I constitute any risk to patients. Suffice it to say that I am regarded as a safe doctor.

There is a peculiar and particular strain which comes from working as a psychiatrist; that is, in having clinical responsibility for patients with the same kinds of illness as my own. This feels like a complex phenomenon: it challenges and uplifts as well as weights and drags. I rationalise my choice and pursuit of career in terms of an altruistic desire to use my own experiences in a way few are qualified to do. It is rewarding, but not easy.

Coping

To cope it helps to understand. My story conspicuously lacked understanding until relatively recently. Now I try to keep an open mind; tolerate uncertainty; live one day at a time, especially when things are not going well; keep counting my blessings. I have always been convinced that mine is a disorder primarily of feeling, with secondary cognitive distortion. I try to be my own cognitive therapist to contain my feelings, and this is a powerful coping strategy.

I take issue with Professor Wolpert that depression, including severe depression, is most closely akin to the emotion of sadness somehow out of control. It is rather the absence of feeling, and the analogy with "malignancy" is conceptually unhelpful.

It is vital to have therapeutic, professional and personal support systems. I have frequent access to a psychiatrist who I trust. The down side has been lack of access to other forms of support in times of illness, when it has not been ideal to be left alone at home day after day. I am thankful to have my husband and family, although family life itself can be a source of stress. I have made little use so far of "users" organisations, although I would mention that a Doctors' Support Network exists for any doctor with present or past mental health problems.

Ways of minimising stress must be incorporated into the stuff of everyday life. Good time management is essential, as the demands of domesticity and professional life have to be juggled, as well as coping with BAD. Obviously, a variety of interests and opportunities to "switch off" outside home and work is helpful.

Awareness and observance of boundaries is protective. These have not always been sufficiently obvious to me. All doctors have to trade off distance from patients through denial of problems with over-involvement. This conflict is prominent in psychiatry and I have felt, at times, particularly affected by it. I tended to err towards over-involvement, especially in the early days whilst getting my professional bearings and also being ill. I am aware that having to cook a meal as soon as I walk in from work can still be a protective mechanism as well as yet another chore.

Finally, I have started to keep a diary, initially as a receptacle for my negative feelings, but through and beyond recovery with more objectivity and pleasure in the act of writing itself.

Conclusion

I have not found the decision to write about myself difficult to make. Others, such as Professor Jamison, have gone before me, and I am in no way diminished as a person by these revelations. I hope that my stance will play a part in changing the defensive, intellectualising attitude still prevalent among doctors, who as a group are beset by mental health problems to an even greater extent than the general public.

I am still adjusting to the different perspective my revised diagnosis conferred. When I am well, I think I understand the nature of contentment: it is to do with accepting what cannot be changed. When I am not well, I cling to hope that some kind of change is possible. The prospects for change, of many kinds, have never been greater.

8   A blot on the landscape

Richard Jameson

Initially so mad that I did not know if I was on planet Earth, let alone in bad odour with the public, I progressed gradually towards sanity and then towards a life in the community. That was 30 years ago, but the stigma still remains – a blot on the landscape.

It is considerably (spectacularly ?) less than when I first fell ill. But the old public misconceptions persist and must be rooted out – misconceptions picked up largely from the lower media and irresponsible word-of-mouth. The doctors have suffered quite as much as the patients – even more so. And yet, who are they? Kind people who see the tremendous suffering here and want to help. However they are branded as a cross between Professor Barmy and Frankenstein. The whole thing is an enormous joke – until you enter the world of insanity and find that it is not a joke at all. Luckily I went up instead of down most of the time. My joy was unconfined. But I have been suicidal too: that was no joke.

It was when I had recovered and was back in the community that the stigma really made itself felt. I lived in constant fear of being found out by employers, by my friends and by any interested party. Between 1960 and 1975 there was not the informed concern there is now. In fact at the beginning there was nothing: no pills, no research, no community care, no interest. It was so bad that my memory has put up the barriers and I cannot repeat the nightmare world I lived in then. It could have happened to somebody else. Of course it was considerably worse 20 years before that. We must congratulate ourselves on having come this far. But there is still some way to go.

As Trustee of an Ealing mental health organisation (poacher turned gamekeeper) I am constantly amazed by the facilities now provided for the user, including a battery of computers on which he can unravel the mysteries of the Internet and, above all, enjoy convivial company over a cup of tea.

The stigma you impose on yourself is one of the worst forms of suffering. It can be so unnecessary. I am or was a loony – so what? You are an arthritic. He is a plumber. We are all human beings. After being officially considered "socially dead", every disabled person is now recognised as a human being. Quite an advance.

Or is this wishful thinking? Are we still in the Dark Ages? Not in my experience. The country has rallied round and we are so much better now than we were. But there are still pockets of prejudice, ignorance and even hostility which must be zapped.

The doctors can do so much, but they are in the front line of attack. It is up to patients like myself to demonstrate the efficacy of the treatment and when it comes to describing the various illnesses, to chase a few cobwebs of misunderstanding away. I am living proof that the system works – unless I am imagining that I have been asked to write this. My gratitude to psychiatrists, nurses, councils and all the social workers is boundless. And what about the researchers and drug inventors, the brain surgeons and the employers who are softening their attitudes?

With great trepidation I went for an interview for a job in a local furniture store and inadvertently spilled the entire beans about my past mental condition to the boss, Mrs Rene Tyler. "Don't worry, love," she replied "We're all barmy in here." I was with that firm for three happy years until it had to close.

The word "schizophrenia" should not immediately and tacitly rule you out at a job interview, as it used to. So much so that I had to withhold the truth. I never lied: I just never told them. I knew I could do the job, and when I was lucky enough to land the job, I did it well. I was with BT for 10 years.

But the spirit of mischief and evil is never far away and for 15 years I fell ill over and over again. It is not the pain, but the inconvenience that I object to: having to restart your career so often that in the end you have nothing you can call a career. And the real love of my life (professional acting) had to go by the board completely. But this is not a hard luck story. I have had a spiffing life and it is not over yet.

For one thing I am writing this article, which is a considerable honour. And appearing on television and radio and in the national press, sorting myself out with every word I utter. I am a great believer in the power of words over the mind. A bad bunch of words can actually make you physically ill, whether you are an individual or a nation. Conversely, marshal your words and you streak ahead.

You have to be able to take a joke. Stigma is often a cruel, destructive joke. Ignorance is equally bad and it is up to the leading health authorities to make absolutely sure that the nation is well aware of the ins and outs of the whole mental situation.

But the horse has bolted. We have already gone a long way towards eradicating stigma. Strong spotlights have been beamed on the ant heap and the little creatures have scurried away. Please leave one or two to go on irritating a bit. Life would be incredibly boring without some mental disorder.

To clear up stigma we have to recognise madness as just another illness, one that should inspire compassion and not ridicule. We have to show that it is 90% curable. And it could happen to anyone. It makes marvelous plots for plays and films, but it is not different to sciatica or lumbago. A disability. Chemicals going wrong in the brain, to be righted by other chemicals. The world of the imagination is extremely powerful, but don't get carried away or, like me, you will get carried away.

Living with schizophrenia

Janey Antoniou

This is a testimony to the stigma that one can experience if one has a mental health problem. To begin with I would like to clarify two things. I feel I suffer from the stigma but am otherwise a mental health service user, and this is one individual's view of the world, others may disagree with what I say.

I'll give a bit of my background, to put what I'm saying about stigma into the context of my life. I was hospitalised for the first time in 1985, but did not know my official "label" until about 1988 when I asked my psychiatrist if he knew of a group of people I could join who were in a similar circumstance to me. He suggested contacting the National Schizophrenia Fellowship. I was shocked by the word and I think that that shows that I had the same preconceptions as anyone else despite the fact that I had been in hospital and knew many people with that diagnosis.

Over the last fourteen years I've had huge problems with illness and have been sectioned several times. I've wandered the streets in my dressing gown and on one occasion was naked in public. I've been taken back to the hospital by the police, with all the neighbours watching me go. To a certain degree – and with a lot of help – I've learned to live with the way things are for me but I have also, in the course of all of this, had to deal with the stigmas of having a psychiatric diagnosis in the community. They seem to fall into several categories.

The attitudes of those in the community

I have a neighbour who used to run inside when she saw me and now ignores me. She will have seen dramatic incidences such as me being taken to the hospital by the police when I've been very ill, and read the sensational headlines in the press. I don't have an issue with her fear of the unknown. The first time I went into psychiatric hospital I was terrified of people around me, but as I was living with them it only took me a day to realise that they were all right really. Later a very good friend of mine told me that it was me who scared her the most on her first admission. Unfortunately my neighbour's fear is such that she chooses not to speak to me, and sadly I think there is nothing really I can do about it. It is this sort of thing that causes the "Not In My Back Yard" behaviour when new facilities for those with mental health problems are suggested.

The pitfalls of employment

Since I had always worked and was able to be open with my colleagues, I don't think I ever fully appreciated how difficult it would be to get another job with the stigma of my "label" hanging over me. Until January 1998 I was a research scientist and I enjoyed it, but in the late eighties I was denied the chance to do a PhD and of promotion because of my health. Now I am unemployed but working freelance and looking for a less stressful or part-time job.

I have every intention of mentioning my psychiatric history if I get an interview but I have not put anything about it on my CV. I also had to persuade one of my referees that he was jeopardising my entire future by mentioning it. It's not that I'm trying to hide anything but I really feel that I have to be there in an interview before I say anything, otherwise the assumptions surrounding mental health problems will ruin any chances I may have. So far I have only been short-listed for one job, and I did not get that.

There are other problems of employment. The employer could make assumptions about sick leave and pensions. For example, a friend of mine's employers were good enough to give her an extra two weeks' sick leave when they heard about her mental health problems, but they took her out of the company pension plan and told her she would have to get her own. Another friend was employed on the proviso that she didn't mention anything to do with her condition to the other workers. I think her employers suspected she might be bullied if they found out.

Treatment and attitudes by mental health professionals

The law and the way the mental health system is set up have caused a huge power imbalance between users and mental health professionals. This has led to a great deal of anger among users. I feel that no real progress will be made until givers of the services and users of the services can sit down as equals and have a discussion about treatments and how they feel about each other more generally.

For me one of the biggest frustrations in having a mental health problem is the way it is perceived by some as making me unable to take decisions about what is best for me. And when I question a decision that's been made nobody listens. While I can understand this when I've been very psychotic and deluded, I resent it in my day-to-day life.

At one stage I was on Haldol depot injections for six months and that was easily the worst time in my life. My brain was functioning all right but my body was so uncomfortable – if I was lying down I wanted to walk around and if I was walking around I wanted to lie down. I was working (but not well) for eight hours a day and sleeping for sixteen. When I tried to talk to the doctor about this he threatened to tell my employers that I was not cooperating with treatment. It was not until I finally said that I didn't care about the job and I was stopping the medication that he realised how horrible I felt.

Now my GP and I have come to a working arrangement that if I want to, he will let me try something new but then I have to stay with it for at least three months before I start complaining. However, I'm very lucky in that I am both educated and articulate; some people are less able to ask for things or explain how they feel and may be intimidated by some professional behaviour.

The issue of respect for those with mental health problems

It seems to me that in this society, for reasons I don't understand, those with mental health problems do not command as much respect as everyone else.

The most blatant example of this recently was the title of the Channel 4 series "Psychos". There is no other disorder or illness that I can think of where mainstream television could get away with titling a drama about it with a derogatory term. It's like calling a programme "Cripples".

Channel 4's argument was that the title reflects what the doctors called themselves in the series. I think that is a non-argument. If a group of people called themselves "cripples" one still would not be able to make a programme with that as the title because the public would find it offensive. There also seems to be a hidden message that psychiatrists can get away with not respecting their patients.

There are many other such examples of disrespect in newspapers, television and in the way people talk. I hope though, that the Changing Minds Campaign run by the Royal College of Psychiatrists and other initiatives can help people to see the reality of mental health problems rather than the stigma.

10 Stigmatisation of dementia

Barbara Pointon

Stigmatisation arises from fear in the onlooker – of dementia itself or of being unable to handle unpredictable and irrational behaviour. There's also widespread ignorance, even among professionals, about the disease and especially about how to communicate when words fail. As no one likes to feel helpless or discomfited, avoidance or exclusion tactics are used. My husband was diagnosed with dementia eight years ago at the age of 51. Here are a few examples of stigmatisation we've encountered.

Social exclusion

We were not invited to special birthday celebrations of family members because they were held in restaurants. I have no doubt it was because my husband's messy eating habits might have given offence. The usual invitation arrived for a Christmas drinks party. But this time it had only my name on it. I didn't go. On another occasion, a different hostess made it clear to me that although we were both invited to a party, "perhaps it would be better if you came up by yourself".

All dementia patients understand more than they can say, but when my husband's ability to speak coherently began to disappear, there were numerous occasions when he became excluded from conversations and not a single word was addressed to him personally. Or he was talked about as though he was not there, even by doctors. Most of our friends and neighbours have been extremely supportive but there have been one or two examples of people pointedly crossing the road rather than having to stop and speak to us.

At this late stage, as well as continuing to chat to him, communication can also be achieved by copying his strange vocalisations, and by eye contact, smiling, singing and stroking. It requires disinhibition, which some visitors understandably find very difficult and so stay away. Yet they are only the same skills they readily employ to communicate with babies.

Social embarrassment

We gave up going to the theatre, concerts or talks because my husband, in his excitement, would occasionally says something aloud and people nearby would turn round with a disapproving "SSsh!".

Because of his visuo-spatial difficulties, he needed help when going to the loo. When there was no disabled facility we had the choice of either my going into the Gents' with him, or his accompanying me to the Ladies'. The startled looks said it all and I didn't want to humiliate him further by trying to explain. To make matters worse, some disabled loos are locked and can only be opened with a special key given out with Orange Badges. But you can only get an Orange Badge if you have *physical* mobility problems and many moderately demented patients remain very active. An example of ignorance in the Town Hall?

At an early stage of the illness, my husband would approach and talk to total strangers, or tag along beside or behind them in the street. Because his outward appearance was just like anyone else's, this behaviour was often completely misconstrued. Once someone raised a hand to strike him.

Ignorance among professionals

During respite care in the mental hospital, I was called to a meeting of doctors and senior nurses because one of the younger staff had made a complaint that my husband had touched her face and T-shirt. This was deemed to be sexual harassment. In disbelief I pointed out that when people are losing their speech, how else can they convey "Thank you" except by touch? I was furious that my kind husband was in effect being labelled a dirty old man.

We have a little grandchild. But my husband doesn't know he's a grandfather because my daughter-in-law's health visitor advised her not to bring the baby anywhere near him. I've tried explaining that persons with dementia seem to have a sixth sense not to harm children or animals, but what's my word against a professional's? I'm deeply hurt by this situation.

Some care staff shout at dementia patients with normal hearing in some strange belief that shouting gets the message across. I'm also appalled by the number of domiciliary and continuing care staff who talk down to people with dementia ("That's a good boy!") or scold them like children ("Don't eat with your *fingers*, Mrs X" when Mrs X can no longer handle cutlery efficiently). A lot more training is required.

Segregation and social isolation

Some friends and family no longer visit my husband now he's in a home because they say he doesn't know who they are. They do not seem to understand that receiving special attention from another human being (recognised or not) is still important to the sick person. Could it be that some visitors want approbation for having taken the trouble to visit and if it is not forthcoming, then they won't bother? Would they adopt the same attitude about visiting in a physical terminal illness?

Some residential and nursing homes ask residents to move out when they develop dementia. Others, like my husband's, promise to keep them to the end, yet when he began to shout a lot, doubts were raised about keeping him. People with dementia are not parcels to be posted hither and thither. As one in five people over the age of 80 develop dementia, staff in all care homes for the elderly should be dementia-trained. Then the stigma of patients being automatically labelled and segregated into EMI units because they are "different" might disappear. Specialist units should be reserved only for those whose behaviour constitutes a real danger to themselves or other people.

Dementia is now where cancer was 15 years ago, shrouded in shame, fear and ignorance. There is still much to be done to "out" the illness and thereby raise public awareness of the devastating effects of it on both sufferers and those closest to them. Until ignorance and fear are dispelled, and people are taught to reach out and find the essential person still in there despite the ravages of dementia, the stigma will remain.

Biographical note

The author looked after her husband at home until recently when he went into residential care. She is now making arrangements to nurse him at home again for the last stretch.

11 An insight into the world of anorexia nervosa, with particular reference to the resulting stigmatisation and social isolation

Rosemary Shelley

Anorexia nervosa is more than just a debilitating illness, more than just a disease; it is a different world, a completely different existence where your inner world is greater than your outer world. It is a way of living that only the sufferer can truly appreciate. It's a dark, isolated world dominated by food, exercise, body image and body weight.

Each day has its set routine, everything is done at rigidly set times and food prepared with military precision, every calorie counted. Time drags, there is physical pain, boredom, social isolation and often despair. Some sufferers want to break out of the anorexic world as they find the existence unbearable; some want to stay, it is their world and they feel safer there than in the "real" world. Some don't know what they want, their brains too starved to make a rational decision to battle against the illness. They stay there forever and that is their life. Welcome to the world of anorexia nervosa.

At the age of fifteen I did not choose to develop an eating disorder, I don't think anyone consciously chooses to starve themselves, at least not in the initial stages. I was just a depressed teenager who felt that I had no control over my life. It was already mapped out for me – GCSEs, A Levels, university, a successful career and then a family – at least that was how it felt. The unfairness of life in general angered me too, the suffering that went on that I was helpless to prevent; war, disease, famine. My hatred at the world and the disliking I had developed of myself over a number of years had festered away with no outlet for the overwhelming anger; that was until I discovered the power of starvation.

No one realised I was anorexic for a number of months, although friends had their suspicions, but soon it became blatantly obvious. It was not a diet gone wrong. I had simply reduced my calorific intake to three hundred a day. Thin catwalk models didn't influence me, I was not interested in what other people around me weighed or looked like. The main thing was that I was in control. I was on a fasting high and content to remain in that state. However, my mood eventually plummeted along with my weight. Soon the cold set in along with the headaches and dizziness. The illness was becoming physical.

Once my family knew about my illness we all thought things would get better from then onwards; little did we know we had ten years of hell ahead of us. The psychiatrist I had waited six months to see only saw adults, we discovered at my first and only appointment. I was sixteen by then. By the time the correct referral had been made it was too late. I had entered the world of anorexia and was firmly grounded there. I would not budge. I was too locked away for anyone to reach me. From being desperate for help I'd become manipulative and deceitful. In my mind the medical profession were a threat because they were trying to take away all I had – my anorexia.

My friends had long given up on me. Anorexia was my only companion. I remained at a very low weight for three years and it was something my friends either could not cope with or just did not have the patience to deal with. I had little to say to them, they weren't part of my world and I was not part of theirs, we had nothing in common. I was only interested in food and weight; rather selfishly I wasn't interested in them because I could not relate to the experiences they were living in their day-to-day lives. I remained at a very low weight until one bleak winter when I decided I had had enough and stopped eating. It was only a matter of weeks before I was hospitalised.

I was not aware of any stigma attached to my illness initially. I think it affected my parents more. They felt the stigma of having an anorexic daughter, which to the outside world meant there were problems within the family to the extent that they could not even feed and care for their own children properly. People must have wondered how they allowed me to walk around in the physical state I was in, but it was my decision to refuse hospitalisation until it was absolutely necessary.

I am more aware of the stigma attached to the illness now. The stigma of being anorexic or having been anorexic is something that is very hard to leave behind. Often friends still treat me like a fragile five-stone anorexic when I'm perfectly healthy. The first thing they comment on is my size, some even enquire about my weight, but I know my value as a person is worth more than any figure on the scales. Meals with friends are awkward. They watch what I eat and how I eat it, yet I am as normal as they are apart from the medical history that follows me around like a ball and chain.

Added to that is the problem of trying to get a job. For "anorexia nervosa" read "unreliable and mentally unstable" – and that is just for a job in the business world. Access to the healthcare profession is even harder. My passion is to go into nursing but I doubt I'll ever be accepted on a course. I've probably got more empathy and understanding than many and I know what it means to suffer, both physically and mentally, but as soon as you declare anorexia on a health questionnaire eyebrows are raised, questions asked and your competence put in doubt.

I know of many people who have been stigmatised by the general public. They have been stopped in the street and asked what sort of impression they felt they were giving to impressionable young girls, others were rudely told to go and get themselves something to eat. Others have even been sworn at or pointed at as if they were some kind of freak. I have experienced that myself along with people talking about me when they think I can't hear. People seemingly fascinated, or maybe appalled, by my emaciated state have even followed me around shops.

For some people the only way out of the anorexic world is to make a suicide attempt, sometimes as a cry for help, sometimes as a genuine attempt. It is after taking overdoses of tablets that I have received most stigmatisation. I viewed it as part of my illness but the medical staff seemed to view it as a waste of their valuable time and a waste of a bed. They didn't want to speak to me, one even tutted in disgust as she passed my bedside. Worst of all, while the other patients have a name I was just a bed number. But then that is what anorexia is all about – counting calories, counting fat units, measuring the figures on the scales, calculating your body mass index. At the end of the day it is all about numbers.

12 The stigma of alcohol dependence – Andy's story

Anon

"People think that wives abusing husbands is a joke – the hen-pecked husband – but I get it and I deserve it. She's had so much to put up with and as long as she doesn't leave again I'll take the beatings, the rows, the fights and the contempt.

I used to like a glass of wine – the odd pint at lunchtime – but now I hate the stuff. It owns me, and every day it lets me know how much I'm its servant – I don't have a job – at first, I would go down to the social with my suit on – a bit of dignity, I thought – but here is no dignity, no respect when you're a drunk. People can tell you know – they see it – no moral fibre, no job, not even a home to call our own.

We never used to have to listen to music from the neighbour's all night, but the old neighbours weren't too keen on the vomit in the drive, the police round night after night or, if not them, the ambulance – where we live now, that's par for the course.

When you're working, when you've got a few quid in your pocket, drink is just something that keeps the wheels going round, but those days are long gone. Our son hates me (and with his mother's eyes), my own sister won't have anything to do with me – if you piss all over yourself and slap her son you can't really blame her – but that's how it works.

I hate the drink – but it's not that. What is worse is what it makes me – you just feel so empty – people look past you, look round you and no-one cares that once you were alright, you had plans, hopes, respect. But you can't respect yourself when the distaste of the world is writ large on every face you see – when your wife stays because of pity and a misplaced sense of duty and when the only person who despises you more comes when you forget to avoid the mirror.

There's nothing wrong with drinking – but there's something wrong with me. Alcohol has ruined my life."

Biography

Andy is a 57-year-old former insurance broker, now retired through ill health, who lives with his wife in a local housing authority flat on the North Peckham Estate. He is an alcoholic, although with a relatively late onset of problem drinking. Although he started drinking at 17, his alcohol consumption did not interfere with the early part of his life – he married, held down a stable job for 26 years, had a child and bought his own house.

Following the death of his mother in 1986, he began to engage in prolonged spells of binge drinking. Although his employers were initially sympathetic, his increased absence from work, poor performance and inconstant attitude led to his dismissal. Although, he obtained a number of subsequent positions, his poor attendance and lunchtime drinking ensured that by 1989, he was virtually unemployable.

Since this time, he has had three drink-driving convictions, two convictions for being drunk and disorderly and one for being a public nuisance. He is now prone to spells of intense depression, has low self-esteem, and his peripheral neuropathy has both restricted his mobility and had an adverse effect on his marriage.

Although he has been successfully detoxed on two occasions, his GP is no longer willing to treat him (regarding his alcoholism as entrenched and self-inflicted), while he himself regards his alcoholism as a lifetime curse. The support he could initially draw on from family and friends has long since dissipated and he is regarded by the few people willing to deal with him to be an incorrigible drunk and nuisance.

Andy has severe liver damage, he is unable to find work as a result of a history of absenteeism and workplace accidents. Of course, he is not helped by having lost his licence (and briefly his liberty) following his third drink-driving conviction. He is now unemployed, his marriage is on the rocks, his wife only sees their grown-up son when he is not around, and his only friend is on the opposite side of the bar. Mercifully, his health deterioration ensures that he will only continue to despise himself for a limited period of time.

13 The stigma of drug dependence – Angela's story

Anon

"You want to know what it is to be an outcast? When I get home from the shops, I don't have a nice little mat with welcome written on it. No, what I have to look forward to is 'Junkie whore' in big red letters across the door. I'm just pleased that the wee one isn't old enough to read yet – but by the length of time the council is taking, she will be before its cleaned. You see, I'm a junkie – it's my own fault – so when my 'respectable' neighbours spray the front of the door, I deserve it. When Stacey was taken into care, her wee heart was broken, but they all look at you and you know what they're thinking 'selfish junkie bitch, can't look after herself, never mind that lovely wee girl'.

She's been taken away from me three times now and I have never deserved it – it only ever happens when that useless toerag gets out of the jail – that's her father by the way. Fortunately, he's in for three years this time, so we won't have any more of his layabout pals leaving their needles lying around, where wee Stacey could get to them.

I said about coming back from the shops earlier on – that's the ones that I'm still allowed to go near – before I got a script, I had to thieve, and its years ago now, but once you're labelled a KT [known thief], you're marked for life. So much for civil liberties. If I get seen on the high street, the police will lift me for nothing – just for being there. And if I do make it into the shops, they never take their eyes off you – you can see them behind the counter, nudging each other – 'keep your eyes on her, she'd steal the coat off your back'.

But the worst is your family – oh so discreetly, they pick up their purses and jackets when you come round, they forget to tell you about parties and christenings, Christ I never even found out about my auntie's funeral till two weeks later. You see, they're scared you'll make a scene – be stoned, beg folk for money for a hit. They really believe that you don't feel it, the hurt, or if they do, that it's your fault.

It doesn't even matter when you tell your own mother that you're getting treatment – all she thinks about is the time you stole her purse, the times you were out of it in the street, the court appearances. They don't understand – my own mother thinks I'm disease-ridden, that I'm an unfit mother, that I'm a dirty little whore – my own mother.

I've tried hard this last couple of years – I'm not thieving any more, I'm well off the game, my drug worker says I'm doing fine. But its hard, they tell you that you should stay away from other users but nobody else wants anything to do with you; they don't understand, they don't trust you, and, as for a job, forget it. It like I have 'junkie' tattoed across my forehead. I regret it – I know I made a mistake, but I'll never be allowed to forget it, nor will my daughter – we're trapped, I'm a junkie for life and everyone tells her that she's got an unfit mother."

Biography

Angela started using heroin at 15 and was injecting by the age of 17. At 18, she gave birth to a daughter, Stacey, who had to be detoxified postnatally. Stacey had a low birthweight and has shown signs of mild cognitive impairment that are likely to be related to her mother's heroin use.

Although currently stable on a methadone prescription and providing heroin-free urines, Angela's stability appears to be related to the absence of her long-term partner, who is also Stacey's father. Currently serving three years for intent to supply heroin, Steve's presence is associated with chaotic periods in Angela's life.

These are the periods in which she is likely to binge on heroin, crack, benzodiazepines and alcohol. She funds these episodes of use through shoplifting and prostitution, and now has a lengthy conviction record. Although the courts are reluctant to take her daughter into care, Angela's inconsistent behaviour means this is now a very real threat.

Angela is subject to anxiety attacks, is plagued by feelings of guilt and loneliness and has attempted suicide on at least one occasion. She is ostracised by her neighbours who are aware of her drug use and of her prostitution, and is unable to break the cycle of condemnation that her drug use and her primary relationship have generated. She sees no way out, because she is cast in a role that is laden with prejudice, incomprehension and fear.

14 The stigmatisation of anxiety disorders

Nicky Lidbetter

Anxiety disorders are extremely common, with one in three people experiencing panic attacks at some time in their life. With such large numbers of the general public affected, it is surprising that as we enter the 21st century, anxiety disorders still carry a stigma. A societal mark of Cain.

The words "anxiety", "stress" and "panic" are so frequently used that in some ways this has had the effect of lessening the severity of anxiety disorders. We all feel "stressed out", or "panicked" because we thought we might be late for work – but this is not what suffering with an anxiety disorder is really about. This flippancy is perhaps one reason why the medical profession, and indeed the general public, do not take anxiety disorders seriously. Sufferers are often referred to as "the worried well" and "neurotic" – in other words, not really ill. The actual level of mental distress experienced by those suffering with anxiety disorders is certainly very much underestimated – who determines whether distress caused by anxiety is any less than that caused by other mental conditions? Despite this, those with anxiety-related conditions still suffer from the same "mental health" labelling process as others, and frequently defer seeking help because of worries about being sectioned, or having a neurotic diagnosis on their records. Indeed many who have sought professional help for their anxiety find their GP reluctant to accept later physical conditions as genuine illnesses once they have an anxiety disorder diagnosis.

Women are frequently believed to be the main sufferers of anxiety disorders and it is suggested that there is some gynaecological link between their distress, often labelled as hysteria, and hormones. Our experience is that just as many men suffer with anxiety disorders, and indeed people of all ages, races, sexualities, classes and cultures are equally likely to be affected by these problems.

Another issue with anxiety disorders is that there is no specific medication at present to treat them. Antidepressants are given as medication, which creates the impression that anxiety is not an illness in its own right, rather a secondary symptom of depression, if it exists at all. GPs often feel powerless when treating anxiety because they feel they are unable to help with these time-consuming disorders. Many do not have knowledge or up-to-date information about various therapies which can be beneficial in treating anxiety disorders, including mainstream therapies such as cognitive therapy. They are frequently unaware of self-help networks in operation in their local area or specialist clinics, which results in anxiety disorder sufferers being left to cope alone with what are often very debilitating problems. Professionals seem generally to lack faith in user-led services, despite there being a wealth of evidence to support the fact that those with anxiety disorders are often best placed to support other sufferers because they can truly empathise with the problems faced. Some professionals may feel in some way threatened by user-led groups; after all they have had years of training, which is undermined if non-professionals are employed in service delivery.

Professionals need to have empathy as it is very hard to understand anxiety disorders without having had personal experience. For this reason, those who have experienced anxiety but are not working in a professional capacity are just as valuable to other sufferers.

Anxiety disorder sufferers are often thought of by professionals and ordinary people alike, and indeed by themselves, as weak, pathetic individuals who should just "pull themselves together". Many perceive that it is the sufferers' bleak outlook that keeps them in the throes of their anxiety. Sufferers are frequently perceived as "attention seekers" or "hypochondriacs" when in fact there are usually very serious issues at the root of any one individual's anxiety disorder, such as abuse, addiction, etc.

For many with anxiety disorders, their problems are further exacerbated by the fact that they are expected to go to services, when often they are housebound through agoraphobia or obsessive compulsive disorder and cannot get out. Many sufferers find they do not have access to a GP because their GP is not prepared to visit them at home, assuming that if they really wanted to they could get to the surgery. To this end anxiety disorders such as agoraphobia are often dismissed and not given the credence that they deserve. The result of this is that those who need therapy and primary care services the most end up being forgotten. Indeed agoraphobia, whilst being a disability in its own right, is rarely recognised as such, particularly by benefits agency doctors and the social security system in general.

Many people with anxiety disorders find that they are misdiagnosed – often receiving a diagnosis of depression and not being referred to appropriate forms of therapy such as cognitive behaviour therapy (CBT). Those who are fortunate enough to be correctly diagnosed and immediately referred for specialist treatment face lengthy waiting lists for CBT, counselling, psychotherapy and hypnotherapy. By the time many who initially present with panic attacks get seen for specialist treatment their condition has often progressed into other anxiety disorders such as agoraphobia which are harder to treat and more resistant to therapy.

Of course another issue specifically around anxiety is that of the diverse nature of anxiety and the ever-increasing number of anxiety disorders. No two sufferers of any one condition have exactly the same symptoms – they may have similarities, but their suffering will be distinct. To this end, treatment of anxiety disorders needs to be more tailored to individual needs. There is often a lack of awareness of the various types of anxiety disorders amongst professionals, particularly those recently given a name such as social phobia, body dysmorphic disorder (BDD), obsessive compulsive disorder (OCD) and emetophobia. Again, a diagnosis of depression is a common outcome of a consultation for sufferers of these conditions.

Anxiety disorders are often seen as an old people's problem, with the view being that as people become older they become more frail, more vulnerable and more susceptible to anxiety. Their anxiety is seen as natural and therefore doesn't warrant treatment. However, the average age of National Phobics Society members is 27, indicating that this is a myth. Indeed we have been receiving increasing numbers of enquiries from parents of children suffering from anxiety disorders ranging from panic attacks to school phobia. It seems clear to us that one way of de-stigmatising anxiety disorders is to work with schools to raise the profile of these conditions, to reassure children that it is OK to have feelings, emotions and anxieties and that these are nothing to be ashamed of. If the next generation sees anxiety as something to be explored and worked on rather than something to be hidden we would be well on the way to combating stigma and opening the door to a healthier society.

15 Living with depression: The reality

Susan Noakes

Depression is an illness which is extremely common in this country. It is estimated that between three and four million people in the UK experience depression at any one time, yet it is possibly the most misunderstood of all illnesses. One reason for this is the word "depression" itself. Depression conjures up numerous connotations. We talk of the weather being depressing; when things go wrong we say we are depressed when we mean we are fed up. Yet depression has specific and clinical symptoms – it is a genuine illness like any other. Many myths and misunderstandings surround the illness. For example, there is a common perception that young people do not suffer from depression and that it is an illness which mainly affects the elderly, who accept the condition as untreatable. Yet depression is the most democratic of all illnesses. It does not respect age, race, culture, wealth, ethnic origin or social status.

With so many people affected by depression, why is there such extreme reluctance on the part of sufferers to talk about their illness? There is a commonly held perception amongst individual sufferers that they are the only ones with the illness, that other people will not understand the condition and out of ignorance will classify them as either mad or dangerous. In Depression Alliance's self-help groups it is surprising how open and willing people are to talk about their symptoms, feelings and fears to total strangers. Comments such as "this is the only place where I feel I can be myself " or "it is good not to have to put on a face but to be able to speak openly and honestly to others" are commonplace. Why do sufferers feel able to speak to total strangers more readily than to members of their own family? Maybe the answer lies partly in the degree of stigmatisation which attaches to depression from both the sufferer and carer perspective. Another popular misconception held by a significant proportion of society is that depression is avoidable and if one suffers it is simply a case of pulling oneself together and getting on with life. There is no realisation that sufferers would "pull themselves together" if they possibly could. Perhaps the lack of sympathy stems from the fact that frequently there are no visible signs of illness to a third party. The "worried well" tag is applied. Sometimes the view is held that someone without depression has more reason to be depressed than the sufferer. This leads naturally to the conclusion that the sufferer is weak-willed and the author of his or her own misfortune. The reality is quite different.

In a weighted poll carried out by Depression Alliance amongst MPs in 1996, only 63% of Conservatives viewed depression as an illness. One was driven to the conclusion that the remaining 37% did not perceive it as a recognised medical condition. Possibly initiatives such as the Defeat Depression Campaign and the National Depression Campaign have assisted in bringing about a change in the public's perception and understanding of depression, and gradually it is becoming viewed as a very real and life-threatening illness.

One of the questions frequently asked of us by people submitting job applications is whether they should reveal their previous history of depression. There can be little doubt that a diagnosis of depression will impact adversely on a job application. Yet there is evidence to suggest that people with depression are highly artistic and creative. There are numerous employment opportunities where such skills could be put to good use.

At Depression Alliance we also see instances where an employee is conveniently moved sideways on returning to work after an episode of depression or otherwise finds promotion prospects firmly blocked. Paradoxically, employment is a most effective form of therapy for someone with depression. It provides them with a structure to the day, avoids isolation by social integration, boosts self esteem in doing something useful and provides independence and choices through a salary which would otherwise not exist. One can, to some extent, appreciate and accept the reservations prospective employers might have on engaging someone with a history of depression. However, it is difficult to comprehend why a person with a poor academic record and a criminal conviction can secure a job interview whilst a candidate with depression and more appropriate qualifications for the position advertised fails to do so.

In Depression Alliance our membership has increased marginally from 2,500 to 3,500 over a period of three years, yet the number of requests for help, information and advice from members of the public has risen dramatically from 14,600 in 1994 to over 70,000 in 1998. It may safely be assumed that the vast majority of people contacting our organisation simply take what they require from the charity and then seek anonymity once more. They specifically shun public recognition or acknowledgement of depression by declining to take membership. One can only conclude that this is due largely to the degree of stigmatisation which attaches to mental health and the perceived fear that membership of Depression Alliance may somehow be transferred to employment records.

There can be little doubt that depression has an impact on the whole family, not merely the sufferer. A carer of someone with depression may also be viewed with suspicion. It is not unheard of for people to enquire whether one can catch depression in the same manner as the common cold. With such ignorance a carer may be perceived as a danger to society who should be avoided where possible. Quite clearly, stigmatisation feeds on fear and ignorance.

The problem needs to be tackled within the primary school setting – it would seem that views can become quite entrenched by the time a person reaches the age of fifteen or sixteen. How this can be achieved remains to be seen. Teachers are already stretched to complete the syllabus within the allotted time and it is questionable whether they have the appropriate skills and knowledge to undertake a mental health education programme.

Stigmatisation may also be compounded as a consequence of poor diagnostic skills by some GPs. The press must also bear responsibility for poor reporting or indulging in sensationalism. In one instance a national newspaper interviewed one of our members who during the course of the conversation mentioned that at times she felt as though she wanted to kill her family. The headline that resulted was "depressive wanted to kill her family". The six words were, of course, taken totally out of context but it made a gripping headline and doubtless helped sell a few more papers. After the article was printed the impact on the sufferer and her family was devastating.

Overcoming stigmatisation requires an effective partnership between all those involved in the health field, either directly or indirectly. The partners include patients, patients' relatives, physicians, psychiatrists, psychologists, pharmacists, politicians and the press. Only then will accurate and reliable information be disseminated to members of the public on the subject of depression. Often articles are written to satisfy the author's personal agenda with little regard for the impact or consequences that might ensue. Misinformation or inaccurate facts are given. Depression is a disease like any other. It does not deserve special attention, ridicule or, indeed, a failure to acknowledge its very existence. Given the prevalence of depression today it is unlikely that there are many people in the UK whose lives have not been touched by the illness to some extent.

16 Schizophrenia: Prejudice and stigma

Cliff Prior

Schizophrenia is a highly stigmatised condition. Prejudice and hostility cause great distress and pain, drive people to avoid care and treatment, even drive some to suicide. The stigma also affects services, for example preventing new facilities being built in neighbourhoods through NIMBY protests, and stopping people in recovery from getting a job.

Is there something new that can be added to this sorry tale? This chapter suggests that repeating the sorts of public education initiatives we have seen in the past will not be enough. Although the public have got it wrong on some of their prejudices about schizophrenia – particularly about violence – the truth is that it really is desperately bad for many people at the moment. The good news is that it no longer need be that bad. Services must improve the reality of life for people with schizophrenia before we can expect the public to change their minds. This improvement is within reach.

Rethink (previously The National Schizophrenia Fellowship) is the charity for everyone affected by severe mental illness, representing both users and their families. It is a campaigning membership charity with networks of mutual support groups, and also the UK's largest voluntary sector service provider in mental health.

Rethink has several public education initiatives underway, ranging from the @ease young people's website and the work with the National Union of Students, to training projects for journalists and media partnerships, advice to TV scriptwriters and training for service users to express their voices in the media. Coverage of schizophrenia is overwhelmingly negative and linked to serious violence. A study sponsored by the Scottish Association for Mental Health (SAMH) in Scotland showed that 66% of media coverage linked mental illness with violence.

The negative portrayal affects professionals and services as well as individuals. Doctors avoid diagnosis as much as individuals and may avoid going into psychiatry in the first place. Poor attitudes lead to a feeling that it isn't worth trying very hard because the outcome will be poor anyway. Appalling conditions in hospitals are tolerated in a way that would be unthinkable in other fields of health care. New treatments are cold-shouldered. Users are done to, not worked with. After all, what's the point of listening to them? They are mad aren't they?

Public attitudes to schizophrenia were captured in a 1997 MORI poll of 1804 adults for Fleischman, Hillard and Lilly. Schizophrenia was the most recognised type of mental illness. However, what people first thought of was split personality. Only when prompted were hallucinations widely recognised as a symptom.

Professionals tend to say that this means the public misunderstand and need educating. However, even people who know someone with schizophrenia – family or a close friend – say that split personality is a characteristic. Interpreting these findings is complex. People may mean unpredictable mood and a changed personality from how you were before – and indeed, poorly treated schizophrenia can be like this.

Responses to other questions show a consistent pattern. Most people are reasonably sympathetic, until it comes to very intimate matters such as whether people would feel happy if their son or daughter was going out with someone with schizophrenia. Those who know someone affected directly are rather more sympathetic. This gives us a strong pointer to the type of public education work that might be successful – person-to-person approaches. Rethink's experience as a service provider, for example, is that neighbours' attitudes to people with a severe mental illness improve when a mental health facility is developed in their street, because they meet real people, and see that they *are* real people.

However, this broadly sympathetic message is still in the context of people believing that the symptoms of schizophrenia are bad news. People who know someone with it believe that even more strongly. This is not a misunderstanding – too often they are right. Poorly treated schizophrenia involves:

- paranoia, often expressed against those closest to you
- emotional withdrawal
- inability to concentrate
- delusions and hallucinations
- frequently, loss of job, home and friends
- the side effects of poor treatment such as rigor, restlessness, shaking, impotence, gross weight gain

We are trapped in a vicious circle, with underfunded unpopular Cinderella services failing people so that outcomes are desperately bad. The public see the results for themselves. The media exaggerate that further, as they do on most subjects. The result is negative attitudes and a belief it is hopeless. In turn, this means mental health care stays a Cinderella service, and that there are few votes to be gained by doing anything about it. And so we go round again.

When we look at the realities of severe mental illness, with over 85% unemployed, 11% homeless and 2.5 times higher mortality, the seriousness of the situation is clear. When we look at mental health services, where 50% of people's first experience of specialist care is a compulsory section, it is clear that services are failing to meet the needs. Carers' experiences are also bad, with most feeling that they are denied information and excluded from care planning.

However, it no longer needs to be that bad. The best modern treatment and care, medical and psychological, delivered early on, coupled with services which provide ready access when things are getting bad, and continuity of care so no-one drops through the net, backed up by social support for accommodation, occupation, money and social contacts, and delivered with the active involvement of the user and their friends and family, constitute a package which can make a vast difference to outcome and quality of life.

The difference between the best and the worst doctors and social services is the difference between recovering a real life and simply surviving. Rethink sees the results of the best care in perhaps one in a thousand people we support, but every year there are a few more, and it can be done more widely. We can shift to a virtuous circle: improving services and care, resulting in improved outcomes, face-to-face contact to show that it can be this much better, leading to better understanding and attitudes.

- *We talk loosely about stigma, when often what we mean is prejudice, because we mean "they" are getting it wrong. "Stigma" means a mark or sign – a negative but perhaps accurate view.*
- *Prejudices can be changed through public education, but stigma can only be changed by changing the reality.*

The public *have* got it wrong about mental illness and serious violence, as shown clearly by the Taylor and Gunn study in 1999. The proportion of homicides committed by people with mental disorder has reduced steadily over the last 40 years, and severe mental illness does not equate to violence. This misunderstanding is the result of media distortion. However, the prejudice about serious violence is fed by the reality of failures in other aspects of mental health care. Rethink believes that the Government have got it right when they prioritise a concerted and long-term programme to improve mental health care. That is what will change public attitudes. However, their spin doctors have got it wrong when they present that policy as a response to a supposed crime wave which does not exist.

Our mission at Rethink is to start by facing up to how difficult life with schizophrenia really is for most people, then moving forward by improving the services and care offered and the real quality of life. We will then help convey those improvements through personal stories and face to face contact. This is an approach we are testing out in a research study in partnership with the Institute of Psychiatry. Phase 1 results are encouraging and are now published.

Mental health professionals should recognise that improving public attitudes is an intrinsic part of their everyday work. If professionals deliver good care, people get better, and the public see that for themselves. Every CPA plan is a public education initiative. It is also important to work with the media, addressing their perspective and negotiating improvements, such as the success in persuading the *Guardian* to use the word "schizophrenia" accurately in their style guide. In Jersey, the Schizophrenia Fellowship turned the anchorman of their local radio station from a critic to a strong supporter, by taking him out to meet people with schizophrenia.

Negotiated improvements need backing up with legal measures. The Disability Discrimination Act is now showing benefits. We also need legal measures to ensure people can get the care they need, as of right. This is being promoted in a joint campaign by the Mental Health Alliance to influence the new Mental Health Act. A petition has already gained over 20,000 signatures, the backing of 50 MPs, the RCN, and unions representing over a million people.

Rethink's job is to help people affected by schizophrenia to recover a meaningful and fulfilling life, to change the reality of life with schizophrenia, and, through that, to change public attitudes.

Reference

Taylor PJ & Gunn J (1999) Homicides by people with mental illness: myth and reality. *British Journal of Psychiatry* **174**: 9–14.

17 From "victim and dement" to patient and person

Clive Evers

Stigma? What stigma? Consider these headlines:

- "Innovation and education"
- "Seaside parties"
- "Major research award announced"
- "Thanks for the Memory"
- "A meeting of minds"

Not much doom and gloom here – all positive upbeat stuff. But yes you're right, they don't come from the *Daily Mail*, *Telegraph* or *Guardian* – they come from the Alzheimer's Society monthly newsletter.

At the Alzheimer's Society, we have a different mind set from the newspapers – we try to convey good news and hope, informed of course by realism. A look at our letters page, mainly from carers, tells a different story – "Silent isolation", "It's sheer exhaustion", "To tell or not to tell?" are themes and issues that still need airing.

I suspect that of all the conditions discussed in this volume, most people would say an inner prayer that they may not be affected by dementia – understandable of course, but still regrettable, for each prayer denies the humanity that will still be within you even if you are affected by Alzheimer's disease, multi-infarct dementia or Lewy body disease. It is important that Alzheimer's disease does not become a stigma. It is a label as well as a disease; when the words are spoken, they can immediately change the way we perceive and act towards the person.

Perhaps one of the most significant barriers to providing good care is our difficulty in recognising the human qualities of those who have become the diagnosed patients. There is a tendency for everyone from doctors and other professionals to friends and family to act differently around people or to avoid dealing with them in a natural way once they are diagnosed. Cognitive deficits, communication difficulties and strange behaviours make most of us uncomfortable, and we may become angry, sad and even frightened. These feelings colour our abilities to see and react to the humanity of the patient. Many patients sense this and withdraw as a result.

It is important to identify and overcome false beliefs and fears about dementia in order to meet the daily challenge of living with a patient. While Alzheimer's involves the slow, irrevocable loss of ability and ultimately even the sense of self, the stereotypical notion that patients lose overnight the ability to think, write, read, talk, work and love is a tragic error.

Changes do occur, but skills and abilities decline at different rates. In fact some skills and feelings remain relatively preserved for many years. When changes do occur, they may require that we modify our behaviour, but how we change and what we say and do can make the patient function better or worse (Cohen and Eisdorfer

1986). What do people with Alzheimer's think about their condition? Well, it is only gradually over the last ten years that anybody has thought to ask them.

Carers

The view had been that carers bore the burden. Carers founded our Society. Carers were the focus of most considerations about help and support. Alzheimer's disease and dementia pose many and complex reactions and challenges. Just a few of these reactions by carers of people with dementia can be seen to have singled them out for special attention.

Grief

Whilst this is normally associated with the loss of a close relative or partner the progressive changes in personality and ability that come with dementia demand multiple grieving. Just when the carer thinks they have adjusted to a new behaviour or the loss of a skill, a further decline or change happens requiring further readjustment.

> *"She is not the person I married: she looks much the same, but she's a different person now. In one sense she's dead already – but still there in another."*

Guilt

It is quite common for carers to feel guilty – about the way they have treated the patient in the past, about feeling embarrassed by odd behaviour, about losing their temper with a sick person, about not wanting the responsibility; guilty for considering placing the person in a home and many other reasons.

> *"She was treated so badly in hospital I vowed not to let her go in again."*

Embarrassment

> *"One of the worst things was when she would run into the street and stop a passer by and ask them to 'get this strange man' – me – out of her house – and we'd been married for over 40 years! She'd be so convincing, which made it more difficult!"*

The behaviour of people with dementia can sometimes be very embarrassing. It is natural to feel embarrassed, although these feelings may fade when they are shared with other carers. Explaining the illness to neighbours usually helps in understanding. But of course at the time the carer will feel marked out by the occurrence.

These and other reactions such as anger and role reversal lead to problems with socialisation. So friends, relatives and neighbours gradually withdraw further, compounding the carer's sense of isolation.

Professionals

It remains remarkable to me that a disease identified in 1907 should only really begin to be responded to by health and social care professionals some seventy years or so later. This is the experience of one of our members:

> *"Elsie and I were married in our 50s and shortly after she had to go into psychiatric care. That was in 1973. Alzheimer's was not as well known then as now, so she was treated for dementia and depression with electric shock treatment, having to go into hospital 4 times a year until they realised it was the wrong treatment (that was in 1988)."*

L Wormald, Carer (August 1999)

Primary care

Perhaps the most intractable professional contribution to the stigma of dementia has been the attitude and response of primary care and GPs. GPs undoubtedly have an enormous range of tasks and responsibilities. It is hardly surprising that they are not all experts in dementia. Moreover, as independent contractors they have been less susceptible to control by management or government directive.

However, the repeatedly dismissive and ageist response to people with possible dementia has been and remains one of the single most important challenges for our Society and I hope for all involved in health and social care planning.

In our primary care report *Right from the Start* carers said that 60% of GPs did not apply a memory test and 42% did not offer any form of diagnosis (Alzheimer's Society 1995). Of those people subsequently found to have dementia, 13% were originally thought by GPs to have depression and 17% to be suffering from "old age".

The same report surveyed GPs themselves about their skills in dementia and their knowledge of local support. Seventy-one percent of GPs felt that they had not had adequate training in the management of dementia. And only 14% referred carers to the Alzheimer's Disease Society.

> "The GP's response to most situations was to put it down to old age. It doesn't create a feeling of confidence or trust. Every situation gives problems because of my parents' inability to help them. Dad's problems as a carer include arthritis of the knee and lower spine, and incontinence makes it difficult to leave the house. Mum has dementia, breast cancer and diabetes."

Mr M Sunderland (1995)

> "Oh that's Alzheimer's. Ha, ha, ha!" and no further comment or explanation was given."

Elsie, 71, caring for her husband

The question of conveying the diagnosis of Alzheimer's disease undoubtedly causes great difficulty and in its own way stigmatises the condition.

Even experts like psychiatrists have this difficulty. In a survey of all consultant psychiatrists working in Scotland in 1997, Dr Robert Clafferty found that 98% said they were willing to tell patients they had depression on the first diagnosis but only 44% of patients with dementia were given their diagnosis.

Another survey of all psychiatrists specialising in old age psychiatry was undertaken by Dr Kirk Rice and Dr Nick Warner in 1995. They found doctors fell into certain groups. Psychiatrists who rarely tell are those who tell less than 20% of their cases and those who nearly always tell are those who tell 80% or more of their cases. They also found great variation in the terminology and words used: some avoided the term "dementia" and used so-called alternatives, like "Alzheimer's disease", "failure of brain cells", "memory problems", or "brain shrinkage". Others told "some appropriate story" or were "economical with the truth". This variation is confusing. There are many examples of good practice in imparting the diagnosis – they need wider dissemination and doctors need more training in how to do this.

These forms of stigmatisation are of course discrete – some would call them discrimination.

Perhaps the worst feature of all is the lack of consistent planning by health authorities for dementia care services. Our report *No Accounting for Health* (Alzheimer's Society 1997) demonstrated that 48% of health authorities had not carried out an assessment of the needs of people with dementia in their area, 79% were not able to identify the resources they spent on dementia in the current financial year, and spending per person with dementia can range from approximately £600 to £1,800 per annum depending on where you live.

No plan, no provision, no problem – and of course this stemmed from lack of central government direction about dementia as a health priority. Over the years it has consistently fallen into the health and social service divide as a result of this lack of commitment. In the past it has been difficult to identify just which division of the Department of Health held responsibility for dementia. Was it the division that dealt with the health of the elderly or with those with mental illness? And what about those younger people with dementia below the age of 65?

Even up to very recently it was only through persistent pressure from our Society that the Department of Health finally agreed to include people with dementia in the national service framework for older people. The very idea of a national framework devoted to the syndrome would of course be like whistling into the wind.

Research

Sometimes stigma emerges unwittingly from research. For example there is a body of research emerging that indicates that people who are better educated have less chance of developing dementia. One study published in the *British Medical Journal* in April 1995 reported a fourfold risk of Alzheimer's disease amongst people with the lowest educational status. There is no shortage of ideas why this may be so. One suggestion is that a common reaction to mental tests amongst older people is to find them intimidating and hence perform badly. This is especially true of those people who have not kept up their skills in reading and writing. However, not every study has found a link between education and dementia, and the link between low social status and dementia may arise from poor physical health and a high rate of vascular dementia.

Some examples of different forms and guises in which stigmatisation can appear with regard to dementia have been given in this brief review.

Public awareness

The good news is that public awareness and understanding of Alzheimer's disease has increased dramatically in the last ten years. This has undoubtedly contributed significantly to reducing if not eliminating the stigma attached to the condition.

In a Gallup poll for the Society in 1989, awareness of Alzheimer's disease stood at 57% of those polled. In November 1994 the world media ripple reporting Ronald Reagan's public announcement of his Alzheimer's provided the biggest boost ever for understanding of the condition.

"My fellow Americans, I have recently been told that I am one of the millions of Americans who will be afflicted by Alzheimer's disease. Upon learning this news Nancy and I had to decide whether as private citizens we could make this known in a public way. In opening our hearts, we hope this might promote greater awareness of the condition. Perhaps it will encourage a clearer understanding of the individuals and the families who are affected by it."

Extract from Ronald Reagan's letter to the American people (November 1994)

Through further work from our Society the 1998 Gallup Poll registered 91% awareness. Partly as a result of this increased awareness we decided the following year to drop the word "disease" from the name of our Society – for public opinion suggests that we have succeeded in conveying the fact that Alzheimer's is a disease of the brain and not the inevitable consequence of ageing.

Earlier diagnosis

Another advance is the gradual shift to earlier diagnosis. There are now many more techniques and methods of investigation that can be used in arriving at a probable diagnosis of Alzheimer's disease during life. Although there is still no single simple test available, advances in psychological tests and brain scanning in conjunction with taking a history means that the diagnosis can be arrived at much sooner than previously.

People with dementia

This means that people with a diagnosis are now approaching our Society directly, whereas previously it was always the carer. So we and other agencies have to develop new ways of working with people who have the disease and of responding and listening to their voices.

Phillip Alderton was diagnosed with Alzheimer's disease in October 1996. He was asked to speak at the Alzheimer's Association Australia 7th National Conference held in Adelaide in August 1997:

> "The specialist did not tell me what I had but said he was writing to my doctor. When I saw the doctor he said: 'I'm sorry to tell you that you have Alzheimer's.'
>
> It may surprise you to know that I was very relieved when he told me the diagnosis. My knowledge of Alzheimers' disease was nil but at least now I had a reason for my forgetfulness. I am now learning as much as I can about it. I do not see it as a problem but view it as a challenge. I will fight it every inch of the way."

Law on mental incapacity

Finally, there are changes afoot in the law on mental incapacity, which we hope will enable us all to have a better say in how we want to be cared for if we lose capacity. For people with dementia and carers these changes cannot come soon enough. They will present challenges for old age psychiatry and all that work in the field so preparation will be essential. But taking control of our care in such situations will again only assist in reducing the stigma associated with dementia.

Consumers in health care

With an increasing emphasis on the role of the consumer in health care this should afford us all with major opportunities for improved responses to patient needs. Indeed the Society has launched a new research grants programme called Quality Research in Dementia (QRD) as a contribution to this. QRD will for the first time give people with dementia and their carers active involvement in setting the research agenda, awarding grants, monitoring projects and getting the results of research into practice (Alzheimer's Society 1999).

Needs of carers

We now know the needs of carers of people with dementia – and direct responses in the form of practical services go a long way to demonstrating that valuable real help and support can be provided. We have published a literature review of these needs (Briggs and Askham 1999).

Active treatments

Much more can now be done in the form of treatments yet so much more could still be achieved. There are two broad categories of active treatment in the care of people with dementia: pharmacological and non-pharmacological.

The expectations of the new anti-dementia treatments are high and may exceed their effectiveness. There is a significant opportunity to develop experience of these treatments through prescribing, and old age psychiatrists are crucial in this process. We also have the knowledge and experience to advise other medical professionals in the use of antipsychotic medication for behavioural problems, which is still widely misused, especially in residential care.

Non-pharmacological approaches such as behavioural therapies are beneficial. We now also have increasing experience of alternative therapies such as aromatherapy, music therapy, sensory stimulation and reflexology. Encouraging and fostering opportunities for their application will usually be positive for patients and carers.

Person-centred care

A major contribution to diminishing stigma is the still developing person-centred approach to dementia care. Pioneered by the late Professor Tom Kitwood and colleagues of the Bradford Dementia Research Group in 1990, this approach shows that with help and support a person with dementia can remain in a state of wellbeing to a far greater extent than many people believe. Much can be done if we are able to keep in contact with that person at the human level.

Conclusion

In conclusion, we hope that continued public awareness, more involvement and focus on people with dementia, the emergence of new treatments and approaches to person-centred care will all contribute to minimising the stigma that is still associated with Alzheimer's disease and dementia.

References

Alzheimer's Society (1995) *Right from the Start.*
Alzheimer's Society (1997) *No Accounting for Health.*
Alzheimer's Society (1999) *Alzheimer's Society Newsletter,* August 1999.
Briggs K & Askham J (1999) *The Needs of People with Dementia and Those Who Care for Them: A Review of the Literature.* Alzheimer's Society. December 1999.
Cohen D & Eisdorfer C (1986) *The Loss of Self: A Family Resource for the Care of Alzheimer's Disease.* Plume.

18 Eating disorders – public perceptions and the experiences of sufferers and their families regarding stigmatisation

Nicky Bryant

Eating disorders are complex illnesses which many people do not understand. They include anorexia nervosa, bulimia nervosa, binge eating disorder and eating disorders not otherwise specified (EDNOS).

The outward signs or symptoms of an eating disorder such as restricted eating, excessive exercise and significant weight loss appear to describe illnesses which can be treated relatively simply – reduce the amount of exercise, increase nutritional intake and adopt a more balanced lifestyle. However, the external symptoms mask a deep-rooted psychological unhappiness and underlying personal distress that are at the heart of many eating disorders. The world holds many fears and pressures for someone with an eating disorder; it presents a situation where they feel out of control, out of place and inadequate.

As a result the person with an eating disorder becomes isolated and trapped in an inner world dominated by food, exercise, body image, body weight, routine and control. In their perception they are not ill, for, as one patient of Charles Lasegue is quoted as saying, "I do not suffer and therefore I must be well." It is this denial of a problem and complete involvement in the anorexic or bulimic world that isolates and excludes their family, friends and loved ones. Many who suffer with an eating disorder are afraid to ask for help and are ambivalent about accepting it.

"Stigmatise" is defined in the dictionary as "to brand as something disgraceful". For many people, the starvation and food restriction of anorexia and the bingeing and purging of bulimia nervosa are looked on as "something disgraceful". "Why don't they just pull themselves together and eat?" and "What a waste of good food", "They are just attention seekers" are comments often heard applied to sufferers of anorexia and bulimia nervosa.

Members of the Eating Disorders Association speak of being stopped in the street and asked what sort of impression they are giving to vulnerable young people, of being looked and pointed at as if they were something out of the ordinary, of parents who are openly questioned about whether they are feeding their children.

The press and media also seem obsessed with portraying eating disorders in a negative light. In November 1997, Accurist watches mounted a huge advertising campaign using a model "chosen because she looked thin". She wore a solid silver wrist watch on her upper arm with the slogan "Put some weight on". This provocatively contentious campaign using the "thin ideal" as a marketing ploy to sell watches only served to further promote thinness as the aspiration for the most vulnerable sections of the population and thus to encourage weight loss. Immediately prior to Christmas, Victoria Beckham, "Posh Spice", was the focus of great media attention and speculation as to whether she had anorexia nervosa because of her thin appearance. For a whole week the papers carried stories about anorexia nervosa and how one could judge if someone was suffering with what are potentially life-threatening illnesses. Public speculation of this nature only serves to increase and reinforce the prejudice and stigmatisation of eating disorders.

Training and employment are other areas where damaging stigmatisation and blatant prejudice against those with a history of an eating disorder has been evident. In April 1994, following the Beverley Allitt case, Dr Stuart Miller was reported in the *Nursing Standard* as saying that any person who has had anorexia nervosa or a similar mental illness "should be barred from nursing". He had apparently drawn up a questionnaire for all those applying for nurse training which was reported to ask directly about disorders such as anorexia nervosa, psychosis or other mental illness. Dr Miller is quoted as saying "Anorexia should be an absolute bar to nurse training because it indicates a deeper personality problem". These comments were hotly condemned by the Royal College of Nursing as "ill informed".

However, many cases of difficulties in obtaining employment or of not being accepted for training and, indeed, of being suspended from work due to a history of an eating disorder are regularly brought to our attention at the Eating Disorders Association. We dealt with four cases relating to employment difficulties as a result of eating disorders in 1999.

The *Nursing Times* of April 1998 carried a story about Corrine Toogood, a qualified nurse who lost a job offer in the NHS, following an Occupational Health assessment. At the medical, Corrine disclosed her history of bulimia and the doctor decided that her appointment "had to be reconsidered due to her medical history". Mrs Toogood took the hospital to an industrial tribunal which decided against her case despite the Chair saying that "The Occupational Health doctor has stereotyped her condition" and "There is no real evidence that the applicant was unfit for the post".

Further guidelines about occupational issues in relation to eating disorders are due to be issued in the near future.

Parents, family and friends are also affected by the stigmatisation that surrounds eating disorders. One member, weighing 5 stone and desperate for treatment, visited her GP to ask for a referral for treatment at a private specialist unit for eating disorders. She was offered no help or support, just the suggestion that she take out a bank loan and go as a private patient. The parents, in great distress and deeply worried about the health of their daughter, issued a complaint against the GP. The complaint acted as a catalyst and the daughter received the specialist treatment and care she urgently needed. The complaint against the GP was followed up with a meeting between the parents, the GP and a conciliator from the Health Authority. After an apology from the GP for the distress she had caused, the family felt that the matter had been closed. Some 5 months later the family received a letter from the practice advising them that the whole family were being removed from the practice list!

People with eating disorders are not mad or attention seekers or disgraceful; they are struggling to cope and survive in a world that overwhelms and terrifies them. They become locked in their rigid, closed and minimal world desperately hoping that someone will come along and unlock the dark door of their self-abuse. They are also terrified of losing their one and only safe and secure friend – their eating disorder.

Stigmatisation arises from a lack of knowledge and understanding of the inner eating-disordered world. We need to extend our hand and offer support and understanding to enable those who suffer with these debilitating and, for some, life-threatening illnesses to move slowly and gently into the outside world. Discrimination only enhances their own strongly held belief that they are not worthy and are totally to blame.

19 Stigmatisation of addiction

David Trotman

Just for a moment, visualise the man slumped across the park bench, clutching a crumpled can of super strength lager; the stale smell of alcohol and urine-sodden trousers permeates the air. Look at the young woman sprawled out in a doorway, a syringe lying at her feet, bare arms showing the track marks of heroin use, and scars of self-destruction.

One starts to visualise the stereotype, the "alkie", the "junkie" – the losers of society; the businessman turned beggar, the schoolgirl selling herself for her next fix. Both are lost in their own worlds of self-hatred, amplified by society's fears, prejudices and lack of understanding.

Here is the tip of the addiction problem facing our society, the few heads that protrude above the parapets of secrecy and guilt that hide many thousands, indeed millions, attempting to equate their habit, their addiction with modern-day life.

Whilst addiction encompasses habits associated with gambling, diet and sex, in this case I refer to substance or chemical abuse alone. We are not dealing with compounds such as vitamins, we are concerned with the ingestion, injection or inhalation of chemicals that will eventually kill, whether used alone or in combination – chemicals such as alcohol, nicotine, heroin, cocaine, amphetamines, benzodiazapines and so on. The list grows as mankind's ingenuity is directed at synthesising new addictive chemicals. This is only surpassed by his or her propensity for manipulating and taking those substances: substances that kill minds, kill relationships, kill love and kill people.

To quote Dr Gordon Morse, author of *Detoxification* and medical advisor to Clouds House, a leading addictions residential treatment centre:

> "Addiction is by all criteria a terminal condition, yet it is the only terminal condition I know where the health professional can help the patient to usually arrest and often reverse the process."

Herein lies the first part of the key to unlocking the negative attitude society has towards addictions. We must look upon it as an illness, not as a situation which "weak-minded" people get themselves into, and thus should pull themselves together and sort out their problems of their own accord.

So, if we have the expertise and a range of treatments that can and do work, why do we as a society, health professionals and public alike, seem to shun the ever growing presence of today's and tomorrow's addiction problems? I'm not discussing resources, personnel, hospital beds and funding here. I know that we are all of one accord, that within the mental health arena we are in dire need of financial investment, indeed rejuvenation. I wish to focus on something more basic, and that is attitude – the simple yet extremely difficult step of understanding, showing concern and a genuine desire to help those who, through varied circumstances, whether of their own doing or not, have brought this situation upon themselves, their families, friends, workmates and locality.

Today we talk openly of diseases such as leprosy, tuberculosis and cancer. Man's prejudice has now been overcome, and in turn has been replaced by understanding and compassion. His ingenuity has been brought to bear, and amazing strides have been made in arresting the progress of these conditions. No longer do we isolate the leper outside the city walls, or shun the tuberculosis patient because his disease reflected poor living conditions and impoverished life style, or draw a veil over cancer, where fear suppressed the move towards public awareness, support and early diagnosis. Thankfully we see the last vestiges of these prejudices disappearing. We can now openly discuss such cancers of the breast, bowel and testicle. Leprosy and tuberculosis are being researched, treated and contained. Understanding and education via quality research enables the commitment to deal with a problem and solve it.

So where have we gone wrong with addiction? What are the consequences, if the public, medical professions and government alike ignore this illness, leaving it to be dealt with by the Criminal Justice System. If this continues, we as a world society are in for a rude awakening, not only from an emotional standpoint but also on a financial basis.

We already know that mankind has had a long standing affinity with recreational drug use: alcohol consumed by ancient Egyptians, Romans and Greeks, coca by the Aztecs, tobacco by North American natives, opium in Asia. However, only mankind has the ability to be seduced by these chemicals so that today we face a pandemic. The UK is not alone in having to deal with this growing problem.

Here are some sobering statistics:

- 70% of violent crime is committed by people intoxicated with either alcohol or drugs.
- 40% of child abuse cases occur following heavy drinking bouts.
- 350 people die from tobacco-related diseases every day in the UK; that is 130,000 deaths per annum.
- There are an estimated 200,000 dependent heroin users in the UK. This figure is increasing by 20% per year, which means that shortly we will have the potential of seeing 1% of the UK population with an addiction to an opiate substance. This is even more significant when we see that the majority of heroin addicts are found within the 26–35-year-old age group.
- In one recent study, the National Treatment Outcome Research Study, 650 heroin addicts committed 70,000 crimes in a 3-month period prior to entering treatment.
- The average spending per day for a heroin addict is around £250. A crack cocaine addict may spend up to £2500 per day.

Current research is now showing an alarming rise in heroin and cocaine use in younger populations (early teens). This is in line with a concomitant drop in drug street prices and growing availability. Much research is now needed to look at short- and long-term effects of synthetic drugs such as ecstasy, new generations of hallucinogens and, frighteningly, the introduction of a very potent, highly addictive smokeable form of methamphetamine. The latter is now causing considerable problems in South East Asia. According to a WHO report, 1.3 million people are addicted to this species of "speed" known locally as Ya Ba.

Where do we stand? I've already stated that the availability of addictive substances to an ever widening age range is growing, prices are falling, but profit margins are such that dealing as well as using is still worth the risk. New products are coming onto the illegal market; old products such as absinthe are making a comeback; cigarette smoking, particularly amongst young females, is on the increase.

Addiction as a disease transcends borders, sex, creed, ethnic group and social class. To confuse the scene more, drug-taking habits and combinations of these (poly-drug use) will vary with respect to time, age of populace and demography. We now deal with a moving target; our need is to fix this target and focus our energies on reducing the risk of our young people becoming enmeshed within the nightmare of addiction.

Whilst maintaining pressure on cutting the supply line, we need to work with people to reduce the demand for these substances. This is one aspect of our work at Action on Addiction; that is to support research in developing effective methods by which we can educate our young, and also to deliver easily digestible information for parents.

Through our work at Action on Addiction we have seen the acute need and chronic lack of practical information and training required by professionals such as hospital clinicians, GPs and nurses, who are seeing a rapid increase in their day-to-day dealing with addiction. Indeed, we hear many accounts of stigmatisation within the medical fraternity toward patients with an addiction. Professionalism may be maintained but attitude changes.

Who gets priority in an A & E department – the workman who has broken his arm whilst on a building site or the "soak" with the same injury falling over the park railings? Who would your GP rather see, the long-term asthmatic teenager or the 18-year-old with a cocaine habit? I find it quite strange that our front-line health professionals at best receive a few hours of "addiction" teaching within their entire training syllabus. I would also extend in-depth training to other professional groups such as ambulance staff, local pharmacists, the police, prison officers, magistrates and teachers, who all need to understand the scale of the problem and the many issues encapsulated within the addictions sphere.

Besides those issues I have mentioned, such as violence, child abuse, theft and death, all carrying their own level of stigma within current society, I extend the list to include suicide and other mental health problems such as anxiety, depression and schizophrenia that may either be a consequence of the addictive process or the precursor and cause for the need to take a perceived chemical escape route.

Another facet of stigma is that it drives the problem inward, so that the patient, the addict, will shy away from requesting help and from the public gaze. The addict's denial of the problem is exacerbated by society's negative attitude to it. All carry a significant prejudice and stigma. Appropriate training and education can overcome this. However, this will take the medium to long term to work its way through the next generation.

In the short term, I believe it is necessary for the media – TV, radio and the written word, as well as icons of society (those in the public gaze) – to discuss and publicise the issues surrounding addiction openly and positively. A programme of enlightenment, not scaremongering, will induce people to discuss addiction and how it may be prevented. For those who have a substance addiction, openness and discussion will bring about a greater understanding and increased support for treatment programmes and further development of therapies.

As a charity we are also researching better and improved methods of treatment which one day will hopefully lead to a cure or cures for addiction. We are beginning to see a general upsurge of positive discussion. Channel 4 recently ran a series of programmes looking at cocaine problems, GMTV have led with morning prime time discussions on alcohol addictions and visits to the Priory Treatment Centre. Indeed, day by day one sees and reads about all aspects of addictions in magazines and newspapers. Dispel ignorance and you erode stigma; get the general population to discuss the issues that count and we can start to bring pressure on Government and seek increased financial support directed at education, prevention and treatment whilst maintaining a positive stance with respect to policing and security.

You may call me a pessimist, but ignore this problem, shun addiction at your peril.

We have to start somewhere. People are recognising this problem although negative attitudes remain: mention of addiction still sees the potential sponsor pull back, when the company directors realise that we support research into treatment of heroin addiction and alcoholism. We have to move forward; here is a condition that can destroy the very roots of society. The irony is that we have the skills, methodology and knowledge to deal with it.

I for one as a father have seen at first hand the damage that drugs and alcohol can do to a person and those around him. That person is my son. Faced with his predicament, our first reaction was fear and flight, but on taking a rational view once the panic was over and our own guilt overcome, we decided to fight. With the modicum of psychiatric care available, with patience, understanding and "tough love", we got through the tears, anguish, smashed rooms, police searches, self-destruction and attempted suicide. He's now happy again and our experience in a positive way has made us much closer. I suppose we were lucky – many are not.

But then again, I'm a simple man trying to be a decent human being. Surely if I can do my bit, I am persuaded that the majority of people can and will overcome the stigma that surrounds substance addiction.

20 The social impact of stigmatisation on users and carers

Melba Wilson

People with mental health problems are amongst the most socially excluded in Britain today. This is largely because of the stigma and discrimination they experience. A significant proportion of people with serious mental health problems are unemployed; mortality rates for those diagnosed with schizophrenia are two-and-a-half times the national average, and two-thirds of media reports misleadingly portray people with mental health problems as violent. People with mental health problems are also denied participation in daily living activities and access to mainstream educational and training opportunities. Mind's Respect Campaign works to reduce stigma by highlighting the problems which people face and by proposing options for a more socially inclusive society through developing models of good practice, applicable in a range of sectors.

Understanding the social impact of stigmatisation on users of mental health services and their carers involves understanding the social and environmental influences which lead to discrimination and exclusion.

Mind works for a better life for everyone with experience of mental distress by:

- Advancing the views, needs and ambitions of people with experience of mental distress
- Influencing policy, education and training
- Improving the development of quality services which reflect expressed need and diversity and

- Achieving equal aid and legal rights through campaigning and education

Current context

In order to begin to understand the impact of stigma on users and carers, it is important to gain an idea of the experiences which many people with mental health problems undergo. The Respect Campaign, which ran from 1997 to 2001 (and is discussed further in Chapter 63), was one of the ways in which Mind took action to reduce stigma and discrimination against people with mental health problems through raising awareness of the effects and incidence of discrimination and thus aiming to create a more equitable life for people with these problems. One aspect of the Respect Campaign involved surveying various constituencies of mental health service users in order to document people's experiences of discrimination. The first of these, *Not Just Sticks and Stones* (Read and Baker 1996), surveyed stigma, taboo and discrimination experienced by people with mental health problems in their everyday lives. It included a sample of 778 users of mental health services. The survey results included the following findings:

- 47% had been verbally or physically harassed in public
- 34% had been dismissed or forced to resign from jobs
- 24% had been refused by insurance or finance companies
- 50% believed they were treated unfairly by health care services

Comments included one from a woman (aged 43) with a diagnosis of depression, who said:

"I work very hard at pulling myself out of a depression and then get threatened and abused by a gang of kids on the way home from my first walk out in weeks. My son is with me. He is also attacked. I lose credibility in his eyes, and in my own eyes. Mud and stones are thrown at us. Hurt and angry, I think: 'What's the point of trying to get better?' "

Another respondent (a woman, 26, diagnosed with reactive depression) noted:

"Last year I was offered a position as a graduate programmer and I was pleased with the prospect of working in industry using the skills and knowledge I had gathered from my time at university. I was devastated to be told a week later that the offer had been withdrawn because my security clearance was not accepted due to me supposedly suffering a mental illness. I suffered from depression because of a terrible relationship, the death of my fiancé and through being raped. I feel disappointed that people still have no understanding of depression, and differing levels of depression. My details are now stored in a database that thousands of companies use, so my chances of gaining employment with other companies are non-existent."

Another Mind survey, *Raised Voices* (Wilson and Francis 1997) asked African and African-Caribbean mental health service users their views and experiences of mental health services, and of discrimination. Fifty-eight percent reported having experienced discrimination in general life because of their ethnic origin. People had been called names and threatened. A number of people were interviewed in detail in the study, and the results strongly suggest that experiences of poverty, unemployment and the feeling of being discriminated against and socially excluded, all contribute to mental health problems.

One person said, of her experience of the mental health services:

"I am loud – that's unacceptable. I dress differently – that's considered strange. I eat different foods – that's frowned upon. My English is not good – they don't try and get an interpreter. I'm discriminated against – they say I have a chip on my shoulder."

(42-year-old woman, diagnosis of schizophrenia)

The final Mind survey in this series looked at "Nimby" ("Not in my backyard") opposition to community mental health facilities, experienced by key service providers in England and Wales. The survey, *Tall Stories from the Back Yard* (Repper et al. 1997), included responses from eight of the largest national housing associations providing for people with mental health problems (response rate 88%); a sample of nine mental health trusts selected to represent a range in terms of NHS region, urban or rural, and level of social deprivation (100%); 213 Local Mind Associations (LMAs) who are providers of services (response rate 47%); and the three other national voluntary organisations who provide mental health services (100%). Key findings included:

- Over two-thirds of all respondents (65% of LMAs, all three voluntary organisations, eight out of nine trusts, and six out of seven housing associations) had encountered opposition to mental health facilities in the past five years.

- In every case and in all areas, opposition faded once projects opened.
- All three voluntary organisations, and eight out of nine NHS Trusts, said opposition had increased over the last five years. More LMAs thought it had increased (39%) than decreased (22%).
- There was no regional variation in frequency of opposition. It happened in affluent suburbs and tough estates, rural Wales and inner city London.
- Local opposition varied from protest letters (57% LMAs), meetings (63% LMAs) to outright violence (19% LMAs) directed at service users, staff and property.
- 63% of LMAs, four housing associations and all voluntary associations delayed opening at least one facility because of community opposition. Approximately 30% of LMAs had abandoned plans altogether. The more optimistic corollary, however, is that 70% of plans still went ahead and, once established, "people got to know people" and the opposition faded.

That is the reality of stigma and discrimination. The effects touch every aspect of the lives of people with mental health problems, including employment, daily living, education and training. It is fuelled in part by prejudicial and ill-informed media coverage, which in turn helps to shape public attitudes towards people who experience mental distress.

Employment

Mental health service users and ex-users are excluded to a large extent from paid work and, as a result, may become or remain poor. The Labour Force Survey (Winter 1997/98) shows that people with mental health problems are less likely than any other group of people with disabilities or health problems to be economically active: 17% are economically active, compared with 41% of disabled people generally. Those who are economically active have more difficulty than any other group in finding a job: a 29% unemployment rate for people with mental health problems, compared with 15% for disabled people generally.

People from black and minority ethnic groups have higher rates of unemployment than their white counterparts. Unemployment rates according to Labour Market Trends June 1996 were:

- white men   9.5%
- white women   6.5%
- minority ethnic men 20%
- minority ethnic women 17%

For Bangladeshi men and women the rates were over 40%. Evidence also points to 62% of young black men (aged 16–24) in London as being out of work (Council of Churches for Britain and Ireland 1997).

There is strong evidence for the adverse effects of unemployment on mental health and the positive effects of work for people with mental health problems. A study of ethnicity and mental health found social position to be an important factor for all ethnic groups and all forms of mental distress (Nazroo 1997).

A study by the Joseph Rowntree Foundation, of black and minority ethnic men and women discharged from psychiatric hospitals in Leeds and Bradford, found that "poverty was a key feature of the lives of both respondents and carers". It reported that "only nine per cent of respondents were in employment, mostly in part-time, low-paid work" (Joseph Rowntree Foundation 1994).

More than a third (38%) of people who responded in Mind's *Raised Voices* survey felt that racism meant that they had been denied employment (Wilson and Francis 1997). Studies repeatedly show that most people with serious mental health problems want to work. American research suggests about 70% of people with serious mental illness identify work as a key life goal (Baron et al. 1996).

Employer prejudice and the lack of support systems oriented to work exclude mental health service users and ex-users from the workplace and barriers in the benefit system compounds the problem. When Mind invited people to tell us about their experience of discrimination on mental health grounds, 69% of those responding said they had been put off applying for jobs for fear of unfair treatment (Read and Baker 1996). They included a man who had more success pretending to have been in prison than in a psychiatric hospital, and a woman who saw a job go to an inexperienced person after she revealed having spent time in a psychiatric hospital. The main areas of change needed to enable people to work (identified by people with mental health problems in a Mind survey on benefits) were health limitations employer attitudes, education, training and qualifications, and benefits and pay.

Mind believes that users and ex-users of mental health services should have equal rights with other employees and job seekers. The disadvantage faced by people who experience multiple discrimination should be recognised in policy and practice. People in emotional distress should have the opportunity to develop personal and vocational skills, to earn and participate fully in society.

Daily living

Discriminatory and prejudiced attitudes have their effect throughout all aspects of people's lives. Seemingly straightforward everyday tasks such as shopping, or applying for a mortgage or insurance, can be made unpleasant or impossible. And the segregated nature of mental health services themselves effectively cuts off service users from the rest of society (Dunn 1999).

Likewise, in education and training, there is little knowledge or understanding of mental health issues in many schools, colleges or universities. Educational bodies do not know where to go for advice and guidance, due in part to the lack of a central body specifically promoting access to education for students with mental health problems (Dunn 1999).

Media

Many users of mental health services feel that media reporting greatly influences how other people perceive them. Philo found that two-thirds of news and current affairs coverage made a link between mental ill-health and violence. Media myths were found to be so potent that they even overrode people's life experiences. People with mental health problems themselves reported feeling "like monsters", because that's how they were portrayed on television.

Mind believes that it is important to work with the media in order to help change the status quo on what and how things should be reported. Again, in the Respect Campaign, we target the media, amongst others. Our "Campaign to Complain" is supported by the Press Complaints Commission and the Royal College of Psychiatrists. It includes 120 individual members (media guardians) who work to exert pressure on the media in relation to the prejudicial portrayal of or reference to people with mental health problems.

Social inclusion

The current government has placed a strong premium on social inclusion – a stance which Mind welcomes. Our view is that purposeful and systematic action can help to bring about a more socially inclusive society, and thus begin to tackle the stigma and discrimination which people with mental health problems experience. Mind's "Creating Accepting Communities" inquiry has recently documented how people with mental health problems are socially excluded.

We have taken evidence from a range of sectors, including statutory and voluntary health and mental health agencies, religious bodies and groups, business, local authorities, black and minority ethnic groups, organisations and individuals, organisations representing people with physical disabilities, the police, professional bodies, and others.

The aims of the Mind inquiry were:

- to find out the extent and the nature of the social exclusion experienced by people with mental health problems in Britain today
- to listen directly to the views of mental health service users and carers on their experiences of exclusion and the ways to combat it
- to hear directly from those working in mental health services how they feel social exclusion can best be tackled; and
- to find out from general employers and providers of goods and services, what help they need to counter the exclusion of people with mental health problems from mainstream society.

The wealth of evidence contained in the report attests to the breadth and depth of exclusion. The report makes a number of recommendations for tackling exclusion. The next phase of this work within Mind is to move beyond simply documenting the incidence of exclusion of people with mental health problems, and instead to proactively seek ways of promoting inclusion within society.

The main thrust of this work will be the development of a model for improving the quality of life for people with mental health problems. The intention is to create a flexible and transferable model, capable of use across sectors – including local authorities, education and employment bodies, as well as public health and mental health services.

The model, which will incorporate clinical and non-clinical outcomes, will develop outcome measures in the areas of (1) preventing discrimination, (2) developing effective partnerships, (3) improving physical as well as mental health and (4) enabling fair access to opportunities. Specific areas of focus will be race and culture, the arts and sport, training and education, employment and neighbourhood and housing.

Mind aims to develop, pilot and evaluate this model over the next few years, in collaboration with a number and range of potential partners. These include representatives in local government, health, education and training, and business, as well as mental health service users and carers.

Mind's social inclusion initiative relates to a central tenet of the government's goal of tackling exclusion and disadvantage, which occurs as a result of stigma and discrimination. The aim of the work of its Social Exclusion Unit has been about recognising and understanding the need to take action to address the multidimensional nature of exclusion. This frames the context in which Mind is developing its social inclusion initiative.

At Mind, we believe this is work which must be undertaken in relation to people who experience mental distress. The aim, in our view, is to move – as users of mental health services rightly argue we must – from a situation which simply chronicles the stigma and discrimination they face to one which actively embraces and encourages change and inclusion.

References

Baron RC et al. (1996) Strengthening the work incentive provisions of the Social Security Act to encourage persons with serious mental illness to work at their potential. Social Security Administration, Washington, DC [Quoted in *Welfare to Work* Policy Document. London: Mind, 1997].

Council of Churches for Britain and Ireland (1997) *Unemployment and the Future of Work: An Enquiry for the Churches.*

Dunn S (1999) Creating accepting communities. *Report of Mind Inquiry into Social Exclusion and Mental Health Problems.* London: Mind: 21, 42.

Joseph Rowntree Foundation (1994) Aftercare of black ethnic minority people discharged from psychiatric hospitals. *Social Care Research* **58**.

Nazroo J (1997) *Ethnicity and Mental Health.* Policy Studies Institute/Grantham Books.

Philo G (ed.) (1996) *Media and Mental Distress.* London: Addison-Wesley.

Read J & Baker S (1996) *Not Just Sticks and Stones.* London: Mind.

Repper J et al. (1997) *Tall Stories from the Backyard: A Survey of "Nimby" Opposition to Community Mental Health Facilities.* London: Mind.

Wilson M & Francis J (1997) *Raised Voices.* London: Mind.

Commentary on Section 2B

Claire Rayner

It is received wisdom amongst many observers today that mental illness carries with it a stigma that is not attached to those who suffer from demonstrably physical conditions. It is something that is frequently complained about by patients and their carers, who maintain that it militates against them in employment, housing and other more subtle ways. There are patients considered by their GPs to be in need of counselling/psychotherapy who flatly refuse to consider it on the grounds that "it will go in my notes and I'll be labelled a nutcase for ever", or that it will damage their chances of getting financial products such as mortgages and life assurance.

There are those who might suggest that such attitudes to the mentally sick are natural in a Darwinian sense, in that fear of those who behave in an alien manner is linked with the xenophobia that protected early man from strangers who might be hostile and the source of pain and/or damage.

However, in some societies, both in the present in some Third World countries and in our own in the Middle Ages, those who demonstrated psychiatric symptoms were regarded with awe rather than hostility or ridicule and were held to be uniquely touched by the society's god or gods. There is evidence of this in the UK; the words "silly" and "holy" were once synonymous. Hence the term 'silly Suffolk' for a county which is blessed with a larger than an average number of shrines and other religious sites.

But what is the situation today? Is a diagnosis of psychiatric disorder a stigma? The contributors to this section all say that it remains a major problem for their constituencies. They display in their presentations the varying effects this stigma has on the members of various self-help organisations. According to Nicky Lidbetter of the National Phobics Society (Chapter 14):

> *"The medical profession and the general public do not take anxiety disorders seriously. Sufferers are referred to as 'the worried well' and 'neurotic' – in other words, not really ill . . . sufferers are often thought, by professionals and ordinary people alike . . . weak pathetic individuals."*

Similarly, this is the view of Depression Alliance (Chapter 15):

> *"There is a commonly held perception amongst individual sufferers that ... other people will not understand the condition and . . . will classify them as either mad or dangerous. . . . In a weighted poll carried out by Depression Alliance amongst MPs in 1996, only 63% of Conservatives viewed depression as an illness. . . . the remaining 37% did not perceive it as a recognised medical condition."*

Two of the contributors go further. They too maintain that the patients they represent suffer from real illness which they cannot control by simple effort of will, and are therefore in need of professional care, and then go on to make their strongest accusations of stigmatisation against doctors. This is the Eating Disorders

Association's view (Chapter 18):

> "Training and employment are areas where damaging stigmatisation and blatant prejudice against those with a history of an eating disorder has been evident. ... Dr Stuart Miller was reported in the Nursing Standard as saying that any person who has had anorexia nervosa or a similar mental illness 'should be barred from nursing' and that '... (it) should be an absolute bar to nurse training because it indicates a deeper personality problem'."

In Chapter 18, Nicky Bryant goes on to describe a 1998 case of a nurse who lost a job offer when her history of bulimia emerged and the occupational health doctor decided her appointment had to be "reconsidered due to her medical history". She appealed against the decision to an industrial tribunal and won.

Addicts, according to David Trotman, for Action on Addiction (Chapter 19), also suffer considerably at the hands of professionals:

> "We hear many accounts of stigmatisation within the medical fraternity towards patients with an addiction ... who gets priority in an A and E department – the workman who has broken his arm whilst on a building site or the 'soak' with the same injury falling over park railings? Who would your GP rather see, the long-term asthmatic teenager or the 18-year-old with a cocaine habit?"

Cliff Prior of Rethink (previously The National Schizophrenia Fellowship) writes in Chapter 16 of the stigmatisation problems of those suffering from schizophrenia. He singles out for particular opprobrium the media perspective on the illness as always linked with violence, quoting a Scottish study that showed 66% of media coverage was linked with violence. He writes too of the casual and highly inaccurate use of the word "schizophrenia" as being a part of the problem. He goes on to make a very powerful plea for accurate use of language:

> "We talk loosely about stigma, when often what we mean is prejudice, because we mean 'they' are getting it wrong. 'Stigma' means a mark or sign – a negative but perhaps accurate view. Prejudices can be changed through public education, but stigma can only be changed by changing the reality."

In Chapter 17, Clive Evers of the Alzheimer's Society presents a view that is a little more positive:

> "We have a different mind set – we try to convey good news and hope, informed of course by realism ... I suspect that of all the conditions discussed in this volume, most people would say an inner prayer that they may not be affected by dementia – understandable, of course, but still regrettable, for each prayer denies the humanity that will still be within you even if you are affected by Alzheimer's disease, multi-infarct dementia or Lewy body disease. It is important that Alzheimer's disease does not become a stigma. It is a label as well as a disease; when the words are spoken, they can immediately change the way we perceive and act towards the person."

That there are, as there always have been and probably always will be, individuals who attract the scorn of their neighbours is a situation that is unlikely to change. It is a reaction that seems to be intrinsic to our natures. The question is how far are we, as a civilised society, prepared to allow such reactions to damage the most vulnerable amongst us? No answer to that question has been provided in these chapters, but at least the question has been asked. Which is surely the first step to finding the answer.

21 The general practitioner's perspective

André Tylee

I will approach this subject entirely from the perspective of a general practitioner who has practiced in Sutton, Surrey for 20 years. I have conducted a "straw poll" of patients seen recently, I will describe some illustrative case histories and I have the results of a local survey of patients' views. I will also comment on GPs' mental health and the way forward, overall, as I see it.

I conducted a straw poll of 17 patients seen one Friday morning by myself in a routine general practice surgery session. I am known by my patients to have a special interest in mental health and consequently see many more patients with mental health problems than the primary care epidemiological studies would suggest. Of the 17 patients I saw that morning, 12 of them were for mental health problems, of which 6 were for depression (one postnatally), 3 for drug and alcohol misuse, 1 for chronic fatigue and 1 for newly diagnosed temporal lobe epilepsy and 1 was a survivor of child abuse.

All of the drug and alcohol misusers were recently discharged from prison for drugs-related offences and were experiencing profound stigma from potential employers. Since the talk, one person has since obtained a job as a chauffeur. The others continue not to find work and therefore cannot break out of the cycle they are in. One patient has spent most of his adult life (he is now in his 60s) in jail, and this is often precipitated by being under the influence of alcohol. Unfortunately, he is attracted to the company of colleagues in a certain public house where he experiences no stigma and is actually seen as a local hero.

The patient with new temporal lobe epilepsy is in his late teens and it has proved difficult to assess whether he also has a psychotic illness. He has a personality seen as strange by work colleagues and has experienced severe and abusive bullying from his work colleagues which precipitated a "breakdown" and perpetual certification from work as well as psychiatric and neurological assessment since.

The survivor from childhood paternal sexual abuse also had work stress, initially simply the quantity of work but latterly a clash with, not surprisingly, a male boss. His verbally abusive manner brought back her childhood experience and consequent depression and anxiety symptoms. She was beginning to experience some work-related stigma and required certification and expressed her desire to find another job.

There were also patients who, when asked in the straw poll about stigma, declared the opposite experience. An ex-policeman recounted the support he had had from colleagues who had covered for him when he was down or stressed. He stated that new policies in the police to replace staff with "civilians" had eroded the supportive nature of the past in his experience.

A shop manager told me how much help he had had from the owner when he needed time off either for his depression or for his wife's severe rheumatoid arthritis.

A housewife told me that her close-knit circle of friends who all had children at the same primary school were totally non-stigmatising and helped with child care. Similarly the 32-year-old woman with chronic fatigue had a circle of friends and felt not at all stigmatised. These examples are important as they provide a balanced primary care-based perspective which is often different from the experiences recounted by people from user groups. A local survey referred to later found that fewer than 10% of primary care-based patients with severe mental illness (SMI) went to user groups. Most felt that this itself can be stigmatising and they did not want to commit themselves to the label needed to join a user group.

Three case studies come to mind. One is a man in his forties who was stressed and depressed only because of a clash with his managing director. Being marketing director he became more convinced the MD was trying to get rid of him. As the GP I can often only hear one side of the story, so I have no way of knowing whether this mounting dislike was for incompetence or just dislike. He became clinically depressed, and only two days after the certificate was issued I received a letter from the MD on two pages asking if he would ever work again and should he begin to consider medical retirement! Needless to say I wrote back to the contrary with an explanation about depression.

Another patient who readily springs to mind is a woman in her forties encouraged for years by her husband to drink to excess. When this in her case turned into alcohol abuse and depression, he completely denied the existence of any problem at all, continued drinking in front of her at home and still does not know or want to know that she is seeing a counsellor from the local alcohol team.

Another stigmatising problem seen in primary care is when old case notes are summarised for medical insurance purposes, loans or in this case a job application. A bright young man in his early twenties got into the interview process for a high-flying post with a bank based in London. He was summarily rejected when he disclosed one previous episode of depression reactive to stress a few years earlier. Employers need to be better educated and encouraged to be less stigmatising.

The user survey I referred to was conducted a few of years ago in seven practices within the then South West London Total Purchasing Pilot scheme. Around thirty patients with severe mental illness in each were interviewed by Kathleen Beresford. Key messages received were that many felt a lack of understanding by front-line reception staff, and employers in particular. They were generally satisfied but like other surveys wanted more time to be listened to and better continuity of care. This confirmed a message received from respondents to a MORI poll conducted for the Defeat Depression Campaign (Priest et al. 1996). In this, people were asked what they would want if depressed. Large numbers considered that their GPs would be unsympathetic or even annoyed. Patients would want listening treatment as most of them believed that antidepressant pills would be addictive. There are clearly a lot of public concerns to take account of, which may partly account for poor concordance rates (Donoghue and Tylee 1996).

It must be remembered that stigma occurs within the profession about colleagues. At present, there are no good occupational health services for GPs. It is very difficult to keep a GP's mental health problems confidential and this must prevent many GPs from presenting. It is well known that GPs themselves have a high risk of mental health problems and this whole area needs to be addressed, hopefully by the anti-stigma campaign.

What is the way forward? Certainly public awareness with the judicious use of celebrities "coming out", but also one's colleagues "coming out" about their own mental health problems, especially in the caring professions. Employer awareness is crucial and occupational health physicians can play a huge role. User involvement in training, especially multi-professional training, will help destigmatise mental health problems, particularly if the front-line reception staff can be involved.

References

Donoghue J & Tylee A (1996) The treatment of depression: prescribing patterns of antidepressants in primary care in the UK. *British Journal of Psychiatry* **168**: 164–8.

Priest R G, Vize C, Roberts A, Roberts C & Tylee A (1996) Lay people's attitudes to treatment of depression: results of opinion poll for Defeat Depression Campaign just before its launch. *British Medical Journal* **313**: 858–9.

22 Ethnicity: Relationship to stigmatisation of people with mental illness

Parimala Moodley

All societies and all cultures stigmatise mental illness. To understand stigma and its effects on people it is necessary to understand people, their heritage and their experiences. Furthermore, stigmatisation will be influenced by the symbolic interpretation of the affliction as well as the form of the illness, the effect on the person's social capacities, functions and individual identity, and most importantly the effect on the family network.

The ethnic minority population of the UK is drawn from across the world. The many different belief systems, cultures and subcultures profoundly influence attitudes towards mental illness and behaviour towards the mentally ill.

This chapter limits itself to a brief consideration of the academic and traditional beliefs of people of Indian, Chinese and Islamic heritage and other factors which may continue to influence the way in which mental illness is viewed. Additionally it considers the position of black and ethnic minority people in a society in which they often feel oppressed and discriminated against, and how this may contribute to the way mental illness is viewed.

Reviews of the three great traditions of non-Western medicine suggest certain common themes in relation to models of understanding mental illness, including stigma. Islamic medicine explains mental illness as due to disturbances of the bodily humours. Mental disturbance was viewed as an illness which was a natural phenomenon with no moral meaning attached to it. A holistic view of the soma and the psyche prevailed. The mentally ill were viewed as a communal responsibility who were honoured as well as being the objects of charity. Academic, professional medicine did not promote the folk beliefs in demons and evil spirits as the cause of madness and insanity. On the other hand, Islamic society in general and Sufism did draw on spiritualism and religious tenets to explain madness. There does not appear to have been any particular stigma attached to mental illness in traditional Islamic society (Dols 1987; Fabriga 1991).

In Chinese medicine there is a very thorough somatopsychic and psychosomatic integration. The cause of mental illness is viewed as multifaceted. This may include possession by spirits, hormones, diet and failure to propitiate the gods or ancestors.

In Chinese society, however, there is said to be an unusual degree of shame and embarrassment when mental illness occurs. The burden of the illness falls on the family, and the behavioural transgressions occurring in mental illness are strongly condemned or proscribed. This may arise from the prevalent culture in which excess emotion is considered unhealthy. The stigma in traditional Chinese society of mental illness has been said to be so strong that it tarnishes family honour and the ancestral lineage (Kleinman 1977; Lin 1981; Ng 1997).

The Indian system of medicine also has a strong integration of mind and body.

There are many models of the understanding of mental illness ranging from the supernatural through astrology to Ayurvedic or Indian classical medicine. As there does not appear to be a separation of psychiatric from physical illnesses, within the Ayurvedic tradition there appears to have been little evidence of stigma. Once again the causes of all illnesses were considered to be multifaceted, including spirit possession, personality, social and environmental causes.

In Indian society at large, the mentally ill do appear to have been stigmatised in a very marked manner not dissimilar to that which is apparent in traditional Chinese culture (Dube 1978; Haldipur 1984; Kakar 1982; Obeyesekere 1977; Weiss et al. 1986, 1988).

The common themes apparent in these three traditions are that:

1. Illnesses were handled in an integrated somatopsychic/psychosomatic fashion. As mental disorders were not separated from physical disorders the Western bias about "being psychiatric" or having symptoms stemming from the psyche was not prevalent.
2. Within the spheres of academic medicine, mental illness was medicalised. Insanity or madness were deemed to be illnesses requiring medical treatment.
3. In these societies in general, there existed more supernatural, religious, moralistic and magical approaches to illness and behaviour. This attracted a strong stigma in some cultures, but not in others.
4. Conditions likely to have stigma attached were chronic, irreversible and relapsing. These were judged to be the results of sorcery and spiritual punishment, or of heredity and constitutional deficits, or of social and moral transgressions.

From the literature it would appear also that within academic medicine in these traditions, people were treated humanely even if they had to be confined for their own safety. Whilst in the academia of the great classical traditions of medicine, mental illness was not especially stigmatised, in society at large the psychiatrically ill were distinctly marked in a social sense.

Within and between all societies there is much variation and ambivalence regarding the valuation of and response to psychiatric illness. These differences, whilst pertaining to the diverse theories that explain illness, are also related to complex cultural, sociological and economic factors. So, for instance, in a society where the cause of the illness is regarded as moral transgression towards ancestors, or social norms or ancestral inheritance of misconduct (as in Chinese), the family may be held responsible, siblings may be excluded from marriage, and there may be intense shame and guilt because the family honour, name and ancestors are tarnished.

Now, whilst societies have evolved and merged and absorbed different ideas about mental illness, various ethnic minority groups in the UK still have some very strong traditional social patterns. Therefore, whilst it may be acceptable to have a Western European model of illness for something like the more physical ailments, of which we believe we understand the causation, it is easier to have a more mixed model of modern Western and traditional ideas of understanding for mental illness – particularly because the current Western medical explanations are not necessarily informative or enlightening and may not accord with the individual's belief systems or health constructs.

Whatever the model of understanding, the consequences for a traditional family, community or society are much more far-reaching, because the social constructs are not nuclear, but communal. Where the person is conceived of in terms of a family or a larger social unit, stigma of illness affects the entire unit and demands a collective response. For instance, all traditional societies set great store by good marriages and the begetting of children. Anything that is likely to affect this such as mental illness will have very significant and far-reaching consequences for the individual as well as all others of that unit. Somatisation has been extensively written about as being highly prevalent in non-Western societies. It is evident and common in the West, but it appears to be more prominent, as a presenting phenomenon, in non-Western societies. In Western culture, where there is a distinction between mind and body, psychological distress should be expressed in psychological terms. If this is expressed in terms of physical complaints it is called somatisation, implying psychopathology. An alternative view would be that where there are both physical and psychological aspects to an illness, there could be an emphasis on the physical aspects of the condition, as opposed to the psychological, consistent with the experience as well as the cultural context. Psychological symptoms, though no less distressing than the physical symptoms, could affect profoundly the individual as well as their network in terms of self-esteem, social status and marriage, i.e. they may be seen as extremely disadvantageous. A number of authors have confirmed that "symptom expression is governed by the perceived stigma attached to psychological problems" (Kleinman 1977; Raguram 1996).

Against this background, if we look at the position of ethnic minority communities in the UK, it is largely a negative and inferior one. Historically, judgements have been made because of physical characteristics which are deemed to be the external evidence or markers for internal deficits, be they small brains, promiscuity, lack of moral fibre, and so on. Even the recent "academic" debates about race and intelligence have caused considerable concern because of the continuing emphasis on particular tests which are deemed to be a reflection of intelligence. The apparent finding that blacks are less intelligent than whites with insufficient emphasis on the inherent biases of such studies are seen as further examples of the negative way that black people i.e. people who are not white, are viewed. We may modify our dress, our language, etc. but we still carry the "stigmata of negritude". So within society people see themselves as being discriminated against and "subjected to multiple oppressions".

People who already see themselves as being stigmatised and discriminated against by the rest of society find themselves in the extremely unfortunate position of being stigmatised by society because they are mentally ill, since this is the position of people with mental illness in society.

Up until now it has been possible, maybe, to draw strength and comfort from one's social and community network, in the face of racism, intolerance, day-to-day as well as institutional slights; but now one is petrified because of the fear of stigmatisation and ostracism from the support network itself. So it is inevitable that there is every attempt at denial and delay in seeking help. Stigmatisation or the fear of it may be an important reason for delaying help-seeking, but it is only one factor and should be taken together with the numerous other contributors such as disenchantment with the mental health system in general.

It has been said that people with mental illness are the most disadvantaged and disabled in society, so where does that leave those who are already at the bottom of the pile and further disadvantaged by mental illness? Ostracised and stigmatised by their own community, does that leave them doubly, trebly or quadruply disadvantaged? The mental health profession has an absolutely crucial role in reducing the negative experiences of mental health service users in general and black and ethnic minority users in particular.

Firstly, we can examine ourselves as a profession and see what psychiatry is doing to perpetuate stereotypes and why we continue to stigmatise those whom we spend our time trying to work with. Denial is a very powerful tool that we use both in regard to how we treat our fellows in society, as well as the people we serve.

Secondly, we, the black and brown and other minority professionals, need to look at our role in perpetuating and colluding with stigmatisation by and within our communities as well as the wider community. We are very aware, largely but not exclusively through personal experience, of the pernicious effects of racism and prejudice. There is a commonly held view amongst the population in general and medical colleagues in particular that psychiatrists are failed neurologists. Additionally, non-Western doctors are deemed always to have come to the UK to become physicians, and having failed, go into the only speciality that would have them – psychiatry. So you are stereotyped as a failure on all accounts – as a person and a professional. Nevertheless, black and other ethnic minority doctors should be in a particularly powerful position, both from their own experiences and their knowledge of minority communities, to help break down some of the barriers to effective communication and to develop a shared understanding. Real dialogue between service users and service providers is imperative if we are to achieve the dream of equitable and appropriate services for all.

Thirdly, there should be respect for different mental health constructs. As the perception of mental illness changes, as society changes, and as people's mental health constructs change, there will be greater acknowledgement of the psychic as opposed to the somatic in all communities, and we are certainly seeing this in the younger generation of ethnic minorities. However, it is necessary to acknowledge that people do have different mental health constructs. If somebody from an Asian background presents only somatic symptoms with no psychic component despite a clear connection to stressful life events, it is not necessary to insist that psychological distress should only be expressed in psychological terms as per the Western view born of body–mind dualism.

"You have to fit into my box: if you don't I will chop off your legs to make you fit".

We need to find a way of working with people which respects their different positions rather than getting into conflicts over our different positions. So much of the confrontation within psychiatry between us and the people we serve is because of the "we know best" syndrome, when in fact we know much about some things and very little about others, i.e. much about the brain but little about the mind.

So, in summary:

- Stigmatisation of the mentally ill occurs in all cultures.
- In some societies there may be historical and socio-cultural reasons which contribute to the negative view of psychological distress.
- Many ethnic minority communities have a vulnerable status in society because of prejudice and racism, and this is further jeopardised by mental illness.
- The loss of status within the immediate community, with the development of mental illness, is further enhanced by their inferior position in society as a whole.
- Mental health professionals, and psychiatrists in particular, should stop stigmatising mental illness.
- Respect for different mental health constructs as well the historic socio-cultural context and the current experiences of the people we serve is essential.

References

Dols MW (1987) Insanity and its treatment in Islamic society. *Medical History* **31**: 1–14.

Dube KC (1978) Nosology and therapy of mental illness in Ayurveda. *Comparative Medicine East West* **6**: 209–28.

Fabrega H. (1991) Psychiatric stigma in non-Western societies. *Comparative Psychiatry* **32**: 534–51.

Haldipur CV (1984) Madness in ancient India: concept of insanity in Charaka Samhita (1st century AD). *Comparative Psychiatry* **25**: 335–44.

Kakar S (1982) *Shamans. Mystics and Doctors: A Psychological Inquiry Into India and its Healing Tradition.* Boston: Beacon.

Kleinman A (1977) *Depression, Somatisation and the "New Cross-Cultural Psychiatry".* Oxford: Pergamon Press: 3–10.

Lin KM (1981) Traditional Chinese medicine beliefs and their relevance for mental illness and psychiatry. In: Kleinman A & Lin TY (eds) *Normal Abnormal Behaviour in Chinese Culture.* Dordrecht: Reidel: 95–114.

Ng Chee Hong (1997) The stigma of mental illness in Asian cultures. *Australian and New Zealand Journal of Psychiatry* **31**: 382–90.

Obeyesekere G (1977) The theory and practice of Ayurvedic medicine in the Ayurvedic tradition. *Culture, Medicine and Psychiatry* **1**: 155–81.

Raguram R, Weiss M, Channabasavanna S & Devins G (1996) Stigma, depression, somatisation in South India. *American Journal of Psychiatry* **153**: 1043–9.

Weiss MG, Sharma D & Gaur RF (1986) Traditional concepts of mental disorder among Indian psychiatric patients: preliminary report of work in progress. *Social Science and Medicine* **23**: 379–86.

Weiss MG, Desai A & Jadhav S (1988) Humoral concepts of mental illness in India. *Social Science and Medicine* **27**: 471–7.

23 Stigma and homelessness

Philip Timms

Introduction

For the 10 years I have helped to provide a mental health service to homeless people in South London, it has become evident that stigmatising attitudes to homeless people exist, not only in the general population but also within the helping professions. This is important for two reasons. Firstly, many homeless people also suffer a long-term psychiatric disorder. Their homelessness adds a burden of stigma additional to that they already experience through having a mental illness. Secondly, it affects the way they are treated by health and social care professionals.

An experience of homelessness and stigma

During the late 1980s, there was a silent, unplanned and uncoordinated series of institutional closures. This occurred both in London and in other major cities, and was separate from the closure of the mental hospitals. It was the large hostels for homeless people that were closing. These had constituted a mixed economy of large, barrack-like institutions since the late Victorian era. Some were charitable, run by bodies such as the Salvation Army. Some were run for profit, by the Rowton House Company. Reception centres or "spikes", the direct descendants of the workhouses, were run by the Department of Social Services.

At the time, I was working in a mental health team providing a service to four such large hostels in South London. The closure programme for one of them demanded that residents be re-settled in a number of smaller group homes in residential roads in the surrounding area. As part of the community consultation, the local council had arranged a public meeting in a local community hall, to try both to gauge the feelings of local people and to give them information about what was being proposed. I had expected to spend a quiet evening on the sidelines, observing consultation calmly taking place. I arrived to find a full house of around 100 people, and a somewhat hostile atmosphere.

What I did not know was that, some years past, an unfortunate child from the area had been assaulted by a resident of the hostel that was being closed. We had expected to deal with questions about drunkenness, but were confronted with the assumption, widely held in the hall, that the residents of large hostels were child-abusers. Research findings that most children who are abused are abused by a family member or someone who knows them were completely disregarded. As far as the local residents were concerned, all hostel users were child abusers, and that was that. This was my first and most dramatic experience of the negative, powerful and unrealistic ideas that can attach themselves to a disadvantaged, easily identifiable and segregated group. The process is currently being re-invented with asylum-seekers.

The establishment of prejudice

How do these ideas develop? The incident described above fits well with Gordon Allport's definition of prejudice as "an antipathy based on faulty and inflexible generalisation. It may be felt or expressed. It may be directed toward a group or an individual of that group" (Allport 1979). In this situation, the population had been assumed to possess the same unpleasant attribute exhibited by one of their number. Moreover, this faulty attribution was inflexible, not amenable to discussion of the evidence against it. Allport listed several domains which can contribute, in any situation, to the development of prejudice or stigma.

Historical/tradition

Allport viewed this as being the single most important determinant of prejudice. Many groups are traditionally stigmatised over generations. In our culture, gypsies, Jewish people, Irish people and homeless people are all easily identifiable disadvantaged groups who have been the butt of prejudice. In the case of homeless people, this dates back to the Tudor period (Beier 1987), when the workhouse system was established. Legislation was punitive and notions of homelessness were often quite bizarre. Homeless people, or vagrants, were viewed as being part of an organised conspiracy – a "corporation", "fraternity" or "company". They were described by different authors as being idle, in league with Satan, inveterate thieves and fraudsters. Perhaps most damaging of all, they were held to be seditious, believing that property should be held in common. In our century George Orwell (1933) described attitudes prevailing in the 1930s. Homeless men were held to be characteristically dangerous, drunk, idle, and to have inflicted their troubles on themselves – to be, in his phrase, "impudent social parasites".

Current socio-cultural ideas

The historical policy towards homeless people had been to segregate them in large, squalid institutions. In parallel with notions of de-institutionalisation in psychiatry, social and housing ideology was in favour of the integration of homeless men into the community. Unfortunately, ideas in the community itself had not developed at the same pace.

Situational

Allport felt that people who lived under the pressure of poverty were more likely to need to externalise their frustrations. This was certainly a relatively deprived part of South London.

Phenomenological, or value-laden words

In this case the name of the hostel had become associated with the negative attributes attributed to local homeless men. So, if you gave your address as the hostel, you would be assumed to possess those attributes, regardless of any unique or personal qualities you might possess.

Person-to-person contact

Allport felt that this was usually the least important factor in generating prejudice. In this instance this would have probably amounted to noticing shabbily dressed and sometimes intoxicated men in the street around the hostel. Direct person-to-person contact would have been infrequent, although the hostel residents were easily visible.

Current attitudes

A telephone survey of public attitudes about homelessness (Toro and McDonnell 1992) suggested that, in the area of the USA studied, attitudes were mixed. On the positive side, the respondents tended to feel that homeless people did not choose to be homeless and that they had a high (30%) rate of mental health problems. They under-estimated arrest rates of homeless people and 58% of the sample said that they would tolerate higher taxes to help the homeless. On the down side, they over-estimated levels of drug use and convictions. Women and younger people were more likely to see fewer personal deficits among homeless people and to see unemployment as more critical. There did not seem to be any relationship between attitudes and political affiliation.

Phelan et al. (1997) acknowledged that poor people have long been stigmatised and blamed for their situation, and examined the assumption that homeless people should be even more stigmatised than the "generic poor". They elicited attitudes by presenting a vignette describing the situation of a domiciled person in poverty, and the situation of a homeless person in poverty. They found that the homeless man is blamed no less and, generally, is stigmatised more than the domiciled man. Moreover, the strength of the stigma attached to the homelessness label was equal to that for being admitted to a mental hospital. In spite of the publicity associating homelessness and mental illness, they found that the stigmas of homelessness and mental hospitalisation were independent of one another. They commented that "the robust tendency to blame the disadvantaged for their predicaments holds true for modern homelessness as well".

Stigma within medicine

As caring professionals, doctors and nurses are supposed to direct their efforts impartially, without regard to social or economic status. Unfortunately, the message from homeless people and voluntary agencies is that they are often discriminated against on the basis of inaccurate labelling, or stigma. There have been continuing problems with the use of general practice services by homeless people. As one homeless person memorably put it: "Doctor, I've got this problem – I'm invisible". In London, Shiner and Leddington (1991) found that many homeless people reported that they were treated badly by GPs, given the cold shoulder by GP receptionists, or just did not like being looked at by other people in the waiting room. Many were registered with a local general practice but chose not to use it. Instead, they would see a doctor or nurse from one of the specialist primary care teams for homeless people, who, they felt, understood their problems better and were prepared to take them seriously.

The same report mentioned problems with A&E departments, mainly around having to wait and then being asked irrelevant questions about whether they had lice or had been drinking. My experience as a community psychiatrist supports this. Two of my patients have had completely unnecessary alcohol detoxifications after presenting to A&E with physical problems. On both occasions it was assumed that, because they were homeless middle-aged men, they were therefore alcohol-dependent. Jeffrey (1979) interviewed A&E staff and found that the homeless were one of several groups regarded as "rubbish", not deserving of their professional attention. Psychiatry is not exempt. Junior psychiatrists are six times more likely to consider homeless people to be inappropriate for admission to hospital, compared with those who have a home (Elwood 1999).

The development of medical stigma

Why should this be the case? Of course, professional people are part of wider society and, outside their special area of expertise, hold many of the same beliefs that are held by the general public. In addition, it seems likely that there is a specific mechanism that is generated by professional care-giving or helping activity with homeless people.

Allport (1979) suggested that the thwarting of a goal-directed behaviour results in a negative reaction, such as a prejudicial attitude:

1. Frustration, or a thwarted goal-directed activity, produces aggression.
2. This aggression may be displaced towards relatively innocent subjects. These may be targeted merely because they are available.
3. Aggression that is displaced onto an innocent subject needs to be rationalised. In this way, the individual can justify his attitude, either to himself or to other members of the group.
4. One way of doing this is to deny the innocence of the targeted subject – to blame them for the problem and thus justify your displaced aggression. A convenient scapegoat is thereby created.

How might this work in practice? Very simply, most care providers still work in an effectively mono-disciplinary fashion. At the point of contact with the patient or client, we have the skills to deal with one area of need. The problem is that homeless people usually present with multiple areas of need which can appear to make pointless any limited intervention in any one area. The doctor or nurse will inevitably feel frustrated and, via the mechanism described above, displace their aggression onto homeless people. It is easier to blame the victim for his or her misfortune than to accept that the structure, of which you are a part, is inadequate. It is, perhaps, particularly easy when there is a large social gap between you and the person you are stigmatising.

Does this, in fact, happen? We know that the majority of homeless people see the A&E department as their first port of call for health services, whether for short-term or long-standing problems (Shanks 1989). This reflects the accessibility generated by the long opening hours and the lack of the need to make an appointment. It is therefore a good setting in which to explore the attitudes of health workers to homeless people. Stuart Cable (1992) did this by interviewing 18 nurses in a Central London A&E department and a series of homeless people and project workers.

The notion regarding multiple areas of need was voiced by one hostel worker, who often had to take residents to A&E. "GPs freak, that's what happens when we send one of our guy's down to see a GP outside. They try to look at one particular problem which they can solve, they're not taking in the whole range of problems". Again, from the hostel worker's point of view "I do expect them to provide a GP service and primary health care", otherwise "The guys just won't bother". So, there is an expectation of a service from the A&E department, both from homeless people and from those who work with them in the community.

However, the A&E nurses clearly did not see providing primary care services as part of their job. "I don't see it as a casualty nurse's place to go providing primary health care, that's for the GP . . . . . You haven't got time for chatting and making numerous phone calls and having conversations about longer-term strategies with people". They reported high levels of frustration as a result. Analysis of the interviews revealed "disregarding, neglecting, ignoring and avoiding as recurrent actions by nurses with regard to homeless people". They tended to view homeless attendees as drinkers and time wasters. This was obvious to one of the homeless interviewees who commented "They see so many people who are alcoholics that they think, because you're down and out, we're all alcoholics, all abusing the system". One worrying feature was that these attitudes seemed to be prominent in more experienced staff. This may reflect the powerful effect of historically established attitudes in any social group, as described by Allport.

Stigma within psychiatry

How does this express itself in psychiatry? One vexed area is that of the NFA rota, which is a common way of re-distributing homeless patients around the consultants in a given area or trust. The problem is that many homeless people actually do have a fixed abode – it just isn't somewhere where they enjoy tenancy rights. It is possible to live in the same homeless hostel for years and still be allocated via the NFA rota. The notion that to be homeless is to be mobile, to be a tramp, results in unnecessary fragmentation of care for homeless patients.

Conclusion

The evidence is fragmentary and anecdotal. It does, however, suggest that stigmatising attitudes held by medical and nursing staff do compromise the treatment of homeless people in mainstream medical and psychiatric services. This is often not merely the effect of general societal attitudes, but is aggravated by attitudes that have become a tradition in settings such as A&E, and are taken on by new staff as they are acculturated within that setting. A powerful reinforcing factor in this is the demand on medical and nursing staff to provide an effective multi-disciplinary, continuing primary care service without the official sanction or the resources to do so.

Obviously, if a homeless person does not feel comfortable in a mainstream service, they will tend to seek some alternative. Shiner and Leddington (1991) comment that "in choosing to use services located within the world of homelessness, people are making a social decision: a decision to minimise the psychological 'risk' to themselves, not a medical decision about which services offer the best level of care".

This will obviously tend to encourage the growth of specialist services and the continuing segregation of homeless people from the mainstream – which will contribute to the maintenance of stigmatising attitudes towards homeless people.

References

Allport G (1979) *The Nature of Prejudice*. Reading: Perseus Books.
Beier AL (1987) *Masterless Men – The Vagrancy Problem in England 1560–1640*. London: Methuen.
Cable S (1992) Identifying the factors involved in the care of the homeless in the Accident and Emergency department: a grounded theory study. MSc thesis.
Elwood PY (1999) Characteristics of admissions considered inappropriate by junior psychiatrists. *Psychiatric Bulletin* 23: 34–7.
Jeffery R (1979) Normal rubbish: deviant patients in casualty departments. *Sociology of Health and Illness* 1: 91–107.
Orwell G (1933) *Down and Out in Paris and London*. London: Victor Gollancz.
Phelan J, Bruce GL, Moore RE & Stueve A (1997) The stigma of homelessness: The impact of the label "homeless" on attitudes toward poor persons. *Social Psychology Quarterly*, December.
Shanks NJ (1989) Previously diagnosed psychiatric illness among inhabitants of common lodging houses. *Journal of Epidemiology & Community Health* 43: 375–9.
Shiner P & Leddington S (1991) Sometimes it makes you frightened to go to hospital . . . they treat you like dirt. *Health Service Journal*, 7 November: 21–3.
Toro PA & McDonnell DM (1992) Beliefs, attitudes and knowledge about homelessness: a survey of the general public. *American Journal of Community Psychology* 20: 53–80.

Commentary on Section 2C

Tom Burns

In a campaign to explore and reduce the stigma experienced by individuals with mental illnesses it would be all too easy to characterise stigma as simply an aberration in a small group of poorly educated or spiteful individuals. This may feel comfortable to those of us dedicated to reducing stigma but does scant justice to the phenomenon, and strategies built upon it would be likely to fail. Diagnosis should precede treatment and we need to recognise the reality of stigma as a pervasive feature in human behaviour. By recognising that it must have a biological basis and probably some evolutionary function we can develop means to reduce its detrimental effects. "Odd" behaviour in any individual will evoke some anxiety in members of the group in humans and in most social animals. Unpredictability or difference of appearance raises concerns of risk – whether from infection or conflict.

Groups where strong social cohesion is essential for personal safety (e.g. fire-fighters, the army) have elaborate rituals to test new members to ensure reliability under stress. Individualism is rejected – and for reasons we all can understand. Stigma towards the mentally ill is an inappropriate and destructive expression of a behaviour pattern that in appropriate contexts is useful and healthy.

The social conditioning of stigma is richly exemplified by Dr Andrè Tylee's report from a typical GP surgery (Chapter 21). Not all mental health problems attracted the same degree of stigma – depressed patients seemed now to anticipate acceptance and support. A policeman with lifelong disabling anxiety was supported and accepted by his police colleagues. He had developed a coping strategy of avoiding front-line duty and working on administrative matters (which his colleagues were happy to relinquish), but reorganisation within the force destroyed his niche and he was soon unable to function, often off sick. Now he felt discriminated against and stigmatised. His colleagues would tolerate his "illness" but not his inability to contribute to the newly configured team.

Even more striking was one of Dr Tylee's patients who felt stigmatised by his psychiatric care but not by his extensive prison record. This echoed the reports of adolescent working class boys in the East End of London in the 1950s, where a police record attracted no stigma at all but admission to a mental hospital led to severe discrimination. It can be argued that this is a realistic appraisal of the biological significance of the two experiences. A prison sentence in such a subculture could simply be a marker for the relatively benign, and certainly short-lived, delinquent phase soon to be followed by settling down. Admission to mental hospital in the 1950s indicated a severe mental illness with potentially long-lasting disability. The entry thresholds for the two institutions are effectively reversed now and the implications (and stigma) consequently reversed.

In Chapter 22, Dr Moodley reminds us that discriminatory behaviour towards the mentally ill has always characterised the three great cultures that she has chosen to present – Islam, China and India. Although many of the revered writings of these cultures display a benign and holistic approach to mental illness, the reality of social behaviour was often mechanistic and rejecting. Her presentation alerts us to the risk of romanticising human behaviour and harking back to a golden age without cruelty and discrimination. That golden age has never existed.

Dr Timms' work with the homeless mentally ill, reported in Chapter 23, confronts stigma in undiluted form. This is a doubly stigmatised group, as Dr Moodley has pointed out it often is for ethnic minority mentally ill patients. The homeless demonstrate the inflation of stigma by distorted and unrealistic assumptions. Dr Timms describes a public meeting on reprovision of a large hostel for homeless men. It became clear that they were stigmatised not only as vagrants, not only as mentally ill, not only as alcoholics – but as paedophiles. These men had societies' most unacceptable images projected on to them. The task of reducing stigma for them is one of education of the public: disentangling myth from the real problems associated with mental illness.

The positive role of education in dispelling myths is undoubted. A study of providing an educational package for local residents when opening a mental health hostel in South London clearly demonstrated greater acceptance of the residents than in a parallel hostel opened without such a package. Not only was there "acceptance" but also positive engagement with the hostel residents. In the same study a local survey of attitudes demonstrated an inverse relationship of tolerance of the mentally ill with age. Younger people were more accepting. Possibly this is because they have been exposed to the mentally ill, whereas their elders grew up in a world where mental illness was shut off behind asylum walls. Whether this is genuinely a cohort effect or simply an age-related difference we will have to wait and see. This author is optimistic that exposure to the mentally ill (despite damaging and distorting tabloid headlines) generally leads to a more realistic and humane acceptance.

24 Stigmatisation of people with schizophrenia

Julian Leff

The origins of stigma

The whole range of psychiatric conditions attracts some degree of stigma, but by far the worst attaches to the term "schizophrenia" and what it conjures up in the mind of the public. Many people, including journalists, interpret the term as denoting "split personality", with associated images of Dr Jekyll and Mr Hyde. Stevenson's novel was actually a sophisticated argument for the recognition that every person is subject to violent impulses, and that we are constantly suppressing these as a result of being socialised. But the aim of splitting them off and becoming a perfectly calm and rational being is illusory. We are all an uncomfortable mixture of the good doctor and the passionate beast. Yet the urge to deny our violent passions and to label them as "madness" is both profound and pervasive. This process of cleansing ourselves of violence and unpredictability is achieved only by attributing these unwanted characteristics to others. The despised other then becomes someone we wish to extrude from civilised society. This was, of course, the fate of hundreds of thousands of people with psychiatric illness who were admitted to the asylums, and often spent the rest of their life isolated from the outside world.

Deinstitutionalisation

In the 1950s the tide of opinion turned, strongly influenced by the experiences of military psychiatrists during the Second World War. Patients began to be discharged from the asylums and the locus of care shifted to the community. The first wave of patients to return to their districts of origin were relatively capable and many could live independently. Some had never been mentally ill but had behaved in ways disapproved of by society, such as having illegitimate children. As time went on and the residual hospital populations shrunk, the patients considered for discharge were increasingly disabled as a result of the creaming off process (Jones 1993). More and more they resembled the popular stereotype of the mad person, showing aggression and sexually disinhibited behaviour (Trieman and Leff 1996). The staff responsible for placement became understandably anxious about resettling patients with these difficult behaviours in ordinary sheltered homes. Consequently, special facilities were established for them. With the exception of this group, the entire populations of the old asylums were discharged to the community, allowing the institutions to close. In England and Wales, 100 of the 130 psychiatric hospitals have disappeared, and with them the most visible embodiment of stigma, the unmistakable architecture of the old asylums; remote, forbidding, and with a palpable aura of incarceration.

Attempts were made to reduce the stigma attached to the asylums by changing their names. One institution we studied began as Middlesex County Pauper Lunatic Asylum, was renamed Colney Hatch Asylum, then Friern Barnet Hospital, and finally, after the hospital was closed and redeveloped as luxury flats, Princess Park Manor. As Andrew Scull has pointed out, "word magic" of this kind fails in its intent since the public are not fooled into believing that the change is more than cosmetic. On the one hand closure of the asylums has removed one source of stigma, but on the other it has brought quite disabled patients back into the community, where they have a high visibility. Early studies of public attitudes, such as that by Una Maclean (1969), found that contact with people with psychiatric disorders tended to soften attitudes. However, at that time the most disabled patients were confined in institutions and it is conceivable that the behaviour and appearance of such people once they are living in the community could reinforce stereotypes. In a more recent survey of Canadian adolescents, Norman and Malla (1983) included a question on whether a person who becomes mentally ill can return to normal. They found that optimism about prognosis was negatively related to social distance; however the correlation between the two factors, although significant, was only –0.13. Surveys conducted in the last decade are likely to reflect the maximum impact of deinstitutionalisation. A study of public attitudes has recently been conducted in Brescia, northern Italy, where deinstitutionalisation has progressed quite far. Vezzoli and colleagues (2001) found that people who had never talked with or met a psychiatric patient had more negative feelings and were less willing to give a patient a job, and most of them thought that the ideal setting for such patients was a psychiatric hospital or a sheltered home.

A survey of public attitudes

Reda (1996) investigated the influence on public attitudes of contact with long-stay patients discharged from two psychiatric hospitals in north London. The study had a quasi-experimental design in which respondents were interviewed in two adjacent streets, in one of which a sheltered home for the discharged patients was located. Surveys of the two streets were conducted before the patients moved in and six months afterwards. It was assumed that neighbours of the sheltered home would have more contact with the ex-patients than residents of the other street, which was parallel to the study street. This proved to be correct since at the follow-up interview half the respondents in the study street reported that they had talked to or seen the residents of the facility, whereas no one in the control street had learned of the sheltered home by the second interview. In both the baseline and follow-up interviews, in response to the question of how they would describe someone with mental illness, a quarter of respondents in both streets said it was difficult to identify such a person, indicating that they did not hold a stereotyped view. The remaining three quarters of the respondents cited a number of characteristics. In both groups difficult communication was the most frequently identified characteristic, followed by strange behaviour, lack of social skills, wandering about, aggression, and abnormal appearance, in that order. Aggression was cited by just over 20% of both groups, considerably less than expected, given the media focus on homicides committed by the mentally ill. At the follow-up interview, attitudes of respondents in both streets showed virtually no change, indicating that exposure to people with longstanding psychotic illnesses had little or no impact on the neighbours. It is of importance that the average age of the discharged patients was 55 and that some of the residents in the street identified the mental health facility as an old age home. It is possible that the public stereotype relates to young men, of whom there were few in this sheltered home.

This survey also revealed some very positive attitudes to community care. When asked whether patients in psychiatric hospitals could live in the community, only one fifth of the respondents considered this to be impossible. Nearly 90% of all respondents were positive about the opening of a mental health facility in their neighbourhood, while over three quarters were willing to offer help to the facility. However, about 60% considered that neighbours required preparation before such a facility was opened. They recommended that the following items should be included in an educational programme:

- Practical skills, for example how to approach a mentally ill person and how to cope with problem behaviours.
- The types, causes, frequency, and degree of seriousness of mental illnesses.
- The services available for the treatment of mental illness.
- The importance of accepting mentally ill people.

These recommendations have been given in detail because they appear to be eminently sensible, and because it is rare for educators to ask their target audience what they want to learn before embarking on a campaign.

An educational programme

The unexpected fund of goodwill existing in the community that was revealed by Reda's survey, and the respondents' request for information, prompted the planning of an educational programme for neighbours connected with the establishment of sheltered homes in south London. These were developed as provision for some of the long-stay patients discharged from a large psychiatric hospital which was closing. In many ways they were comparable to the patients studied by Reda in her research in north London. The two homes involved in the evaluation of an educational programme were in two different districts, but took very similar groups of patients. A coin was tossed to randomly select one of the streets as experimental and the other as control. A survey of neighbours' attitudes was conducted in both streets at baseline and one year after the patients had moved in. An adaptation of Reda's survey questionnaire was used as well as other instruments. An education programme was run in the experimental street, while the control neighbours received no information about the sheltered home or its occupants (Wolff et al. 1996a–d).

In the experimental street 146 immediate neighbours of the sheltered home were sent an invitation to a reception to be held in a local church hall. Of these, 16 attended the reception. Attenders were offered food and drinks and were given a pack of information leaflets about mental illness, schizophrenia, community care policy, and supported houses in their district. Staff from the supported home and research staff were present. A video was shown which had been specially filmed for the programme. It lasted about 20 minutes and included the following: the history of community care and evidence for its beneficial effects on patients, explanations by staff of the contrast between life in the psychiatric hospital and living in the community, accounts by local residents and tradespeople from another area of their experiences with discharged patients, and a description by a former patient of his move into supported accommodation. After the video, people were given the opportunity to question the staff.

Following the reception, neighbours who did not attend were offered the information leaflet and copies of the video to borrow. Neighbours were invited to a barbecue and two other social events in the house to meet staff and patients. About 15 people attended the social events, while 20 arranged a discussion with a member of staff around the information pack, and a further 20 saw the video and read the leaflets without engaging in the discussion.

The baseline survey of the experimental and control streets revealed very similar attitudes to those found by Reda, including a fund of goodwill. The majority of respondents (60%) said they would make friends with neighbours who had a psychiatric illness, and 90% had no reservations about working with a mentally ill person. The follow-up survey showed that the education campaign resulted in only a small increase in knowledge, but had a significant impact on lessening fear of the mentally ill and attitudes of rejection. In the home in the experimental street most of the patients reported having social contact with their neighbours on a regular basis, and two patients each considered three of their neighbours to be friends. By contrast, the control patients reported no social contacts with neighbours. Thus this small-scale focused campaign achieved its aim of reducing fear of the mentally ill and hence stigma, to the extent that the patients began to integrate socially into their community. There is a danger of idealising the concept of community, which was revealed by comments made by the residents who attended the reception. One of the main reasons they gave for appreciating the occasion was that it gave them the opportunity to meet their neighbours!

Mental illness and violence

The process of deinstitutionalisation has been accompanied by an increasing focus by the media on homicides committed by mentally ill people, even though most of these tragic events have involved patients who have never spent more than a few weeks as inpatients. As confirmation of this, a five-year follow-up of 670 patients discharged from two psychiatric hospitals in north London recorded assaults on the public, other patients and members of staff by 13 patients, amounting to 2% of the sample (Trieman, Leff and Glover 1999). If the long-stay population of asylums being resettled in the community contains only a tiny proportion of assaultative people, why is the closure of the psychiatric hospitals associated by the public with dangerous consequences? The strength of this association is reflected not only in the bad press given to deinstitutionalisation, but also in vociferous protests by groups of residents against sheltered homes being opened in their streets. If a home is opened despite this opposition, the angry protests soon die down as it becomes obvious that the new residents pose no threat to their neighbours. It appears that there is a persisting image of mental hospitals as secure containers for violence and unbridled sexuality, with the attendant fantasy that unlocking the doors will release these feared behaviours among the defenceless public. Wolff et al. (1996a) found that women with young children expressed more fear of the mentally ill than other groups in their community sample, even though attacks on young children by psychotic patients are extremely rare.

As a response to these negative public attitudes, resettlement programmes are usually conducted as inconspicuously as possible in the hope of avoiding any opposition. Our experience has shown that while slipping patients into the community sideways may circumvent protests by activists, this strategy fails to mobilise the goodwill that exists in every neighbourhood. Localised campaigns have the potential to reduce irrational fears and hence stigma, and to facilitate the development of social relationships between patients and their new neighbours. Without this, patients can readily remain as isolated in the community as they were behind the high walls of the asylums.

References

Jones D (1993) The TAPS Project. 11: The selection of patients for reprovision. In: Leff J (ed.). Evaluating community placement of long-stay psychiatric patients. *British Journal of Psychiatry* **162** (Suppl 19): 30–5.

Maclean U (1969) Community attitudes to mental illness in Edinburgh. *British Journal of Preventive and Social Medicine* **23**: 45–52.

Norman RMG & Malla AK (1983) Adolescents' attitudes towards mental illness: relationship between components and sex differences. *Social Psychiatry* **18**: 45–50.

Reda S (1996) Public perceptions of former psychiatric patients in England. *Psychiatric Services* **47**: 1253–5.

Trieman N & Leff J (1996) Difficult to place patients in a psychiatric hospital closure programme: The TAPS project 24. *Psychological Medicine* **26**: 765–74.

Trieman N, Leff J & Glover G (1999) Outcome of long stay psychiatric patients resettled in the community: prospective cohort study. *British Medical Journal* **319**: 13–16.

Vezzoli R, Archiati L, Buizza C, Pasqualetti P et al. (2001) Attitude towards psychiatric patients: a pilot study in a northern Italian town. *European Psychiatry* **16**: 451–8.

Wolff G, Pathare S, Craig T et al. (1996a) Community attitudes to mental illness. *British Journal of Psychiatry* **168**, 183-190.

Wolff G, Pathare S, Craig T et al. (1996b) Community knowledge of mental illness and reaction to mentally ill people. *British Journal of Psychiatry* **168**: 191–8.

Wolff G, Pathare S, Craig T et al. (1996c) Who's in the lion's den? The community's perception of community care for the mentally ill. *Psychiatric Bulletin* **20**: 68–71.

Wolff G, Pathare S, Craig T et al. (1996d) Public education for community care. A new approach. *British Journal of Psychiatry* **168**: 441–7.

25 Stigmatisation and suicide

Simon Armson

Setting the scene

What does stigma mean? The *Collins Concise English Dictionary*, Third Edition, defines stigma as "a distinguishing mark of social disgrace". There are important links between the way individuals and society, as a whole, approach both mental illness and suicide, and these can, and should be, tackled by us all. The "anti-stigma" campaign currently being conducted by the Royal College of Psychiatrists and the "Challenging Stigma" emphasis for World Mental Health Day 1999 work towards reducing the stigmas associated with mental illness and, within this, suicide.

These campaigns coincide with an increased focus on suicide and mental health by the UK Government. The White Paper "Saving Lives – Our Healthier Nation" sets an ambitious target "to reduce the death rate from suicide and undetermined death by at least a fifth by 2010" – this target will be all the more challenging because of the stigma attached to suicide. It is planned to implement this initiative through a three-way partnership involving individuals, communities and Government. Voluntary organisations will have a crucial contribution to make towards achieving this target. In addition, the long awaited National Service Framework for mental health will look at how quality local services can be provided to meet national standards of care for those people suffering from mental illness. It also recognises and acknowledges the stigma that has been attached to mental illness and suicide and how this can lead to discrimination and to social exclusion for sufferers. This is a huge issue for the Government to tackle but The Samaritans is pleased to see the positive steps that are being taken to address the problems of mental illness and suicide and that a clear focus has been put on the need for working in partnership with the various sectors. The Samaritans will be wanting to play a part in this process.

The history of suicide and stigma

In understanding the stigma of suicide, we need to track back in history. Until 1961, suicide was a crime, hence the term "to commit". Suicide was decriminalised in England and Wales in 1961 and, more recently, in the Republic of Ireland in 1993. Suicide in Scotland has never been a felony. Therefore, it is fair to say that the stigma associated with suicide could have part of its roots in its criminal past. It could also be the result of religious beliefs and the fundamental incomprehensibility experienced by some when considering that most radical denial, of the gift of life itself. Allen (1977) pointed out that "Historically, society's attitudes toward suicide and the suicidal act reveal a wide range between a rational one of acceptance, an irrational one of superstition, and a hostile one of punishment".

Throughout history, religion has played an important part in influencing the stigma attached to suicide. Initially, Christianity was relatively accepting of suicide. In the fifth century, St Augustine pursued a number of arguments which are still valid today, including the suggestion that suicide was a greater sin than anything it could be avoiding, and that life was divinely ordained by God and so must be experienced.

From the beginning of the fourteenth century through to the eighteenth century, it seems as if attitudes towards suicide began to become more relaxed. In some circles, suicide was once again not seen as a sin but as an acceptable option. European governments began to change their laws, and in 1824, England's parliament passed a law allowing a person who died by suicide to be buried in a churchyard, although only between 9 pm and midnight (Werth 1996). Werth tells us that the nineteenth century saw the introduction of a new way of approaching suicide. This was a move away from viewing it as a theological, moral, philosophical and legal issue to one that was seen as a social, medical and psychological problem capable of statistical analysis. This continued into the twentieth century, with assessments taking place to ascertain the link between mental illness and suicide. Blumenthal and Kupfer (1986) suggested that there were a number of areas that influence suicidal ideation and behaviour: psychosocial milieu, biological vulnerability, personality and family history, and genetics.

As well as attitudes changing over time, attitudes to suicide vary considerably in different cultures. For example, we will all be familiar with the practices in Japan where hara-kiri used to take place in order to avoid capture or disgrace and, in India, where suttee by a Hindu woman was expected when her husband died.

Current attitudes

It is attitude that lies at the root of stigma. To a certain extent, personal attitudes about the sanctity of human life and attitudes to death are all influenced by cultural norms, beliefs and religious teaching. However, personal attitudes and professionalism need to be kept separate, so allowing an objective approach to an individual being treated by a professional.

A number of studies have taken place assessing the attitudes of professionals who deal with people who attempt suicide or who have suicidal thoughts. Many of the earlier studies (e.g. Patel 1975; Ghodse 1978; Goldney & Bothill 1980) found that ". . . more negative feelings were expressed towards suicide and parasuicide than towards any other medical emergency, and . . . that hospital staff . . . were hostile and unsympathetic to the typical overdose".

The attitudes of staff in the A&E departments of hospitals are often reported as being negative towards those who attempt suicide. However, in an intervention study of deliberate self-harm assessment by accident and emergency staff carried out in 1997 by Crawford, Turnbull and Wessely, it was ascertained that the impact of a limited amount of specific education on the quality of psychosocial assessment of a self-harm patient did correlate with the quality of care provided (Crawford et al. 1998). It also found that communication between the A&E staff and the hospital's parasuicide team improved. With the Government's emphasis on primary care, general practitioners are seen as an important resource for people suffering from depression or who have suicidal thoughts.

One of the initiatives that The Samaritans is currently working on is the Doctor Patient Partnership and The Men's Health Forum, which is aimed at helping men cope with their feelings; thus it is hoped that a reduction in the incidence of suicide in this group will result. This initiative aims to encourage better communication between patients and health care professionals offering vulnerable patients information about where they may turn for intervention and support.

Looking beyond the medical and nursing professions, research carried out by Leane and Shute (1997) in Australia in 1997 studied the knowledge and attitudes of Australian teachers and clergy to youth suicide (Leane and Shute 1998). These professions are often regarded as "gatekeepers for distressed young people" (this role was confirmed in the research). It was concluded that teachers and the clergy could play an important role in suicide education and prevention.

In the USA, Sawyer and Sobal (1987) reported that negative attitudes towards suicide were found among frequent church attenders and those with strong religious preferences. Some active churchgoers still appear to regard suicide as a moral evil.

A few studies have been carried out to examine the attitudes of teachers. In a survey of Tennessee school principals carried out by Peach and Reddick in 1988, almost all respondents regarded young people as not having the right to suicide. In other research, school personnel were found to be uncomfortable around the issue of suicide and even trained school counsellors preferred to refer students to outside agencies. A quick review of some of the literature relating to attitudes towards suicide reveals a mixed and changeable picture.

The role of the media

The media play an important part in public education generally. This includes the impact of reporting mental illness and suicide. Concern over how individual suicides are reported in the media has arisen from studies which have suggested a risk of imitative behaviour, particularly amongst adolescents and young adults. In a study of presentations for self-poisoning following the portrayal of a paracetamol overdose in the medical television drama *Casualty*, 20% of the patients interviewed said the programme had influenced their decision to take an overdose and 17% said it had influenced their choice of drug (Hawton et al. 1999). Although the evidence is conflicting, and in many cases lacking, there is cause for concern that inappropriate depiction of suicide can influence the attitudes and behaviour of the audience or readership. Equally, it is clear that positive explanation of the issue in a sensitive way can help to educate and destigmatise the issue of suicide.

Therefore, the media play a vital role in forming opinion and attitude and thus reducing stigma. But this has to be done with great care so as to avoid the risk of simply making the problem worse.

In 1997, The Samaritans held a symposium aimed at promoting discussion on the effects of the media's portrayal of suicide and attempted suicide on those bereaved by suicide and society as a whole. This resulted in the publication of The Samaritans media guidelines on the portrayal of suicide.

The role of the coroner

The coroner also plays a part in the stigma attached to suicide. When investigating a death that might have been self-inflicted, a coroner must prove, beyond reasonable doubt, that the person who has died intended to take their own life in order to return a verdict of suicide. The inquest is often attended by the press, it will involve witnesses and relatives and will include post-mortem reports and suicide notes (if one has been left). It can be an extremely harrowing experience for bereaved relatives where the stigma of suicide is at its most stark.

Many coroners are very aware of the sensitivities of those bereaved by suicide and will go out of their way to do all they can to respect this. This can ease the distress of bereaved relatives, but more because the stigma of suicide has been avoided rather than overcome.

The vision and work of The Samaritans

The Samaritans has been working since 1953 to befriend those people passing through a crisis and in imminent danger of taking their own lives. The focus for our work is our Vision:

"Fewer people will take their own lives because:

- *Samaritan befriending is always available at any hour of the day or night for all those passing through personal crisis and at risk of dying by suicide*
- *Samaritans provide society with a better understanding of suicide, suicidal behaviour and the value of expressing feelings that may lead to suicide."*

The second part of The Samaritans Vision is where the main focus for this part of our work lies.

A few years ago, The Samaritans commissioned some research to look at the taboo of talking about suicide. It revealed that, in too many instances, this taboo is very strong and, in particular, exists among those who may be at greatest risk.

The research was based on the results of a telephone survey of 1,000 adults from a representative cross section of society and some qualitative research groups. One of the questions asked was: "People who attempt suicide are only thinking of themselves – do you agree or disagree?" More than a third of the sample agreed with this statement, with older people least likely to disagree.

However, 42% agreed with the statement "People who attempt suicide deserve more sympathy than they get" and 60% agreed that "Suicide is not an easy way out".

The Samaritans, together with other professional and voluntary organisations, is trying to increase the public's awareness of the signs of suicide risk and/or depression, to promote the importance of mental health, to offer support to those passing through crisis and in imminent danger of taking their own lives, and to challenge intolerant views by promoting the value of listening and talking.

The Samaritans believe in working in partnership with organisations which will enable us to reach those people within society who are at highest risk of suicide. Examples of such partnerships are with the Prison Service and the Rural Stress Information Network (RSIN). The Samaritans is also currently embarking on research with Oxford University which will look at adolescents and suicide. An example of this work is the recently published youth pack for schools, which aims to promote a sensitive and accepting atmosphere in which young people can learn more about themselves and others.

Conclusion

There is little doubt that both suicide and the feelings that may lead towards it are still heavily stigmatised within society today. If this is to change the need for constructive partnerships cannot be over-emphasised. For its part, The Samaritans is keen to make a significant contribution towards this end.

References

Allen N (1977) History and background of suicidology. In: Hatton CL, Valente SM & Rink A (eds). *Suicide: Assessment and Intervention*. New York: Appleton-Century-Crofts: 1–19.

Blumenthal SJ & Kupfer DJ (1986) Generalizable treatment strategies for suicidal behavior. *Annals of the New York Academy of Sciences* **487**: 327–40.

Crawford MJ, Turnbull G, & Wessely S (1998) Deliberate self harm assessment by accident and emergency staff – an intervention study. *Journal of Accident and Emergency Medicine* **5**: 18–22.

Ghodse AH (1978) The attitudes of casualty staff and ambulance personnel towards patients who take overdoses. *Social Science and Medicine* **12**: 341–6.

Goldney RD & Bottrill A (1980) Attitudes to patients who attempt suicide. *Medical Journal of Australia* **2**: 717–20.

Hawton K, Sumkin S, Deeks JJ et al. (1999) Effects of a drug overdose in a television drama on presentations to hospital for self poisoning: time series and questionnaire study. *British Medical Journal* **318**: 972–9.

Leane W & Shute R (1998) Youth suicide: the knowledge and attitudes of Australian teachers and clergy. *Suicide and Life-Threatening Behavior* **28**: 165–73.

Patel AR (1975) Attitudes towards self poisoning. *British Medical Journal* **ii**: 426–30.

Peach L & Reddick TL (1988) An assessment of selected educators' understandings of adolescent suicide. Paper presented at the Annual Meeting of the National Social Science Association, Tennessee.

Sawyer D & Sobal J (1987) Public attitudes toward suicide: demographic and ideological correlates. *Public Opinion Quarterly* **51**: 92–101.

Werth Jr JL (1996) *Rational Suicide? Implications for Mental Health Professionals*. New York: Taylor & Francis.

26 Cinematic portrayals of psychiatrists

Anthony Clare

Introduction

Most people never encounter a psychiatrist in a professional setting. As with mental hospitals, the public's perception of psychiatrists is formed at second-hand. A powerful influence, perhaps with television the most powerful, is the cinema. Over a century that has seen both the cinema and psychiatry strengthen their grip on the imagination, the creativity and the experience of individuals and society, the portrayal of psychiatrists on screen has been a mixture of positive and negative, harmful and helpful, good and evil.

Psychiatrists, as seen through the eyes of film makers, are at one and the same time omnipotent and useless, progressive and reactionary, compassionate and destructive, perceptive and blind. A particularly popular representation of the psychiatrist is as a deeply flawed psychologically disturbed individual who cures through empathy or destroys through malevolence. Female psychiatrists are almost invariably portrayed as histrionic and dependent, as likely to be cured by love as therapeutically effective. Psychiatrists seeing themselves portrayed on screen should take a careful look. Whatever the image, caricature or miniature, affectionate or hostile, however paradoxical or stereotypical, the image shown there is the image patients see. More recent portrayals, affected by a developing collaboration between psychiatrists and film and television writers and scriptwriters, suggest that a more realistic and balanced portrayal is beginning to emerge. In this chapter, some of the more persistent cinematic stereotypes of psychiatrists are explored.

Since the appearance of the first psychiatrist in the movies – the harried superintendent of Dr Dippy's Sanatorium in 1906 – there have been hundreds of cinematic psychiatrists portrayed by Hollywood in particular and world cinema in general, right up to and beyond the remarkable and repulsive Dr Hannibal Lecter played mesmerically by one of this country's most respected and since knighted actors, Anthony Hopkins. Given the enormous influence of the cinema, and particularly its appeal to young people, should we, the more mundane and real-life counterparts of our celluloid colleagues, be perturbed, gratified or unconcerned by how we are portrayed? In this context it is worth noting that many people have no first-hand experience of psychiatric hospitals or of psychiatrists. Their only visual image of both is likely to be derived from television and the cinema. Is the sum total of the many and varied portrayals of psychiatrists a beneficial and largely positive portrait or is it a contributory, stigmatising factor in the public perception of psychiatry, psychiatrists, psychiatric illness and psychiatric treatment?

Cinematic portrayals

There is no clear-cut unambiguous portrait of a psychiatrist that emerges from the cinema. Part of the picture that does emerge is inherited from the psychiatrist's history as asylum superintendent, purveyor of grim, grisly and largely custodial treatment. Part of it derives from psychoanalysis, and cinematic portrayals influenced by this school have contributed to one of the most potent contemporary images of the psychiatrist as an excavator of the mind, an amalgam of the fictional detective Sherlock Holmes and the very real, archaeologically minded Sigmund Freud. Part again is provided by the notion of the psychiatrist as every bit as disturbed as his/her patient, reflecting one of the stigmatising views of mental illness, namely that it affects and contaminates anyone who becomes too intimately connected to it. The mad psychiatrist, like the mad patient, is wild, dangerous, unpredictable and in need of restraint and custodial control. There is also a part of the portrait which shows the psychiatrist as incompetent, a naive and silly fool faced with the awesome complexity of the human mind.

Many psychiatrists have not much liked what they have seen of their portrait within the contemporary cinema. Irving Schneider (1987) writes of "the invented profession" which from time to time resembles the real profession of psychiatry but which for the most part has "created its own nosology, treatment methods, theories and practitioners". Gabard and Gabard (1987) comment similarly, observing that "practitioners of psychiatry have seldom found reason to applaud the image of themselves appearing on the screen". They suggest a typology of cinematic psychiatrists which includes the faceless psychiatrist, the active, the oracular, the eccentric, the emotional, the sexual and the social agent. Each of these categories has a good and a bad representative. Schneider has a more simple classification – dividing psychiatrists into Dr Dippy, Dr Evil and Dr Wonderful.

The mad and the bad

The "mad" psychiatrist is a well-established cinematic stereotype and overlaps with the bad or "evil" one. A particularly dramatic example of the seriously disturbed psychiatrist is provided in Brian de Palma's film *Dressed to Kill*, in which the central figure is a homicidal transvestite practitioner played by Michael Caine. The mad psychiatrist can either be calculating or comic. The serial killer Dr Hannibal Lecter in *The Silence of the Lambs* and the lecherous quack Dr Fritz Fassbender in *What's New Pussycat* may appear to have little in common yet both are quite unbalanced. Each in his own way reflects two widespread stigmatising beliefs – that psychiatry attracts the unbalanced and the unbalanced flourish in psychiatry. In *What's New Pussycat* Peter O'Toole seeks help from a Central European analyst, played by Peter Sellers, to enable him to curb his philandering and settle down and marry his latest flame, Carol. However, his analyst has on his mind the subject which psychiatrists are supposed to be preoccupied with, namely sex. O'Toole interprets the craziness of Dr Fritz Fassbender as evidence of his professional genius!

Before I turn to the stereotype of Dr Evil let us consider the opposite side of the coin, Dr Wonderful. After the antipsychiatric period of the 1960s and 1970s which saw films such as *One Flew Over the Cuckoo's Nest* and *A Clockwork Orange*, there has been a resurgence of the oracular, caring and impressive part-detective, part-confessor who was such a feature of Hollywood's golden era of cinematic psychiatry, namely the 1940s. One of the most influential psychiatrists from this golden age is Dr Jaquith in the 1942 film *Now Voyager*, played by Claude Rains. According to Gabard and Gabard (1987), *Now Voyager* did much "to domesticate and demystify the image of the psychiatrist in America". Dr Jaquith runs a clinic, Cascade, which resembles a country manor rather than any ghastly asylum, also much loved by Hollywood movie makers. Dr Jaquith dispenses talk rather than tablets and at one point in the film is able to give a humane, idealistic and confident account of what it is that psychiatrists do – talk, listen and guide.

More recently, the cinema, reflecting developments in modern psychiatry, has taken on board the need to marry the biological and the psychological. In the Oscar-winning film *The Prince of Tides* Barbra Streisand plays Dr Lowenstein, a female, Jewish psychotherapist involved in treating a young woman who has just made a serious suicide attempt. She dispenses Largactil as well as psychotherapy and sees her role in terms both of excavating the cause of her patient's agony and keeping her alive. True to form, where there is a female psychiatrist involved there is a romantic interest; in this film, instead of falling in love with her patient, she does the next best thing and falls in love with the brother.

What makes *The Prince of Tides* of interest, in addition to the fact that it portrayed a psychiatrist dispensing drugs who was nonetheless humane and compassionate, is that it reflects a struggle of stereotypes. The suicidal patient is shown shackled to a bed. The psychiatrist appears willing to reduce the calming medication but leaves on the shackles. There is reference to a team. But most striking is the fact that this psychiatrist is not the cool, detached, urbane, almost god-like figure of such films as John Huston's *Freud; The Secret Passion* or Richard Gere's analyst in *Final Analysis*. She loses her cool, swears and makes plain that she is eclectic when it comes to choosing a treatment that will help her patient.

There is no shortage of female psychiatrists in the movies, according to Laurel Samuels (1985), who catalogued some of the most famous. Almost invariably they are portrayed as corrupt or effective but inadequate as women. Equally common is their tendency to fall in love with their patients, often curing them and themselves in the process. One of the most celebrated films to portray the love affair between female psychiatrist and patient was the 1945 romance-thriller *Spellbound*. Ingrid Bergman, a young psychiatrist in a fashionable sanatorium, falls in love with the highly disturbed Gregory Peck. At one point in the movie, Bergman's training analyst observes: "Women make the best psychoanalysts until they fall in love. Then they make the best patients."

The psychiatrist as manipulator, as priest, as pervert, as lecher, as stricken, tortured soul – these are just some of the screen images that have seduced Hollywood. And when it comes to therapy, the winner is – catharsis. The excavation of buried, traumatic memories, for fairly obvious dramatic reasons, is the treatment to which again and again movie makers return. In another Oscar-winning film, *Ordinary People*, catharsis appeared again, and with it a portrayal of a psychiatrist as such a likeable, humane, approachable, jargon-free and unpretentious person that psychiatrists shown the film at an annual meeting of the American Psychiatric Association reportedly indicated that this is the kind of psychiatrist they would most like to be! Indeed, Judd Hirsch's portrayal of the sensitive, caring and fallible Dr Berger served, in the words of Gabard and Gabard (1987), "to reverse the antipsychiatrist tradition and in a sense to bring back the old pattern of reconciliation". Dr Berger is casually dressed, incompetent with machinery, has a cluttered desk, gives off a slightly addled aura and is not above hugging his patients, albeit male, and being quite blunt and confrontational. One reason that doctors and patients liked Dr Berger is that he appears to be the kind of psychiatrist one might wish to see when feeling vulnerable and isolated. He touches a cord. The part played by Judd Hirsch reminds one of the psychiatrist described by a manic depressive patient as follows:

"*I remember sitting in your office a hundred times during those grim months and thinking, what on earth can he say that will make me*

*feel better or keep me alive? Well, there was
never anything you could say, that's the
funny thing. It was the stupid, desperately
optimistic, condescending things you didn't
say that kept me alive; all the compassion and
warmth I felt from you that could not have been
said, all the intelligence, competence and time
you put into it; and your granite belief that mine
was a life worth living. You were terribly direct
which was terribly important, and you were
willing to admit the limits of your understanding
and treatments and when you were wrong. Most
difficult to put into words but in many ways the
essence of everything. You taught me that the
road from suicide to life is cold and colder and
colder still, but – with steely effort, the grace of
God and an inevitable break in the weather – that
I can make it."*

(Goodwin and Jamison 1991)

That anonymous patient, I have since learned, was Kay Redfield Jamison, who has since made her own superb contribution to ending the stigmatisation of the mentally ill by writing one of the truly great autobiographical accounts of psychiatric illness (Jamison 1996).

A somewhat different and more recent stereotype, a contemporary updating of Dr Dippy, is the narcissistic psychiatrist. In *What About Bob*, Richard Dreyfuss plays a psychiatrist plugging his book (and family) on Good Morning America, but there is a complication in the shape of Bob, one of his patients. A more disturbing version of the psychiatrist more engrossed with himself than his patients is seen in the film *Safe*, where a brief interview involving a depressed housewife reveals a psychiatrist who is distant (note the enormous desk), insensitive, intimidating, uncaring, unempathic and, it is strongly implied, useless.

But the malevolent, dark forces seen to lurk within psychiatry continue to find representation within the cinema. One of the most powerful conflicts between the good and the bad is shown in the film version of Pat Barker's novel *Regeneration*, in which the wondrously decent and humane Dr Rivers, played by Jonathan Pryce, is exposed to a demonstration of the use of electrical treatment by a cold, insensitive monster of a colleague in reversing the hysterical mutism of a young soldier brought back from the front in World War I. The genre maintains its remorseless appeal, reaching its apogee perhaps in *The Silence of the Lambs*. The character of Hannibal Lecter embodies several of the seemingly ambiguous and ambivalent elements of the movie psychiatrist. He is intellectually brilliant, capable of boring into the most secret recesses of the mind. He is articulate, observant, dry, detached and watchful. He is a voyeur and manipulator. But above all he is a cannibal. This psychiatrist will literally eat you. Those terrifying fears that many patients have of psychiatrists, that they will read their mind, take them over, render them helpless and dependent, cannibalise them, are personalised in the role of one of the most influential, magnetic and legendary cinematic psychiatrists of them all.

Conclusion

Most people never encounter a psychiatrist in a professional setting. As with mental hospitals, the public's perception of psychiatrists is formed at second-hand. A powerful influence, perhaps with television the most powerful, is the cinema. Over the century that has seen both the cinema and psychiatry strengthen their grip on the imagination, the creativity and the experience of individuals and society, the portrayal of psychiatrists on screen has been a mixture of positive and negative, harmful and helpful, good and evil. Psychiatrists, as seen through the eyes of film makers, are at one and the same time omnipotent and useless, progressive and reactionary, compassionate and destructive, perceptive and blind. Psychiatrists seeing themselves portrayed on screen should take a careful look. Whatever the image, caricature or miniature, affectionate or hostile, however paradoxical or stereotypical, the image shown there is the image patients see.

References

Gabard K & Gabard GO (1987) *Psychiatry and the Cinema*. Chicago: University of Chicago Press.

Goodwin FK & Jamison KR (1991) *Manic-Depressive Illness*. Oxford: Oxford University Press: 769.

Jamison KR (1996) *An Unquiet Mind*. New York: Alfred A Knopf.

Samuels L (1985) Female psychotherapists as portrayed in film, fiction and nonfiction. *Journal of the American Academy of Psychoanalysis* **13**: 367–78.

Schneider I (1987) The theory and practice of movie psychiatry. *American Journal of Psychiatry* **144**: 996–1002.

27 Imagining the nineties: Mental illness stigma in contemporary cinema

Peter Byrne

Representations of people with mental illness have continued to be plentiful in mainstream films of this decade. The decade began with a number of comedy films which centred on the stereotypical mental inpatient: dishevelled, distracted and invariably amusing. There are fewer examples of the portrayal of mental illness as indulgence or a product of narcissism. The commonest representations show ill people as sad pathetic creatures, struggling in a world that has become too cruel for them. The recent glut of mental illness films from Australia and New Zealand have extended this from melodramatic sympathy into metaphor. The psychokiller film has endured unchanged, with awards for the most ludicrous, but more positive has been the recent trend of satirising these films within the horror genre itself.

Humour

Early in *Crazy People* (1990), Emory Leeson (Dudley Moore) is brought to the Asylum because of his strange behaviour causing his colleagues concern. What he sees are the images and behaviours of "comedic lunacy": the man on the stairs laughing to himself, a group outside playing volleyball without a ball, and an elderly "normal-looking" woman disclosing that she is William Holden. His reaction is a contemptuous one, commenting that he hopes there isn't a singles night – an ironic comment given the means of his salvation isn't Psychiatry (is it ever?), but a relationship with fellow patient Kathy (Daryl Hannah) in the true "love conquers all" motif of psychiatric films. With this film, we can categorise *The Dream Team* (1989), *Loose Cannons* (1990) and *What About Bob* (1991).

It is also interesting to see how when dealing with manic depression, the humour of the mania is overwritten at the expense of the depression. In *Mr Jones* (1993), Richard Gere's mania provides almost all the key scenes in the film, there is no real discussion of his low moods (unlike the original script) and audiences learn the cure for his condition is to fall in love with his female psychiatrist. Unlike this film, *Don Juan DeMarco* (1995) registers itself in the realm of fantasy. Despite what appear to be grandiose delusional claims, his psychiatrist (Marlon Brando) listens attentively and resists the hospital's ethos of speedy disposal of their charges.

Two questions arise for anyone who wishes to examine these films: what constitutes satire, and when does the humour become part of the stigmatisation process? *As Good As It Gets* (1997) treads a fine line (literally), but some of the dialogue (unrepeatable here) in *There's Something About Mary* (1998) is offensive. We must drive a balance between poe-faced objections and the need to challenge offensive stigmatising portrayals. Many will have difficulty with the cruel satire of *The Idiots* (1998) and *Mefune* (1999). Stigma existed for centuries, and silence has often delayed its passing: if these films provoke discussion, then they are to be welcomed.

Indulgence and pretence

There can be no better example of narcissistic anxiety than the screen persona of Woody Allen. In *Husbands and Wives* (1992), his anxiety is rooted in his need to impress, and desire for, Juliette Lewis in a scene where she has lost the only copy of his novel. It is not just that his suffering has its roots in his own vanity, but it is somehow appropriate to these shortcomings. By *Deconstructing Harry* (1998), dubbed by some as a return to his "cinema of complaint", the Allen character has become acutely aware of his neuroses, and gives into them as impulsively as he follows other libidinous urges. *Analyse This* begins with Dr Sobel (Billy Crystal) listening to his weeping patient, recently deserted by (yet another) boyfriend. He fantasises that he yells at her, with a vicious pull-yourself-together tirade. Relative to other stereotypes described here, true pull-yourself-together moments have been rare of late. *Primal Fear* (1996) concludes with acquitted murder suspect Edward Norton's admission he was faking Multiple Personality Disorder all along.

The poor things

Shine (1996), an Australian film about a previously unknown pianist David Helfgott, was a critical and commercial success. Two divergences from his real life story stand out. Firstly, Helfgott maintains that he never suffered from depression in his life. Secondly, it was his psychiatrist who rescued him from the back wards to perform in her piano bar, but why spoil a good "love conquers all" storyline? In one scene, a montage of his famous victory in London merges into a session with electric shock treatment: his fingers are shown in close up, playing an imaginary piano until the dreaded shock kicks in. It is as if the shock treatment has sapped his creativity.

Another Australian film, *Sweetie* (1989), portrays the animosity between Kay and Sweetie, sisters from a dysfunctional family. The predominant atmosphere is one of melodrama, with occasional flashbacks inferring that Sweetie's behaviour is rooted in overindulgence as a child. When we first meet her, she has broken into her sister's home. Kay describes her as "a bit mental". They each inhabit an underworld, a mixture of comedy and tragedy, where neither has the skills to make it. Its director, Jane Campion, also made *An Angel at My Table* (1990) about artist Janet Frame and her misdiagnosis of schizophrenia. The Asylum is seen in an identical way in each of *Awakenings* (1990), *Fisher King* (1991), *Benny and Joon* (1993), *Clean, Shaven* (1993) and *Twelve Monkeys* (1995). The last four films were set in modern times, and need to update their images of grim Bedlam-like, psychiatric institutions.

Returning to New Zealand and Australia, *Heavenly Creatures* (1994), *Angel Baby* (1995), and *Cosi* (1996) deal with schizophrenia and delusional states. These films, along with the three discussed in this section, make up a significant proportion of these countries' film output. Film academics and psychiatrists will speculate on this. It may be coincidence, film borrowing from film, or a metaphor for finding one's place (as a film industry or a country) in the world. It could also be the impressive mental health promotion ethos of these countries.

Psychokillers

Having discussed well-made comedies and serious films, we leave the ridiculous until last. Maniacs are still at large, in cinema at least. The decade began with commercial success and critical acclaim for *Silence of the Lambs* (1990), a "psychological" thriller which turns on the fact that the "crazed" genius, Dr Lector, knows the killer (Buffalo Bill) personally. 1990 was a good year for these films: *Basket Case 2*, *Child's Play 2*,

Disturbed, *Friday 13th: 8*, *Halloween 5*, *Howling 6: The Freaks*, *Maniac Cop 2*, *Nightmare on Elm Street 5*, *Psycho 4*, and *Stepfather 2*. All these films relate the homicidal behaviour of the killer(s) to mental illness: in *From Dusk Till Dawn* (1996), Richard Gecko (Quentin Tarantino) experiences auditory hallucinations early in the film, and is clearly marked with mental illness. One film *Clean, Shaven* (1993) started as a genuine attempt to portray an individual's experiences with schizophrenia. His hallucinations were distressing, provoking self-harm, and his delusions were centred about young children, apparently wishing them harm. Psychosis was paired with dangerousness, and schizophrenia was lost among the high body count. The British film *Butterfly Kiss* (1994) portrays a woman with schizophrenia and is a hybrid of British social realism and the psychokiller film. *Scream* (1997), and (not without irony) its sequel, provides an antidote to the horrors of the films just listed, albeit in a horror movie whose humour centres on the absurdity of the psychokiller genre.

In this short piece I cannot discuss every film of the 1990s with mental illness themes, but I have shown some trends.

28 Whither psychiatry?

Sir David Goldberg

Future events are moulded by inventions that simply have not yet been invented, so we cannot possibly say what they are going to be. There are two ways of handling the problem of predicting the future. The first is to take a run at it, and predict the future by trend lines. In 1975, I was asked to predict what psychiatry was going to be like at the millenium. I went back to 1875, and collected measurements each 25 years on the numbers of people identified as lunatics and psychiatrists respectively in England. With 4 data points, it would surely be a simple matter to predict the 5th!

Unfortunately, both the predictions that I made were wrong, as events took an unexpected turn. My only correct prediction was of a new and effective psychological treatment for depression: this several years before cognitive behaviour therapy was described. However, that was a lucky guess, based upon my optimistic view that clinical psychologists would achieve great things once they cut themselves loose from doing tests at the request of psychiatrists.

The alternative is to make certain assumptions about possible future changes, by asking what the drivers of change are, and what might prevent change occurring. These can be divided into technological drivers, and social and political drivers.

Technological drivers

Information technology

It seems likely that in a fairly short time the distinction between television, telephone and personal computer will disappear, and more and more people will have access to the internet. The advent of the internet has already caused people to go "doctor shopping", and it is to be expected that doctors and other therapists with unusual skills will market these to a wider audience. There is already software capable of making diagnoses, and other software giving information about best therapeutic practice. It will not be long before such information is generally available, so that users will be able not only to diagnose themselves but also to obtain information about the best treatments for their disorder, and the availability of such treatments. Thus, doctors will find that the treatment they give is being monitored by their patients. These changes will be accompanied by newer and improved versions of computer-assisted treatments, so that the vast numbers of patients with common mental disorders at present without treatment will have access to improved forms of treatment, without the stigma of having to see a mental health specialist. There will be intelligent systems to assist prescribers making the supervision of drug treatments both safer and more rational. These advances can be expected over the next five years.

Brain imaging

The most dramatic changes in our knowledge of mental disorders can be expected when investigators begin to combine imaging technologies with other technologies, for example electrophysiological data or neuropsychological data. They are already beginning to do this. There is a real prospect of redrawing the boundaries of mental disorders with such information. The most likely area is psychosis, where at present we differentiate between psychoses of short duration and established psychoses, calling only the latter schizophrenias. I predict that once better data are available, such distinctions will become academic. Although they were originally designed to avoid stigmatising people with a label of schizophrenia, I predict that once the distinction is lost the label of schizophrenia will become less stigmatising. However, one cannot predict what the new classification will look like – only that it will be different. Psychoses accompanying drug dependence may come to be seen as similar to puerperal psychoses; merely a releaser of a schizophrenia-like psychosis. Once more, such changes can be expected in the next five years. Similar changes may be expected in the classification of depression: we may be able to distinguish between subtypes of depression which at present are all confounded into a single group based upon possession of critical numbers of depressive symptoms. A better understanding of dementia may also lead to earlier diagnosis.

The Human Genome Project

This seems less likely to produce major breakthroughs in knowledge of mental disorders than imaging, since even when a gene or set of genes is identified, the problem of devising a treatment remains. The search for better pharmacological agents cannot begin until this stage has been reached: even over 20 years, it may still not be possible. DNA testing for susceptibility to alcohol and hard drugs is more likely: possibly in 10 years, probably in 20. However, a knowledge of the genetic markers for disease may lead to a better selection of patients to enter clinical trials. It should also be possible to investigate susceptibility to side effects by DNA testing, although the clinical usefulness of this is not that great. The effects of the Human Genome Project on the stigma of mental illness is debatable. It might increase it, despite the optimism of the geneticists. Insurance may be more difficult to obtain, and marriage prospects may be reduced, for those carrying morbid genes. Perhaps the next stage of research into proteomics should now be planned.

Neural transplantation

It seems likely that genetically engineered stem cells will replace fetal tissue for transplantation, since there will always be problems associated with the use of fetal tissue. Developments are likely in Huntington's disease as well as Parkinson's disease; with repair of spinal injury a more distant target – perhaps 15–20 years.

Neuropharmacology

It is particularly difficult to forecast progress in this area, as most of the discoveries in the past 50 years have been made while drugs were being developed for other purposes. It is a safe bet to predict that side effects of known psychotropics will continue to be reduced, and this has the advantage that uptake of the drugs improves. It is also likely that an agent for treating Alzheimer's disease will be discovered using techniques of molecular biology, once the basic mechanism has been finally elucidated. A cocaine blocker is also fairly likely to be produced, which might lead to modulation of both substance P and cortisone-releasing factor: clinical trials will determine the future utility of this approach.

Social and political drivers

Cost containment

Looking to the future, we can expect that the rich and super-rich will continue to purchase one-to-one treatment from the specialist of their choice, and will tend to receive expensive treatments that will depend largely on their choice of expert. The indigent poor in developing countries will continue to exist, and will often receive no treatment at all, as at present. As services improve, their only access to treatment will be from local medical clinics, from attached community workers.

That leaves the large majority of the population, who are either receiving statefunded or insurance-funded care. These will find it progressively harder to obtain expensive items of medical service like the latest operation or the newest drug, or indeed to have long stays in hospital.

Governments of whatever kind are keen to limit health expenditure: we complain of serial reductions in our mental health budgets, Americans bitterly complain about managed care; in each case, the government is desperate to limit health expenditure in the face of expensive new drugs, expensive new high-tech procedures, and increased longevity. Whatever the rhetoric about the mentally ill, only public safety sets limits on financial stringency. The main difference between countries is not state-funded versus privately funded care, but the amount of GDP that is devoted to health.

Manpower issues – psychiatrists and psychologists

Although numbers of psychiatrists have been rising progressively since the de-institutionalisation of the mentally ill, there is no reason to suppose that these trends will continue. Indeed, from the standpoint of cost containment, they almost certainly will not, although they will probably level out. Psychiatrists are expensive, and relatively difficult to manage. However, they do accept responsibility when things go wrong, although such a responsibility is becoming progressively more difficult to discharge. As the purchasing functions pass from health authorities to primary care groups, it is inevitable that resources will be drawn away from the hospital services and into primary care. Unless mental illness services adapt themselves to the needs of primary care purchasers they will find themselves confined to a small laager, dealing only with the disruptive and the dangerous. Only the intrinsic fascination of the subject is likely to continue to attract doctors to practice it.

Psychologists are rather less expensive, and have skills which are in great demand. They work in a range of medical settings, and it is likely that their numbers will continue to expand in the foreseeable future. However, a relatively small proportion of the burden of care of those with severe mental disorders falls to their shoulders, and they are unlikely to want to accept a greater proportion of this burden.

Numbers of hospital beds

These will still be needed in any scenario of the future. The required number is determined by two factors – the inception rate of psychotic illness in the local population, and the availability of residential alternatives in the community for those whose illnesses do not remit within a few weeks. The future availability of home-based treatment and "crisis care" in more domestic settings may well provide an alternative to admission to a hospital ward. Hostels with 24-hour nursing care may replace most long-term hospital-based care.

Nurses

At present we have a national shortage of nurses, as new roles cause demand for their services to increase. It seems likely that nurse practitioners will soon gain restricted prescribing rights, and will be benefited by an intelligent computer program which matches symptoms to pharmacological agents, counsels against polypharmacy and escalating doses, and responds to possible interactions between drugs. The likely arrival of such workers provides a direct challenge to the escalating numbers of psychiatrists. There are now more practice nurses than GPs, with an ever-increasing range of responsibilities. It is likely that part of the task of providing mental health treatments will fall to them, probably assisted by computer-based treatments.

Only a minority of community psychiatric nurses – about 10% – have been trained in evidence-based treatments such as family interventions and simple cognitive behavioural skills – the limitations on the university system are such that it will take about 10 years to remedy this skill deficit. A new class of worker is required.

Community care workers

It would not be difficult to provide a training that contains both social work skills and some modified nursing skills. Such training might be taken up by some of the many graduates who at present cannot find work – for example, psychology graduates. Such workers are already employed in the voluntary sector, but the training they are given needs to be thought through and improved. There needs to be a clear career progression for those wishing to take additional training to a higher level. The staff establishment needs to come first, with a pay structure.

Pooled funding

The financial burden of many forms of care – for the mentally ill, for learning difficulties, and for the elderly – falls partly on the health service, partly on local authorities. If local budgets were pooled, and put under a common management for each of these services, it might be possible to produce the community facilities, and the trained staff, who will be needed in a future service. There would be a separation of functions between nurses employed by the health authority and social workers employed by the local authority: advantages of this include breaking down administrative and clinical barriers and producing a more integrated service, avoiding the build-up of patients unnecessarily detained in hospital beds when they could be in the community, and the faster development of a cadre of "community care workers".

Prevention

In general, primary prevention is more difficult than secondary prevention, as the causal chains producing mental disorders are, at best, only partly understood. At present, conduct disorder in childhood can be prevented if parents are offered "parent training"; there is some evidence that educational interventions during primary school can prevent later drug dependence; the excess of cerebrovascular disease causing dementia in males of low social class could be prevented by better control of blood pressure, weight and smoking behaviour in adult life; there is accumulating evidence that those with a genotype predisposing them to schizophrenia can sometimes be prevented from developing it by avoiding cannabis; and there is suggestive evidence that subclinical depression can be prevented by self-help materials, either computerised or in manual form.

Where relapse prevention is concerned, there is good evidence that appropriate psychotropic drugs can prevent subsequent episodes of depression, bipolar illness and schizophrenia, and good evidence that cognitive behaviour therapy can prevent future episodes of depression. It is difficult to predict the additions to this list, and real difficulties are inherent in the fact that many of the social conditions conducive to mental disorders are difficult to control.

The services in the world now are much more acceptable to patients and their carers than the services that were available just after the Second World War ever were, and technology offers enormous hope to the future development of innovation and the efficient administration of optimal effective treatment.

Conclusion

The world is a more exciting one than that in which I started my journey. The harm done to patients by long stays in mental hospitals has been well documented, and it has been greatly reduced. There is now an admirable tendency to care for patients whose illnesses do not respond to treatment in as normal an environment as possible – this can only be good.

Patients are likely to receive treatment more quickly, to be given drugs which suppress many of the unpleasant symptoms, and to be treated in places that are less likely to produce the defect symptoms associated with total institutions. Many thousands of people receive treatments today who would not formerly have had treatment at all. Across the world, primary care services are improving, and doctors are becoming more aware than they once were of psychiatric problems. All this is very good, and still further improvements are likely in finding drug treatments with fewer unwanted side-effects, as well as even more effective psychological interventions. We stand on the threshold of further advances in both neuroscience and information technology: both will yield further improvements. We are able to do more, for more people, than ever before. These forces of change are inexorable, and constitute the main reason why my prediction about the future is an optimistic one. Despite my reservations, in many important respects services for the mentally ill will continue to improve.

Commentary on Section 2D

Mark Salter

What shapes our contemporary images of mental illness?

Our images of mental illness come second hand. As Clare observes in Chapter 26, few of us ever experience psychiatry personally. Instead, our beliefs and opinions about mental illness – and the behaviours that arise from them – derive from a endless stream of images created by other people. This ability, this need, to contain and communicate thoughts and feelings in symbolic terms is one of the defining features of our species; at no other time in our history have we found ourselves so awash in such a turbulent sea of images. We pride ourselves on the sophistication with which we create these images, yet in our portrayals of mental illness and its treatments, there remains a great disparity between the ever-evolving complexity of form and the unchanging simplicity of content. Whether in print, on stage or on screen, our depictions of mental illness, psychiatry and psychiatrists almost invariably return to the well-worn basic themes of tragedy, horror or comedy.

The philosopher Bertrand Russell made the point that what people really want is not knowledge but certainty. Much of the function of the human nervous system, or mind, seems geared toward this end. We have evolved to detect change, not constancy. Change carries with it uncertainty, and with uncertainty comes discomfort. It is our own irrationality that brings the greatest discomfort; the idea that we may do strange, unpredictable things for no discernible reason is one of the most frightening ideas of all, in part because it reminds us that the problem may lie within us. It is this fear that sustains the stigma of mental illness, and many of our images of mental illness involve an attempt to control this fear. We try to explain the inexplicable by categorising it, stereotyping it, labelling it or inventing stories about it. The need to build narratives in order to explain our world is powerful, and our stories do not need to be true in order to bring comfort. Once we feel as though we have an explanation for something, we feel safer, and the simpler the explanation the better.

These themes of mockery, horror, dramatisation, false explanation and over-simplification recur throughout almost all of our contemporary images of mental illness, and are reflected in all of the papers in this section. Thus, as Clare and Byrne explain, in Chapters 26 and 27, in the movies, it is either love or a sudden cathartic surge of some other emotion that provides the quick, simplistic "cure", rather than months of painstaking – and very uncinematic – struggle towards change. In Chapter 24, Leff tells of how Robert Louis Stevenson's original and sophisticated account of human nature is boiled down into a crude Manichean tool with which we may easily identify the good "us" and relocate the bad "them" elsewhere. Madness is usually depicted as something that happens to someone else – somewhere else and, for centuries, that somewhere else has usually been behind tall brick walls. The asylum will remain a familiar location in our minds long after the walls of the real asylums have come down.

How can we alter our images of mental illness for the better?

Leff provides an insight into the surprising things that can happen when these falsely comforting walls, mental and physical, are taken down. One study that sought to measure changes in local attitudes after the opening of a psychiatric care hostel encountered a significant fund of goodwill among the general public. Intriguingly, it also found that an educational package aimed at altering understanding of mental illness did not need to increase knowledge in order to be effective. There are important lessons here, with both humanistic and cost implications; large full-scale public education efforts may not be the best way to win minds or target resources – better instead to work on people's fears "focally and locally". Another lesson seems to be not to underestimate the sophistication of the general public. We are not fooled by mere changes in name alone. Just because we are fed a steady stream of simplistic, often grotesquely unrealistic, stories, it does not mean that we are unwilling or unable to embrace more sophisticated ideas and images. Armson's historical résumé of attitudes towards suicide in Chapter 25 shows how our attitudes can evolve, describing a shift from an ancient, moralistic way of thinking towards a more complex scientific, sociomedical approach.

Humans have, for the greater part of their civilisation, construed and responded to mental illness in an essentially moral rather than scientific way. If we are able to incorporate the results of social and medical enquiry into our symbols and stories of mental illness and its treatment, it seems reasonable to hope that, in time, our culture will move onto a more enlightened and less stigmatised view. This has already begun to happen in other areas of life, such as disability, race and sexuality. If mental illness is to join this list, then all parties will need to take risks that may not seem to be part of the work to which they are accustomed. Workers in the mental health field will need to find new ways to excite the interest of the image makers in the results of their work. The image makers, on the other hand, will need to take the risk of trying something new, untested and more complex on us, its customers. Clare shows that this is possible, citing a cinematic example where complex, metaphorical and apparently paradoxical ideas co-exist within a single story; a film where the psychiatrist is both custodial and compassionate. Rather than the pendulum of understanding swinging between two simplistic "explanations" of psychiatry, the viewer is encouraged to form a more accurate and sophisticated impression: drugs and talking treatments are not an "either or" situation. Byrne hints that this use of imagery in the drive towards a more enlightened view of mental illness is well under way in some parts of the world. Some of the most sophisticated and thought-provoking cinematic portrayals of mental illness have come from Australasia and Scandinavia, parts of the world where vigorous attempts have been made to promote the idea of mental health.

What promise for the future?

There is no doubt that imagery can play a powerful role in harnessing the energy contained in Leff's "fund of goodwill" and so change the stigma of mental illness for the better. Mindful of Goldberg's caveat in Chapter 28 about the limits of prediction, it seems certain that technology will continue to provide ever more ingenious ways to make us watch, listen and think about the complex problems of our lives. The challenge lies in ensuring that our imagery is up to the task. The science which Goldberg and Armson regard with such optimism can only provide us with tools and raw materials; it is very much up to the hearts and minds of all of us to complete the job. It will not be an easy one. Voltaires and Kubricks are born rarely and it will require people with just this intensity of talent to transform Redfield Jamison's haunting words into instantly recognisable images.

The more we can draw themes and stories of mind into the public arena, the greater our chances of success. Goldberg hints at one way to achieve this. In his description of the mental health work force of the future, he conjures the idea of a new breed of mental health worker – part nurse, part social worker, part psychiatrist. What if a thorough, practical grounding in methods of the media and the imagery of stigma were also incorporated into the training of such a worker? Psychology has never been as popular as it is today. Incorporating its discourse into the images of our time will be one of the great challenges that face the both the carers and the image makers of the twenty-first century.

Part 3

The origins of stigmatisation: Stigmatisation as a survival strategy

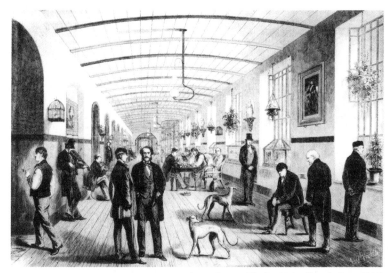

A men's ward in Bethlem Hospital, *c.* 1860

29 Personal responses to a lack of shared perception

Mary Eminson

Introduction

The ideas which I shall outline below arose from a personal response to the Royal College of Psychiatrists' Stigma Campaign. The campaign is founded on the assumption, well supported by research, that stigmatisation of the mentally ill is prejudicial to them and detrimental to all aspects of their treatment in mental health services, and to their role as members of society.

It is important to emphasise the strength of my own commitment to combating such negative effects, and to changing the behaviour of the majority towards the stigmatised minority. However, in order to bring about change, some exploration of the reasons for such stigmatisation may be necessary. In this task, there are some analogies with tasks undertaken during the course of my normal clinical work, which is with children, adolescents and their families. In clinical circumstances where relationships between parents and children have developed negative qualities, and criticism and scapegoating of a child is occurring, it is essential to unravel the reasons for the psychological processes which are deplored, if an appropriate and effective remedy for the adverse effects of these processes is to be found. In this context behaviour change can be token and ineffective in bringing about real and long-lasting changes in the quality of relationships, if not accompanied by some understanding of how pejorative labels came to be applied to the child. I shall consider the possibility that such an analysis might also be useful when a particular group in society is criticised and scapegoated.

It is beyond my scope or expertise to consider the roots of and reasons for stigmatisation generally, but an outline sets the context for the one area that I shall explore. Amongst the reasons predicated for stigmatisation of the mentally ill, Hayward and Bright (1997) summarised four themes. First, there is the perceived dangerousness of mentally ill people, with a sense of personal threat which is thought to accompany this. Second, there is the attribution of responsibility for their sickness to those who are mentally ill, as if they somehow deserved it and brought it on themselves. Third, mental illness is seen as having a poor prognosis, being difficult to treat and therefore embarrassing: to be shunned and avoided as an irreversible form of illness. A final reason postulated for stigmatisation is the disruption of social interactions which is threatened by the effects of mental illness; a general dislike of the uncertainties of interaction with the mentally ill. Clearly these explanations are of very different kinds, relating to very different areas of the stigmatiser's functioning. Issues of social role are of course those which were explored in detail by Goffman (1963). I wish to consider further the way in which the "majority culture" member ascribes a role to the stigmatised person. This could be considered to include the issue of their dangerousness in the broadest sense: clearly one extreme of social role distortion is the threat to one's physical safety resulting from interactions with a stigmatised person.

One way of explaining the attribution of stigma to those whom we perceive as dangerous or uncomfortable to be with is from an evolutionary perspective. Put succinctly, Darwinian notions of evolutionary psychology would suggest that, at its fundamental level, one basis for our attribution of stigma to a mentally ill person relates directly to the drive for species survival. The mentally ill person may be seen as both a "less good bet" genetically for sexual reproduction and a possible source of immediate danger and risk. When explored in the abstract, such arguments are persuasive, but making links between this explanatory model and the less all-encompassing psychological and socio-cultural explanations for stigmatisation is difficult to achieve. In attempting to explore the way the "biological" responses might arise I shall suggest that initially we need to explore the extent to which perceptions can be shared between those who are mentally ill and mentally healthy, which might be relevant to survival, dangerousness and social role.

Lack of shared perception as a key to stigmatisation: anecdotal evidence

Whilst I alluded earlier to a possible analogy between clinical work and the campaign against stigmatisation, my initial thoughts arise primarily from feelings experienced as a member of the public rather than from my role as a psychiatrist. I shall describe anecdotes which arose in the course of ordinary life outside my work. These relate to occasions when I encountered individuals who were clearly mentally unwell, without my previously being aware of this.

The first example occurred in the street where I lived, a row of terraced houses where one Sunday afternoon I was approached by a neatly dressed elderly lady who walked into the communal yard and seemed surprised to see me. She explained "My son's just flitted in round here [i.e. he has just moved in] and I've got the wrong entry." It was a street of virtually identical houses and it was not unlikely that a stranger would mistake one yard entrance for another. I explained that no-one had moved in near me. The old lady left, but returned ten minutes later using exactly the same phrase. I felt slightly perplexed and escorted her out of the yard, looking around for a removal van. Again she walked off. When twenty minutes later she returned, yet again, using identical phraseology, my growing unease hardened into certainty that this lady was suffering from dementia. I asked her more direct questions and established that she was very confused, her initial statement being no more than a social patter, to conceal the gaps. At this point I experienced a sense of profound relief; I no longer had to worry about how to make sense of this situation, but knew that I should take some initiative beyond what is normally socially acceptable behaviour with strangers: this included asking if I could look in the lady's handbag, find her address and contact a relative.

On the second occasion, travelling with friends, I was upstairs on a night bus in the city, when a young man began to talk about what he thought he could hear: people downstairs who might be threatening violence and mugging passengers and the driver. There had recently been a spate of such attacks late at night and the young man was clearly alarmed, which in turn alarmed us. However, as the minutes went on there appeared to be increasing discrepancies between what he said and what we noticed, although it was difficult to verify the truth of his statements whilst the bus was travelling. Eventually, after several minutes I decided to talk to him directly and it became obvious that in fact the young man was describing an inner experience of frightening voices, rather than responding to something that was happening around us.

Once again my experience was of relief, both because I no longer needed to listen for possible frightening voices, nor did I need to be fearful about the possible muggers, but also because I was able to respond appropriately, helping him to think about who would help him cope with these distressing experiences.

The common thread between these two critical incidents was an increase in anxiety and perplexity during the course of the interactions, whilst I attempted to align my own perceptions with others', and a sense of profound relief once I appreciated that this was impossible. The relief appeared to be based first of all on realising that their perceptions and mine had no necessity to agree, and secondly on greater confidence, perhaps because of my training as a psychiatrist, that I knew how to talk to the people concerned and how I might act to assist them.

Whereas intellectually, from a species perspective, shared perceptions may be one of the parameters by which we judge a person's suitability as reproductive material, there may be more immediately relevant survival value in the sharing of perceptions. I suspect however that my sense of relief when appreciating the severe disturbance of perception experienced by both of these people also included a diminution of the value I placed on them in terms of their usefulness to ensure my survival. Perhaps, as a survival strategy, we may be inherently prone to divide the world into those who share our perceptions and those who do not: into those who are "with us" and those who are in a significant way "not with us". Basing our actions as individuals on the actions of those who are confused, deluded and misled in their perceptions, who are responsive to inner experience rather than external reality, is essentially risky. At a species level those with distorted perceptions are of limited use to us and indeed may actively lead us astray, whether on the plains of Africa or on the night buses of Sheffield.

Tolerance of lack of shared perception

If species (or personal) survival is one reason for distancing ourselves from those whose perceptions are severely disrupted, may the same psychological mechanisms be brought into play to a lesser degree in dealing with those with less severe, less perception-distorting mental illness? Personal experience would again suggest that this is the case.

In conversation some time ago with a friend who was said to have recovered from her recent depressive illness, similar processes occurred. Whilst we were planning a brief outing together my friend became concerned about the possible thoughts and attitudes of other people we might meet, who might be critical and hostile towards us; worried that she was not "pulling her weight" in the planning and anxious about the risks of the trip, including car parking and other practical matters which I judged to be easily surmountable. Eventually it occurred to me that my friend's recovery from depression might be less complete than I had assumed, and that her depressive cognitions about possible hazards and others' thoughts and attitudes were causing her to make a distorted appraisal of the activity we were to undertake. I recognised that this did not prevent us from remaining friends, nor did it lead me to discount my friend's views entirely, but I was aware that I attributed less weight to her views in relation to the planning of the trip: I did not attempt to synthesise our judgements. I experienced what I now recognise as a familiar set of responses: a sense of relief once I appreciated that it was not necessary for me, intellectually, to share her appraisal of the risks. We were able to continue planning with a lack of shared perceptions about certain key areas.

I believe we use these mechanisms, of checking the accuracy of others' perceptions before relying on them, in all sorts of benign circumstances. Our tendency to distinguish between those who are "with us" and those "not with us" before we rely on someone's judgement is part of a range of responses: we may suspend our judgement of people as being not "with us" for relatively long or short periods, and we commonly reverse our decisions. For example, when friends or relatives are drunk, or under the influence of drugs, we readily discount their version of the world and their appraisal of it without rejecting them totally.

Two further examples of altered states merit attention in what I am suggesting is a spectrum of our perceptions of those who are "not with us". A very commonly recognised experience of more long-lasting distorted perception is when "in love". Most readers will be able to summon personal experience of the state of being "in love" (often described in popular literature and song as "madness") in which their appraisal of the loved person, which seemed realistic and unbiased at the time, now seems in retrospect quite bizarre, even embarrassing, when seen from the safe perspective of the present.

A second, commonly acknowledged, altered state is being "mad with grief", a well-tolerated state in Western and other societies. In general, extremes of emotion at times of bereavement are accepted and condoned as understandable breaches in rationality. A rather remarkable example was of a man visiting the UK as part of a campaign by relatives of murder victims against capital punishment. A newspaper report of Bud Welch, 55-year-old father of one of the victims of the Oklahoma bombing in 1995, is quoted (Pallister 1999). Mr Welch describes his responses when he learned his 23-year-old daughter Julie had been murdered in the bombing, "Revenge and hate were the first emotions . . . I didn't even want them tried. I wanted them fried." The account continues "I now know why people who are charged with crimes such as that [murder] have to wear bullet proof vests, because people like myself would kill them." He gives a time scale of his responses: "After about five weeks I decided that I wanted a trial to find out the truth. But I still supported the death penalty for another eight or nine months." Mr Welch then concluded this would not bring his daughter back, and "recognised it [his own murderous impulse] was revenge and hate – and that it was revenge and hate that killed Julie." Mr Welch now views his initial reaction as "a form of temporary insanity." There seems little doubt, despite Mr Welch's threats of violence, and the danger to others inherent in his wish to harm the bombers during his "temporary insanity", that generally this account would be viewed with tremendous sympathy, and without the sense of fear and terror in the reader that might be experienced in relation to those threatening such acts from a different emotional context and with a more immediate personal threat.

Theoretical frameworks

These examples of our tolerance of distorted perceptions are used to reintroduce some ideas from Hayward and Bright (1997). They suggest that much research on stigma is unhelpful because it fails to take into account the *context* in which the stigmatiser finds the stigmatised person. Much existing research is based on a model of person perception, itself based on units of information. Hayward and Bright's contention is that this fails to replicate decisions made in real life. For example, what we know about a person is a collection of facts and judgements. "If we know Jane we may know that she is attractive, that she likes drinking tea, that she is a smoker, and tends to be rude and abrupt in her manner. We make value judgements about each of these facts. We like her attractiveness, dislike her rudeness and smoking, and are neutral about her tea drinking. We will judge Jane on a combination of her qualities: her gestalt." Thus, much research based on the meaning of the label "mental illness", when employed out of context, is misleading – for example, asking "unit of information" research questions, such as "If you were going to sit next to somebody in a plane, would you like to sit next to somebody who is mentally ill?" This results in most people answering "no", and including the mentally ill person in the category of those whom they would not want to sit next to. However, after a period of conversation with their neighbour on a plane, if most individuals happen to discover that the person suffers from a mental illness, most are not concerned at all, and make no effort to avoid sitting with them: the context in which the judgement is made would alter the results of asking the question. The authors point out that the mentally ill themselves, if asked the "seat on a plane question", also hold stigmatising views of the mentally ill. Psychiatric patients assume like any member of the public that "the mentally ill" in question are those who are much more disturbed than themselves.

It has been argued that some forms of stigmatisation of the mentally ill may be explained by the need to share perceptions in order to maximise opportunities for individual and species survival. Could it be that, in relation to this and other aspects of social interactions, our responses to the mentally ill may be tempered by contextualisation, by a lack of a sense of threat and by confidence in how to respond to the person whose perceptions we cannot share? Furthermore, if stigmatisation of the mentally ill is a spectrum of responses rather than an "all or nothing" phenomenon, then there may be utility in examining ways in which stigmatisation of other groups is tackled and addressed in the light of the "distorted perception" hypothesis, *not* in order to combat the basic, biologically driven conclusion that the person is "not with us", but to find ways to temper subsequent responses.

Combatting the stigma of mental illness by methods used with other stigmatised conditions

Susan Sontag's 1978 essay *Illness as Metaphor* explores the metaphorical meanings of cancer and the projections ascribed to cancer and cancer sufferers, using comparisons with other illnesses (especially tuberculosis). Her essay is a blistering, coruscating account of attitudes to what was, in 1978, a highly stigmatised illness. Re-reading the essay, one is struck by changes in social attitudes and how diminished is the stigmatisation of cancer today by comparison with some twenty or so years ago. There may be much to be learned from studying how the de-stigmatisation of cancer has come about, and there are many different methods and mechanisms: these will not be explored here, with one exception. Sontag proposed in her initial sentences that amongst the correctives for the position she was describing was for each of us to acknowledge our potential membership, at some time and in some measure, of the stigmatised group, the cancer sufferer. For example:

> *"Illness is the night-side of life, a more onerous citizenship. Everyone who is born holds dual citizenship, in the kingdom of the well and in the kingdom of the sick. Although we all prefer to use only the good passport, sooner or later each of us is obliged, at least for a spell, to identify ourselves as citizens of that other place."*

Is it possible that, using this analogy, by acknowledging that each of us has a membership at some time and in some measure, of the "not with us" group, i.e. mentally ill, that we might reduce our stigmatisation of those who suffer particular forms of this sickness?

Uncertainties remain in my own mind as to whether we can use the same mechanisms to extend our tolerance and sympathy to those who have chronically perception-distorting illnesses as we can to those who we recognise as having currently distorted perceptions but who are likely to return to sharing most of our perceptions. How much continuity is there between our appraisal of those at the distant end of the spectrum, many of whose key perceptions are distorted (e.g. by schizophrenia or dementia), and our appraisal of those whose perceptions we are aware are distorted for only a short period and by known and familiar factors (e.g. being "mad with grief")? Be that as it may, possible remedies may be depictions of the mentally ill in contexts which increase our sympathy for them and our understanding that they are able to fulfil many social roles in a normal fashion, even though we cannot rely on the accuracy of their perceptions. Presentations of the mentally ill, as part of families, sharing activities in an unstigmatised way, carrying out ordinary social tasks, whilst not being expected to undertake activities which might be affected by their distorted perceptions, may offer a potential way to include the mentally ill within our concept of personhood, without denying the reality of their distorted perceptions.

References

Goffman, E (1963) *Stigma. Notes on the Management of Spoiled Identity.* Englewood Cliffs, NJ: Prentice Hall.

Hayward P & Bright J (1997) Stigma and mental illness: a review and critique. *Journal of Mental Health* **6**: 345–54.

Pallister D (1999) Spare the life of my loved one's killer. Murder victim's families speak out against the death penalty. *The Guardian*, 9 October: 19.

Sontag, S (1978) *Illness as Metaphor.* Harmondsworth: Penguin.

30 Shame, stigma and the family: "Skeletons in the cupboard" and the role of shame

Paul Gilbert

Stigma is recognised as a serious impediment to well-being and social relationships. Goffman (1963) argued that stigma was a social mark of a devalued self-identity; a social judgement on those deemed inferior or worthy of rejection. Stigma is often another term for discrediting negative stereotypes, forms of prejudice and discrimination. Corrigan and Penn (1999) have reviewed much of the evidence showing that people with mental illness are subject to intense discrimination. They are less likely to be offered employment, accepted for loans, or wanted as neighbours, friends or sexual partners. Interestingly, when social ostracism and rejection happens between school children we call it bullying.

This paper will look at possible evolutionary reasons for stigmatising. Before doing so we can first clarify various related terms, especially shame and humiliation. These are given in Table 1.

Table 1. Relations of stigma to shame and humiliation

Stigma	Socially agreed attributes worthy of devaluation, and/or social avoidance *Typical social behaviours – devaluation, shunning, exclusion, or rejection, persecution*
External shame	Evaluation by self of others' evaluation of self: 'Others see me as' unattractive, flawed, bad or inadequate *Typical behaviours – avoidance*
Internal shame	Evaluation of self by self: "I see myself" as unattractive, flawed, bad or inadequate *Typical behaviours – concealment*
Humiliation	Devaluation or power abuse by others, but seen as unjustified or unfair *Typical behaviours – revenge*

While *stigma* relates to group values and social sanctions, shame and humiliation are related to internal experiences of the self; one *feels* ashamed or humiliated. Shame is a common experience of being stigmatised or having such traits (Lewis 1998). However, humiliation, with its more aggressive profile, is also a possible outcome when a person believes that their stigma is unfair and unjustified (Gilbert 1997, 1998a). The relationship between these constructs is shown in Figure 1.

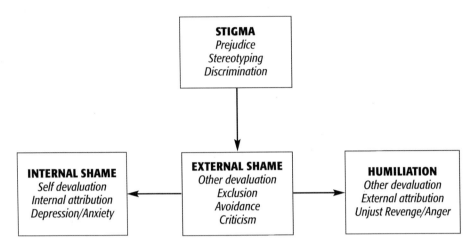

Figure 1. Relationship between stigma, shame and humiliation.

External shame relates to an awareness that others disapprove of the self, and one is thus seen as a 'devalued' individual. Such traits vary from those of criminality, race, religion and mental illness. In our research we have developed a scale to measure external shame. This scale asks people to rate how much they believe others see them as inadequate or defective, and look down on them. In both student and clinic populations such beliefs are significantly correlated with feeling personally inferior to others, internal shame, depression, social anxiety, interpersonal problems, submissive behaviour, and (in students) homesickness (for a review of some of these studies see Gilbert 1998a). Pinel (1999) coined the term *stigma consciousness* to refer to the self-awareness that one is subject to stigmatisation.

Internal shame relates to self-evaluations and feelings about the self. These include internal attributions and a sense of self as devalued compared to others. In extreme cases it can lead to self-dislike or even hatred – one wants to be rid of that 'bad or flawed' aspect of the self.

Humiliation relates to a sense of injustice and desire for revenge for being treated in a certain way, e.g. with discrimination or contempt.

Not surprisingly, people try to conceal possible stigmas from others. There are many sad stories of how far people and families will go to try to conceal from the public gaze that they or a member of their family has a stigmatising mental illness or have been subject to stigmatising experiences (e.g. sexual abuse and rape). Recent research, however, has shown that the act of concealment itself can be psychologically and physiologically costly because it affects what people reveal to others, increases fear of detection, interferes with interpersonal behaviour and maintains negative self-evaluations (Pennebaker 1997; Smart and Wegner 1999).

Evolutionary origins of stigma

There are various possibly interconnected evolutionary reasons for the emergence of stigma as a divisive process in social groups. The evolution of mental mechanisms and social behaviour is driven by genetic self-interest. Individuals are inclined to invest in certain kinds of relationships but shun others because this has had advantages in the past. There are, however, many different types of social relationship that require commitments and investments which are related to key biosocial goals and tasks. Thus animals, especially primates, have evolved to secure their reproductive interests by: (a) avoiding various natural dangers in the environment; (b) selecting, attracting and maintaining access to sexual partners; (c) care of offspring and related kin; (d) selecting, attracting and developing alliances with cooperative others; (e) competing with potential rivals for resources. Stigmatising practices can relate to each or all of these domains, and we can ask what might be the benefits of exclusion/rejection or avoidance of some members of a social group. There are at least five possibilities:

- *Danger avoidance and fear* – those who are seen as possible agents of contamination and/or whose behaviour is dangerous or threatens the group order.
- *Genetic poor bets* – damaged offspring or kin.
- *Sexual poor bets* – those seen as unattractive as sexual partners.
- *Cooperative poor bets* – those who are seen as likely to be net takers rather than contributors – poor reciprocal altruists.
- *Desire for superiority* – in order for some to be superior and make claims on resources, others must be rendered inferior (social hierarchy related).

Danger avoidance and fear

Disease danger

Many animals will avoid or reject and even attack those who are diseased in some way. Jane Goodall (1990) has studied chimpanzees in the wild for over thirty years. When a polio epidemic struck the Gombe Valley a number of animals lost the use of their arms and/or legs. Those so affected were avoided by the others, even though before their illness they had been active and well known members of the troop. Healthy animals seemed fearful of the ill and paralysed.

In human societies too, history is replete with examples of social avoidance of the sick and deformed. For both human and other animals there is probably an evolutionary strategy to avoid possible contagion. However, as Lazare (1987) notes, medical practices can contribute to stigma. For stigma to be applied there is usually also a connotation of *inferiority*. Lazare states that patients are often at high risk of experiencing shame and humiliation in the medical encounter because they are presenting parts of themselves not normally shown to strangers and because in illness these parts can be abnormal, in smell, shape and texture or potential contagion. As he says (p. 1645),

> "As if the humiliation of disease, treatment and dying were not enough, there are medical and lay terms assigned to various conditions that may be intrinsically shaming: hypertension, heart failure, coronary insufficiency, failed back, lazy eye, Mongolian idiocy, and incompetent cervix."

We should not forget that some treatments themselves are associated with disfigurement (e.g. cancer treatments), deformity (e.g. breast removal) and stigmatising movements (e.g. antipsychotic drug side-effects).

Physical danger

Individuals who are seen as unpredictable or hostile are clearly avoided if they are regarded as dangerous. This is a simple survival strategy of course, but in humans stigmatising is a way of keeping those regarded as dangerous at a distance.

Value danger

Those who threaten the social order and its hierarchy and/or become traitors are heavily stigmatised, e.g. behaviour therapists becoming analysts! Stigma is used to stabilise group unity and conformity. Indeed, the issue of group stability and conformity may underwrite much stigma.

Genetic poor bets

Although many families are very caring of offspring who are ill, deformed or behaviourally odd, in low-resource environments these are children who may elicit less investment from their parents and kin and be treated less favourably than those who are seen as good reproductive bets.

Reproductive or sexual poor bets

Animals who show signs of disease, are weak or are outside the norm in some way usually do poorly in attracting sexual partners. Physical attractiveness or ability to control resources is often a key to sexual success, and those who are "not up to it" can be rejected. In human society the physically ugly and deformed are likely to more stigmatised than the physically attractive (Ectoff 1999), even though there is nothing dangerous about these conditions. And those who are inferior to the extent that they cannot control resources (e.g. due to a mental illness) are also more likely to be regarded negatively.

Cooperative poor bets

Cooperation (and reciprocal altruism) is a central behaviour in human social groups, and many forms of social relationship are based on exchange. For exchange to take place people must be seen as relatively reliable and trustworthy. Stigma is especially prevalent in contexts where individuals are seen as unlikely to be good reciprocators or are cheaters. For example, those who engage in criminal acts are clearly not reliable and may be dangerous. Exploitative behaviours are highly stigmatised in groups.

Although there is no research evidence as far as I know, I suspect that one of the most typical reasons that people with mental ill health are stigmatised is because they are seen as unreliable, that is they will not be able to fill their roles as well as the mentally healthy. If people have traits that lead them to work excessively then, although at some level this behaviour may be seen as dysfunctional to them and their families, this is rarely a stigmatised trait. However, if they get burnt out and depressed then they may be stigmatised with little recognition of previous "good work". In general, contributors and "value endorsers" are approved of and esteemed while those who are seen as net takers, dependent or potentially disruptive to the group are more likely to be accorded low status and stigmatised.

Desires for superiority

This aspect of stigmatising is related to what Buss and Dedden (1990) call the "Derogation of Competitors". As noted above, this is the typical way bullying occurs in school children, especially in girls (e.g. via name-calling, encouraging others to demean and exclude the bullied).

Individuals within groups often seek to increase their share of resources. One way of doing this is to seek to belong to a prestigious group. The boundaries that define and separate ingroup from outgroup or high from low status subgroups can therefore be various. They may be made on the basis of race, gender, age, profession, economics, locality, or religion – or not being able to perform desired roles. Since superiority (with special access to resources) is the aim, *group practices must discriminate to avoid a collapse into equality*. Pratto et al. (1994, p. 741) argue that:

> "Ideologies that promote or maintain group inequality are the tools that legitimize discrimination. To work smoothly, these ideologies must be widely accepted within a society, appearing as self-apparent truths; hence we call them hierarchy-legitimizing myths. By contributing to consensual or normalized group-based inequality, legitimizing myths help to stabilize oppression. That is, they minimize conflict among groups by indicating how individuals and institutions should allocate things of positive or negative social value, such as jobs, gold, blankets, government appointments, prison terms, and disease. For example, the ideology of anti-black racism has been instantiated in personal acts of discrimination, but also in institutional discrimination against African-Americans by banks, public transit authorities, schools, churches, marriage laws, and the penal system. Social Darwinism and meritocracy are examples of other ideologies that imply that some people are not as 'good' as others and therefore should be allocated less positive social values than others."

So, according to this view, stigma can be a positive process by which the elite seek to maintain their position and the various benefits of status (acclaim, prestige, power, material resources) that go with it by an active process of stigma subjugation.

Family cycles of shaming and stigmatising

There have been many efforts to understand the inter-generational transmission of shame in families. For example, Lansky (1992) pointed out that various unresolved emotional conflicts, and mental illness in a father (e.g. alcoholism, narcissistic disorders) can lead to poor parenting. Such fathers can have poor frustration tolerance and are liable to aggressive and shaming behaviour (showing high expressed emotion) or else to withdraw. Not uncommonly, a particular child can be the target for negative projections. The essence of Lansky's view is that unresolved shame and stigma in parents seriously increases the chances of similar problems in their children.

Perhaps one of the best known treatises on the inter-generation of family shame cycles has been presented by Fossum and Mason (1986). They point out that within shaming families there are often poor boundaries, perfectionism, excessive criticism, intrusiveness and/or withdrawal, and authoritarian parenting styles – all of which can lead to difficulties with affectionate intimacy. Such interactional patterns undermine a child's sense of self-esteem, personal attractiveness and trust in others. As Fossum and Mason make clear, these interactional patterns can become part of the family style, are carried from one generation to the next and are reflected in the nature of close relationships. Moreover, the inability to deal with conflicts without shaming is one reason why people find maintaining relationships difficult. Thus marital and family therapists will often have to help families deal with conflicts arising from excessive shaming and blaming.

Other sources of stigma

There are of course many other social and psychological processes that influence stigmatising practices. For example, there is the issue of responsibility. People who are seen as gratuitously exhibiting certain socially disapproved of traits are more likely to be stigmatised than those who are helpless victims. Not so long ago mental illness was seen as character weakness, punishment for sin, or the effect of pacts with the Devil.

And stigmatisation can involve moral judgements for good or bad (it is wrong or unjust to stigmatise people who are ill, it is morally right to stigmatise people who disrupt the social order or values). Moral crusades can often involve stigmatising those who do not fit the desired social order or values.

Feelings towards the stigmatised

It is not inevitable, however, that the stigmatised are treated with hostility or contempt. A common feeling for illness-related stigmas could be pity. Nonetheless even a pitying or compassionate orientation to the stigmatised may still lead to keeping a distance, an indirect form of discrimination, e.g. people may feel sad or sorry for a mentally ill person but still don't want him living next door.

Consequences of being stigmatised

As noted above, personal shame can be a consequence of feeling that one possesses a stigmatised trait or attribute. Over the course of human evolution influencing others by appearing attractive to them and stimulating positive emotions has been a key to social success. So we want to be *desired* as a lover, *chosen* for the team, seen as *worthy* of research grants. These tactics have largely overtaken aggression in everyday life though aggression is still a means of exerting control over others. These tactics can be detected in Table 2.

Table 2: Variation of status enhancing and maintaining strategies

Strategy	Aggression	Attractiveness
Tactics used	Coercive Threatening Authoritarian	Showing talent Show competence Affiliative
Outcome desired	To be obeyed To be reckoned with To be submitted to	To be valued To be chosen To be freely given to
Purpose of strategy	To inhibit others To stimulate fear in others	To inspire, attract others To stimulate positive affect in others

Adapted from Gilbert P & McGuire M (1998) Shame, social roles and status: the psychobiological continuum from monkey to human. In: Gilbert P & Andrews B (eds). *Shame: Interpersonal Behavior, Psychopathology and Culture.* New York: Oxford University Press: 99–125. With permission.

Internal shame can arise from the belief that one cannot elicit others' positive emotions but will elicit instead anxiety, anger, contempt, disgust or ridicule. These can be located in many domains of our being, e.g. our bodies, behaviours, feelings and associations with others. The effect of shame is to increase a sense of inferiority as well as negative affects such as depression and anxiety. Thus mental illness can be "a double whammy". Not only is one ill but one is unattractive too and thus shamed. This considerably increases the stress of mental illness both directly and indirectly and contributes to symptoms. There are now a variety of techniques to treat shame-based syndromes (Gilbert 1998b).

Confronting stigma

Corrigan and Penn (1999) point out that there have been three basic ways that groups confront stigma. These are *protest*, *education* and *contact*. However, all these can be a two-edged sword.

Protest can be used to deter the media from perpetrating negative stereotypes of the mentally ill or lobbying MPs or the general public. The down-side of protest is that it does not necessarily promote more positive attitudes, and may lead to suppression of stigmatising behaviours that can have a backlash. Protest can also be used to counter unrealistic images and social practices that can contribute to stigma and shame. One thinks, for example, of the media's excessive portrayal of thin as beautiful, and motherhood as happy smiling babies.

Education involves providing information on mental illness. As a general principle education works to reduce stigma in cases of fear and ignorance. However, as Corrigan and Penn (1999) point out, a lot depends on what exactly is taught and how. Teaching people about the symptoms of schizophrenia proved far less effective in reducing stigma than targeting information on the potential dangerousness. Moreover, education and protest can help to reduce stigma but it can also drive it underground (e.g. racism).

Contact with people who are stigmatised and avoided can do much to reduce prejudicial attitudes. However, again much depends on the quality of the contact. Bad experiences can increase stigma.

Finally we should note that there is much we as professionals can do to help in this area. First, by researching carefully what kind of social interventions are destigmatising and by becoming more involved with protest and education. Second, by stressing the treatability of many conditions. People are far more likely to come forward for help if they know they can be helped and the treatable are less likely to be stigmatised than the untreatable. Also, by becoming more aware of the possible stigmatising effects of treatment (e.g. the side effects of antipsychotic medication). Third, we could involve people far more in treatment processes and decisions. Fourth, we need to work more with advocacy groups. Fifth, we must recognise that sadly, one or too bad experiences can undermine much hard work. An early release from hospital followed by someone being assaulted or killed can do much to reinforce stereotypes and fear.

And lastly we must do all we can to put our own house in order. Many professionals are fearful of revealing that they themselves have a history of mental disorder. Too often we take the view that mental illness occurs only in others. Even though the medical profession has amongst the highest levels of mental health problems (e.g. depression and suicide) in the postgraduate professions, there is still a great reluctance to come forward for help. So we need a much more compassionate approach in our own camp.

Conclusion

Stigma is a social process of discrimination, shunning and exclusion. There are a variety of social reasons for it, some of which may be rooted in our evolutionary history and pursuit of genetic self-interest. This tells us of the power of stigmatisation, and to reduce it we need to give careful thought to our best means of campaigning against it.

References

Buss DM & Dedden LA (1990) Derogation of competitors. *Journal of Social and Personal Relationships* 7: 5–47.

Corrigan PW & Penn DL (1999) Lessons from social psychology on discrediting psychiatric stigma. *American Psychologist* 54: 765–76.

Etcoff N (1999) *Survival of the Prettiest: The Science of Beauty.* New York: Doubleday.

Fossum IRH & Mason MJ (1986) *Facing Shame: Families in Recovery.* New York: Norton.

Gilbert P (1997) The evolution of social attractiveness and its role in shame, humiliation, guilt and therapy. *British Journal of Medical Psychology* **70**: 113–47.

Gilbert P (1998a) What is shame? Some core issues and controversies. In: Gilbert P & Andrews B (eds). *Shame: Interpersonal Behavior, Psychopathology and Culture*. New York: Oxford University Press: 3–38.

Gilbert P (1998b) Shame and humiliation in the treatment of complex cases. In: Tarrier N, Haddock G & Wells A (eds). *Complex Cases: The Cognitive Behavioural Approach*. Chichester: Wiley: 241–71.

Goffman E (1963) *Stigma: Notes on the Management of Spoiled Identity*. Englewood Cliffs, NJ: Prentice Hall.

Goodall J (1990) *Through a Window. Thirty Years with the Chimpanzees of Gombe*. London: Penguin.

Lansky MR (1992) *Fathers who Fail: Shame and Psychopathology in the Family System*. Hillsdale, NJ: Analytic Press.

Lazare, A. (1987) Shame and humiliation in the medical encounter. *Archives of Internal Medicine* **147**: 1653–8.

Lewis M (1998) Shame and stigma. In: Gilbert P & Andrews B (eds). *Shame: Interpersonal Behavior, Psychopathology and Culture*. New York: Oxford University Press: 126–46.

Pennebaker JW (1997) *Opening Up: The Healing Power of Expressing Emotions*. New York: Guilford.

Pinel EC (1999) Stigma consciousness: the psychological legacy of social stereotypes. *Journal of Personality and Social Psychology* **76**: 114–28.

Pratto F, Sidanius J, Stallworth LM & Malle B (1994) Social dominance orientation: a personality variable predicting social and political attitudes. *Journal of Personality and Social Psychology* **67**: 741–63.

Smart L & Wegner DM (1999) Covering up what can't be seen: concealable stigma and mental control. *Journal of Personality and Social Psychology* **77**: 474–86.

31 Intrapsychic mechanisms

Patricia Hughes

The endeavour to understand the phenomena and causes of mental illness is undermined by the popular media, who often portray mentally ill people as wilfully immoral or violent, unpredictable and inhuman. This media misbehaviour is a flagrant example of stigmatisation, but stigmatisation is widespread in society, and at times most of us are probably guilty of a degree of the unthinking prejudice which characterises it. One way of understanding the motivation behind such thinking and behaviour is to look at our need for safety, not only physical but also psychological. We all have expectations and established ways of relating to the world which can be flexible and adaptive but can also be rigid and defensive, especially when we are anxious, and feel threatened. From childhood we learn strategies to protect our self-image and self-esteem, and these may include disavowing some of our own feelings and characteristics and attributing them to another person. This is especially likely to happen when the recipient shows something of the projected characteristic. People with mental illness are thus an easy target for seeing our own feelings of incompetence, aggression or need in another person, and for treating them with hostility or contempt. Projection is not only harmful for the recipient, however, but also for the person who projects, who thereby loses something of his own personality, which is no longer available to him for understanding and developing himself and his relationships.

In Ted Hughes' poem, 'God Help the Wolf after Whom the Dogs Do Not Bark' (*Birthday Letters*, 1998), written to his wife, the troubled, talented, mentally ill Sylvia Plath, the particular character of stigmatisation is evoked, describing the contempt and derision, and the active relationship between the stigmatisors and the stigmatised which maintains the shame of mental illness.

Science versus superstition

Psychiatrists for all their faults do think seriously about why people become mentally ill, and how we may understand and classify mental illness. Popular superstition, often whipped up by media excitement, often demonstrates a simple classification system: they are not human or they are morally weak. Either mental illness is depicted as spontaneously arising brain disease – frightening because the person is deemed to have such a damaged brain that he is no longer human, lacking normal constraints and entirely unpredictable – or by implication the illness is seen as a quasi-moral failure to control feelings and behaviours. These caricatures are not new, but it is peculiarly disturbing to see them used by literate writers and producers not to educate but to excite readers and viewers. The result is no doubt increased profit, and also a reinforcing of stigmatisation.

Moral weakness and the less-than-human

People who lose control of their feelings, thoughts and behaviours are often seen as culpable in their misfortune, while people with physical illness are more likely to elicit sympathy. Those of us unfortunate enough to suffer a serious episode of depression, for example, often conceal it from colleagues where we will comfortably admit to a coronary artery problem. Mental illness has long been seen as a moral failure to control emotions. In the 18th century the Frenchman Francois Boissier de Sauvages wrote "The distraction of our mind is the result of our blind surrender to our desires, our incapacity to control or to moderate our passions" (Foucault 1965).

Two hundred years ago Esquirol in France, the Tukes in England and Reil in Germany protested their outrage that the insane were thrown into prison with criminals (Foucault 1967). Yet although we do have better provision for many people with mental illness, the problem remains. A survey of prisoners on remand showed that around two thirds of people in prisons currently suffer from mental illness (Brooke et al. 1996), but resources to treat them are impoverished. This situation is widely recognised, yet there is apparently little will in our society to provide therapeutic care rather than punishment. Could it be that many of us really suspect that the mentally ill are responsible for their condition? The circle of blame and "justified" punishment of the mentally ill continues both inside and outside the judicial system.

Anthropologists and social scientists describe how disadvantaged groups may be de-humanised, and even characterised as animals (Thomas 1983). At different times, advantaged English writers have characterised the poor, Africans, the Irish and women as subhuman. Inevitably, at most times and in most countries the mentally ill have been a target for this (Foucault 1967). Once seen as less than human, ill-treatment is justified: we have rationalised – however irrationally – our behaviour. Fellow feeling is suspended, and we can offer less with a relatively clear conscience. In addition, both as part of the de-humanising process and as a result of it, disadvantaged people become ready receptacles for projections of various unattractive feelings and behaviours.

Both the wish to blame and the process of dehumanising are observable social phenomena; as rational people we may want to better understand how this state of affairs comes about. Before I discuss the particulars of intrapsychic mechanisms I will offer three assumptions which we make when we try to explain human behaviour. These are:

- that human behaviour is motivated
- that there are commonly occurring motivating factors
- that there is some kind of mental structure which explains the phenomena of how stigmatisation occurs

Motivation in human behaviour

Ted Hughes' poem referred to above alludes to states of mind, to intentions and motives. A fundamental kind of psychological thinking is that human behaviour – our own and that of others – is motivated, and we interpret behaviour as arising from motives, including beliefs and desires (Hopkins 1991). At its simplest we see a person walk to a tap, fill a glass with water and drink it. We interpret the behaviour as meaning that he is thirsty and wants a drink. We interpret motivation, albeit more speculatively, for more complex behaviours without an obvious associated physical need: "She has agreed to give a talk because . . . she wants to be helpful / she enjoys public speaking . . ." This interpretive and explanatory thinking underpins psychological theories of how the mind works. It assumes there is mental activity which explains and gives meaning to observable behaviour.

Safety as a motivating factor

Human motivation is highly complex and often highly individual. However, there are certain motives which may be regarded as universal, and at least in part biologically determined. Darwinians tell us the need for safety is a powerful motivating factor for all higher animals (Deacon 1997), and the importance of safety in understanding human behaviour has been elaborated by psychoanalysts (Sandler 1985) and developmentalists (Bowlby 1969). Infants have inborn (genetically determined) behaviours which promote safety; as they mature, the genetic propensity is enhanced by their learning behaviours which increase safety, and not only in infancy but throughout life humans seek relationships which offer a sense of safety. And a part of my sense of safety comes from my self-image, which is closely related to my self-esteem.

A sense of psychological safety may depend on my having a self-image where I am in control of my life and feelings, where others respect me. Conversely, I would feel unsafe with a self-image of helplessness, with feelings or behaviour out of control, of irrational or incompetent behaviour, or of a self in despair. I would feel particularly unsafe in the role of a person shamed and exposed by public observation of these feelings and behaviours.

People with mental illness sometimes have feelings and behaviours out of control, may behave irrationally, and may at times be incompetent, but they do not have a monopoly on these feelings and behaviours. What do we do psychologically which allows us to stigmatise the mentally ill as deserving fear and contempt, while we are relatively able to escape identification with these shaming characteristics?

The mental map: mental representation and expectation

Let's return to the model of the mind which seeks to give meaning to behaviour. How does this come about? Psychiatrists believe that the brain and neuropathology are important in understanding behaviour, and it is well established that brain change may cause symptoms and change behaviour and conversely that behaviour of all kinds is accompanied by brain activity. However, a thorough knowledge of how the brain works may explain the origin of some mental pathology, but does not provide a fully satisfactory explanation of human behaviour, either among those described as "mentally ill" or among those whose behaviour is socially sanctioned even if irrational or cruel.

We are individuals in terms of our personality and sense of self not only because of genetic differences, but by virtue of experience stored in our brains. This includes experience in the external world, and stories, dreams and imagined activities. Mental representation of experience is based partly on historical record, partly on the child's interpretation of it at the time, and partly on some revision since the original event (Hughes 1999). Experience is laid down by associations which are often social and cultural, but which are neurally encoded. Researchers from various backgrounds including neuroscientists (e.g. Luria 1980), cognitive scientists (e.g. Johnson 1997) and psychoanalysts (e.g. Sandler 1985) describe mental representations as including representations of self and the other, with a linking emotion. Such mental representations of self in the world give us a repertoire of roles we can fill, and offer complementary roles to those we relate to.

Now mental representations are not a recording of history; many changes may take place between the historical record and how we represent subjective experience. So if there are characteristics in ourselves that we do not like, or which have caused us pain, we may internally attribute them to another person.

- Jane's mother has a chronic illness and is often depressed and emotionally unable to respond to her child. Jane adapts by denying her own needs and being careful not to make too many demands on her fragile mother. Internally, she has attributed her own need for care to her sick mother, and is sensitive to the fact that her need for attention and care are too much for her mother. Jane acquires a mental representation of a scenario of a vulnerable person with limited resources who may collapse completely if over stressed, and a needy other whose hungry demands may damage the person she depends upon. This particular representation may not be relevant until Jane is again in a situation where dependency is an important part of the relationship.

Mental representations give us a "map" to approach new situations with expectations which shape our behaviour. Often we revise expectations on the basis of new observations, but when we are anxious we are more likely to cling to preconceptions. We may thus interpret current perceptions in the light of these preconceptions and may react with relatively rational thought.

The concept of psychological defence mechanisms

Psychological defences are a response to threat to our psychic safety (Sandler 1987). A threat to safety may be internal or external. It may be an environmental threat or an internally generated feeling which disrupts our sense of well-being or self-esteem, or an impulse likely to damage our equilibrium. There is nothing intrinsically wrong with using psychological defences: they are a normal part of how we cope with the world. We all have experiences in life which cause painful emotion, and we all have wishes and impulses at odds with our views of how we want to be, which may also cause us anxiety or discomfort. Naturally we want to be rid of such unpleasant feelings and find various ways to reduce them. A psychological defence may be a simple behaviour, like avoiding a situation where we anticipate being anxious, or it may be a conscious psychological manoeuvre, like actively suppressing a painful memory, or it may be unconscious, like forgetting to go to a tedious meeting. Sometimes solutions are adaptive, sometimes maladaptive.

Projection as a defence

The agreeable black and white world of childhood, where bad people are truly bad, and get their just deserts, and good always triumphs, is still a tempting option for adults. One measure of maturity is an awareness that we have both creative and destructive feelings, that our needs and attachments are complex, and that successful relationships require negotiation between our own needs and wishes and those of other people (Klein 1975). Maturity allows us to recognise and accept the aggression, envy, and depression in ourselves. Such recognition and acceptance makes it more likely that we can control and use such feelings constructively, so that aggression is expressed as healthy assertiveness, envy as stimulating competition, and depression as greater awareness and acceptance of our limits. If we are excessively frightened or shamed by these feelings and cannot accept them, then we are likely to find a way of getting rid of them.

Mental representations include a representation of self and other, with a mediating emotion (Luria 1980). All the roles represented are part of our behavioural repertoire, and at different times we may enact either the self role, or an identification with, for example, a parent.

Jane grows up with a mental representation of an anxious child with a worn-out mother. Now married, she finds herself at times feeling anxious but afraid to make demands on her partner, and she is hypersensitive to seeing him as tired by her needs.

As a mother herself she is also identified with her own mother, and sometimes feels afraid of the demands of her young child. The actual situation is coloured by her internal model and its associated anxieties, and unawares she gives both partner and child behavioural cues that they possess the characteristics that she unconsciously anticipates. She thus shapes their behaviour and the relationships.

When anxious or stressed we may automatically and unconsciously project a role from a mental scenario, attributing the unwanted role to another person and keeping oneself in a complementary role. So we can project feelings we find unattractive or shameful to the disadvantaged, including the mentally ill, feel sorry for them or even contemptuous, and thereby distance ourselves from them.

A projection is more likely to "stick", that is to be accepted by the other and to persist in the perception of the projector, if the recipient has something of the characteristic which is being projected (Sinason 1986). So if I project my aggressive feelings on to my aggressive colleague and then act afraid of her, she is even more likely to bully me. And if I project my aggression, fear of being out of control, and sense of incompetence on to people with mental illness, and give them behavioural and social cues that they are all these things, and then patronise them and treat them with disdain, then they are even more likely to continue to demonstrate these behaviours.

The cost of projection towards people with mental illness

This is stigmatisation obviously, with all the shame and pain for the stigmatised person. And society may self-righteously use the implication of moral inferiority to justify failure to adequately resource treatments for mental illness and to support staff in a stressful job. It may be used to justify discrimination in employment and accommodation. Projection has a deleterious effect on the stigmatisors too. Rather than coming to terms with our own vulnerabilities, or changing aspects of ourselves which we do not like, we use a precarious solution which depends on our having an external figure to contain what we do not want. In addition, fear and shame about our own shortcomings is intensified by the contempt with which we treat the mentally ill, and it becomes even more difficult to acknowledge our own depression, irrational thoughts and self doubt.

Conclusion

In summary, I propose that we project certain of our own unwelcome characteristics on to people with mental illness, who are ready recipients, in part because they show behaviours and feelings which we may have in smaller or larger measure, but which we are relatively able to conceal, and which are socially deemed to have a different meaning because we are not "mentally ill" (Rosenhan 1973). These characteristics are likely to include a sense of incompetence or failure, irresponsibility, irrational and aggressive behaviours, feelings of despair, and perhaps dependency, and a need for care. People with mental illness do of course show all of these things. But so do we all. The fact that their incompetence, self destructiveness and despair are public, and that they have been designated as "the mentally ill", makes them ideal receptacles for the incompetence, aggression and despair of individuals and of society.

Projection of unwanted parts of our personalities is harmful to those who receive the projections, and depletes the personalities of those who project. The recipients, as I have tried to explain, are even more likely to demonstrate the projected characteristics because of the overt and subtle behavioural cues they get which indicate that for example, they are incompetent.

References

Bowlby J (1969) *Attachment and Loss,* Vol. 1: *Attachment.* London: Hogarth Press.

Brooke D, Taylor C, Gunn J & Maden A (1996) Point prevalence of mental disorder in unconvicted male prisoners in England and Wales. *British Medical Journal* **313**: 1524–7.

Deacon T (1997) *The Symbolic Species: The Co-evolution of Language and the Human Brain.* Harmondsworth: Allen Lane.

Foucault M (1965) *Madness and Civilisation.* New York: Pantheon.

Hopkins J (1991) The Interpretation of Dreams. In: *The Cambridge Companion to Freud.* New York: Cambridge University Press.

Hughes P (1999) *Dynamic Psychotherapy Explained.* Oxford: Radcliffe Medical Press.

Hughes T (1998) *Birthday Letters.* London: Faber and Faber.

Johnson M (1997) *Developmental Cognitive Neuroscience.* Oxford: Blackwell.

Klein M (1975) The psychoanalysis of children. In: *The Writings of Melanie Klein.* London: Hogarth Press. [Original work published in 1932.]

Luria AR (1980) *Higher Cortical Functions in Man,* 2nd edn. New York: Basic Books.

Rosenhan DL (1973) On being sane in insane places. *Science* **179**: 250–8.

Sandler J (1985) Towards a reconsideration of the psychoanalytic theory of motivation. *Bulletin of the Anna Freud Centre* **8**: 223–43.

Sandler J (1987) *From Safety to Superego.* London: Karnac.

Sinason V (1986) Secondary mental handicap and its relationship to trauma. *Psychoanalytic Psychotherapy* **2**: 131–54.

Thomas K (1983) *Man and the Natural World. Changing Attitudes in England 1500–1800.* Harmondsworth: Penguin.

Commentary on Part 3

Sheila Hollins

My response to the fascinating chapters in this section is influenced by my background both as a psychiatrist working with adults with learning disabilities and as the parent of a young adult with learning disabilities. All three authors, in exploring our need to understand where stigma originates, suggest that the avoidance of danger is a key factor in the behaviour of the majority. Paul Gilbert in Chapter 30 suggests that in seeking safety we distance ourselves from those who are different, or who have broken rank. In this way we shame and exclude people whose social role is disrupted thus turning them from victims into culprits. Pat Hughes reminds us in Chapter 31 that our defence mechanisms are our normal response to any threat to our psychological safety, and of course these may be conscious or unconscious, adaptive or maladaptive. The authors also all write about the importance of language, the pejorative way in which words are often used and the ways in which language can influence our behaviour. In different ways they drew our attention to the characteristics of professional, particularly psychiatric, relationships with patients or users.

In Chaper 29 Mary Eminson reflects on some of the distancing devices we use, and draws our attention to Sontag's (1978) distinction between "the kingdom of the well, and the kingdom of the sick". I was asked to consider whether there are common forces at work in the stigmatisation of one group compared with another. Is there a double risk for those who have a dual diagnosis such as those people with learning disabilities who also have a mental illness? How does a disorder or experience affect an individual's personhood; how does it inhibit or facilitate individual achievement and social inclusion within a particular cultural context? Gilbert suggests that there are different processes for different conditions. Goffman (1963) answered these questions by suggesting that stigma was created and expressed in the encounters between normal people and those who have an undesired difference. Such stigmatisation changes a person's social identity and encourages negative attitudes in other community members. We must also be aware that the meaning of disability varies with differences in cultural values and practices, and social and economic organisation.

People with learning disabilities and those who represent and advocate for them do not like to be too closely associated with mental illness, even though there is a higher prevalence of mental illness in this group. Indeed, since the early 1990s in the UK, the term "learning disability" has been preferred to the term "mental handicap", which had often been confused with "mental illness". Learning disability was not included in the Royal College of Psychiatrists Stigma Campaign because the inevitable association with mental illness was seen by Mencap and other advocates as too risky. This suggests that a double stigma is operating. Many of the things discussed at the seminar could, however, have been said about people with learning disabilities.

Von Balthazar, a Swiss philosopher and theologian writing in the 50s and 60s, in trying to make sense of the Holocaust, suggested that fear of difference was a fear of one's own group being displaced eventually by those people who are different to oneself. He hypothesised that beauty signifies love, and that the perceived most beautiful face is an amalgam of all the faces we have seen. He wrote extensively about the way in which beauty and goodness are seen as synonymous, that people who are not beautiful are excluded and can be assumed to be the ones who will be sent to hell. Gilbert reminds us that it is a human characteristic to want to be chosen because we are attractive to others. Research by myself and colleagues has been exploring the way in which people with learning disabilities are included or excluded from rituals in our society, particularly funeral rituals. People with learning disabilities are not usually invited, and I think that says something about the extent of their perceived difference.

I recently participated in a collaborative policy academy in Washington DC, which was organised by the President's Committee on Mental Retardation. The aim of the Academy was that the participating teams would model inclusion in the search for more effective policies in learning disability. The "England" team included users and carers, managers, policy makers, clinicians and others. Some of the professional members had difficulty initiating conversation, social interaction and explanations to the three users. By the fourth day the experience of sitting alongside three people with learning disabilities in that setting changed their understanding and their attitudes, not just their knowledge. One participant reported that he had thought it was a good thing to have users there because it showed that we were serious about inclusion, but that this would mean we would have to prepare our papers more carefully. He had thought that this would slow us down, so that we would not get as far, but that is not what happened in practice. He had thought that we were engaged in an intellectual process, when in reality we were engaged in a process that allowed us to hear what people were saying to us, and this speeded things up.

How do those of us who are professionals rate as ordinary community members? Hughes challenged us to think about our own need to care both in and out of role, and Eminson gave us two very good examples of that. It is difficult to know how to be a psychiatrist when you are not the psychiatrist but simply the relative or the neighbour of someone who is ill. How deskilling it can be when we are out of role. If we move towards a more equal relationship, is there a risk that we will lose some of our professional power or effectiveness?

We were challenged to think about whether we should be more political. I think that it depends at what level one is being political. Community development can be quite a political activity, and we should certainly engage in that. The language that we use can be political, for example if we use the language of empowerment, and our present government's language of inclusion. To practise inclusion, however, is not an intellectual activity, it means sitting down beside people and listening to them. Perhaps the process of narrowing the gap between professionals and patients will itself be a powerful way to diminish stigmatisation.

References

Goffman E (1963) *Stigma: Notes on the Management of Spoiled Identity*. Englewood Cliffs, NJ: Prentice-Hall.
Sontag S (1978) *Illness as Metaphor*. Harmondsworth: Penguin.

Further commentary on Part 3: The tendency to stigmatise

Arthur Crisp

This time-honoured propensity has probably served mankind and its ancestors well in protecting the species and ensuring personal survival. Such biological mechanisms as those subserving immediate survival, the quest for food, reproduction and related territorial needs are presumably its foundation. Moreover, the crudity of categorisation and labelling of related perceived possible threats needs, constitutionally, to be safely over-inclusive, before juggling the consequent options of relating to, coming to dominate, fleeing from or ignoring the source.

In recent social history such core matters as race and political persuasion, diseases such as leprosy, cancer and AIDS, and various physical handicaps have all triggered this process. One can see, with just these few examples, how idiosyncratic are the concerns evoked, e.g. perceived immediate physical danger, excessive demands for change, death and infection. Many factors influence the natural history of such stigmatisations, for instance changing familiarity, better general control over the perceived threat, assertiveness of the minority group concerned, and changing societal and personal value judgements.

Throughout this time, the stigmatisation of people with mental illnesses has prevailed, with rare exceptions. Western man has brought his particular perception to bear. Mental illnesses have some unique properties. They express themselves primarily through cognitive, affective and behavioural symptoms and signs; those very dimensions that make us what we are as individuals. The afflicted person may be perceived as identified with, and not separate from, the illness (Alison-Bolger 1999). Psychiatry itself adopts this perspective with many mental illnesses as it attempts to explain links between the illness and the individual's development, their personality and their relationships. This biopsychosocial model may be widely applicable, but it is often restricted, in the public's mind, to mental illness. Perceived negative aspects of the illness then readily attach themselves to the afflicted person, as also happens, for instance, with physical illnesses regarded as self-inflicted. Secondly, unlike many other stigmatised groups (e.g. the physically disabled, with their ramps, rumble strips, Olympic Games and back-up legislation), the mentally ill rarely fight their corner. The nature of their illnesses, whether characterised for instance, by inertia, egosyntonicity or cognitive breakdown, militates against it. Meanwhile, one of the features of the recent "Changing Minds" campaign survey (Crisp et al. 2000 and Chapter 3 of this volume) has been its attempt to secure public opinion concerning six or seven mental illnesses. Sufficient of the public clearly recognises differences between these illnesses, and this is reflected in the differing negative opinions expressed concerning each of them.

The literature on this subject is patchy. It has tended to focus on schizophrenia and depression, and much of the best has recently emanated from Australia, where related and well organised anti-stigma campaigns have run through much of the last decade. A Department of Health commissioned literature review on public attitudes to mental health/illness concluded that the experience "does not bring a strong sense of understanding, but rather of acknowledgment – that we do think of those with mental health problems in this discriminatory way" (Department of Health 1999). The authors suggested that "the origins of fear and dislike of those with mental health problems may well from a deeper spring in society". The report implies that greater understanding at this level may be a necessary next step if change is to occur. The ways in which we have come to apply our natural capacities and instincts to the tasks of relating or not relating to those of us with mental illnesses in our given and changing cultures and with our existential concerns would seem to provide the arena for this quest.

The self-interest hypothesis

Haghighat (2001) has presented a "self-interest" theory as providing the basis for our proneness to stigmatise. "Self-interest" could be advanced as a reason for much human behaviour. So far as stigmatisation of people with mental illnesses is concerned, "self-interest" in its broadest sense is a useful unifying proposition serving a range of purposes from protection of self-esteem, reinforcement of mental defence mechanisms, through to protection of socio-economic status and potential for economic exploitation. Haghighat attaches most importance to the licence it provides for socio-economic exploitation. He reviews literature which reflects the breadth of vision he wishes to bring to bear. Within "Constitutional origins", which oddly he distances from genetic influences, he cites the work of experimental psychologists which supports notions of the need safely but broadly to categorise potential threats and thereafter, if confirmed, to load them with other negative attributes. He considers "Psychological origins", and the chosen literature consolidates the notion that, defensively, we need to identify scapegoats and thereafter to condemn and avoid them. Thereafter he proposes that stigmatisations, whether they be of another race, fellow competitors or people with mental illnesses, are weapons in socio-economic competition. He seemingly sees no biological substrate to this theme, but pauses briefly to present possible independent evolutionary influences, serving species rather than personal self-interests. Could our present-day attitude partly be fuelled by our ancient need to distance ourselves from "poor reproductive bets" and those who are "sexually unattractive" (Gilbert and McGuire 1998)? More certainly, the severely and chronically mentally ill may be perceived as "poor economic bets" when it comes to considerations of reproduction and its more immediate social consequences. He concludes by advancing the plausible proposition that, "the fundamental basis of all stigmatisation is pursuit of self-interest", which society naturally comes to enshrine.

If we propose that our repertoire of responses has evolutionary biological origins we can then consider how they have been harnessed to serve man's present self-interest when confronted by those with mental illnesses in his midst. For instance, the "Changing Minds" campaign national survey shows that people with schizophrenia and the addictions in particular are perceived by the majority of the public as dangerous, and therefore are likely directly to evoke ancient considerations of control or flight. That perception is of course generally exaggerated and its fuelling is another matter for consideration. Adverse and selective media attention, lack of diagnostic clarity and co-morbidity are some of the factors that have led people to perceive those with schizophrenia as much more dangerous than they are. Sontag (1988), writing within the context of having cancer herself, stated ". . . diseases acquire meaning (by coming to stand for the deepest fears) . . . . It seems that societies need to have one illness, which becomes identified with evil, and attaches blame to its 'victims' . . . . Any disease that is treated as a mystery and acutely enough feared will [also] be felt to be morally if not literally, contagious". Finzen and Hoffmann-Richter (1999) suggest that schizophrenia, in recent years, has taken on this mantle to an ever greater extent from cancer and AIDS which Sontag was writing about. Haghighat's emphasis on self-interest expressing itself importantly in terms of economic exploitation can apply to all mental illnesses, although he does not identify any particular ones and may mainly have had schizophrenia in mind throughout much of his discourse.

In contrast, the campaign survey reveals the theme of perceived self-infliction, especially in respect of the addictions but also in those afflicted with eating disorders, who, however, are not also seen as dangerous. Similar literature over the years has revealed this same association in the public's mind (Department of Health 1999). It raises the problems of "free-will" and "choice", which Haghighat does not address. Perhaps we can only cope with this dilemma by not discussing it. Belief in it is often the cornerstone of our self-image, at least in the Western world; it is also the basis of law and order in society. Max Hamilton used to comment, "Free-will is something we believe we have, but we equally believe that we can predict how others will behave". In psychiatry we constantly seek determining explanations for both form and content of mental illnesses. At the same time, we usually operate as if our patients have choice, though we may also know that sometimes their decisions, e.g. whether to engage in the prospects of change, will depend upon the context (such as experience of stigmatisation, legal constraints, transferences within therapy). Meanwhile, this dilemma may be at the heart of people's tendency to blame such groups of patients in particular. Haghighat considers that psychological mechanisms may be at work here, though he stops short of examining their relationship to the stigmatiser's own personality and its robustness or otherwise in respect of defences against personal dysphoria (see Chapter 31). Yet, as with responses to dangerousness, it accords with his self-interest hypothesis.

Two of Haghighat's main thrusts have to do with the view (e.g. Littlewood 1998) that we may be prone to take advantage of the mentally ill by exploiting them economically. This could be linked closely to our ancestral origins and those commonplace natural behaviours of attempted territorial domination and its purposes. Haghighat himself examines causation categorically. Although ultimately he extols a monistic philosophy, he does not, for instance, seriously attempt to explore interactions between psychological and sociopolitical perspectives.

Interventions

Haghighat concludes with an inventory of interventions which he hopes might collectively provide opportunities to mute the self-interest that drives our stigmatisation of, distancing from and otherwise our exploitation of the mentally ill. Several of these fit comfortably with the campaign's survey finding that the public overwhelmingly perceives people with all mental illnesses as difficult to communicate and empathise with. Such perceptions and expectations promote distancing, social exclusion and ignorance. An association between prejudice and ignorance has long been demonstrated, though the nature of that relationship is unclear. Haghighat commends educational programmes and is aware of their limitations in reaching out to people's deep fears. He sees the potential value of familiarity with people with mental illnesses, providing it is accompanied by the necessary social skills. He applauds, though he is also sceptical of, the work of Wolff and his colleagues (Wolff et al. 1996) and Leff (see Chapter 24), who have begun to develop and evaluate neighbourhood induction programmes. In this connection, a community psychiatric nursing initiative in Glasgow is also noteworthy (Kaminski and Harty 1999).

But Haghighat's main hope appears to be that mankind will grow up and adopt a more fraternal caring society, throwing off his biologically driven competitive nature and evolving along correct ideological lines. However, he describes also the chaos into which we are thrust these days through endless bombardment with information and our increasing geographical mobility – and acknowledges that, under such circumstances, we may become defensively prone to ever coarser negative compartmentalising and labelling processes. Mankind has always had the capacity to be more cruel than nature requires. Along with his belief that fraternal ideologies will triumph over the law of the jungle, Haghighat identifies the need to curb undue competition and freedom to exploit others in the interests of the entire community. Much law and custom are designed to do just that. But justice and compassion in particular are not the prerogative of the State. Such morality can also have other springs. Toleration of the mentally ill has occasionally been more evident in ancient civilizations. Theologians (Lewis 1943) have sometimes equated social and scientific evolution with moral decline, i.e. cognitive development without the corresponding affective maturation and related increase in self-awareness that Haghighat reminds us is the key to personal growth. Befriending the mentally ill today is importantly a voluntary activity, doubtless with origins as diverse as those fuelling social exclusion of the mentally ill. There is agreement that, above all, we need more than ever to search for and respect the uniqueness of the individual apart from his/her illness; yet also recognise the contributions to civilisation that have sprung from such associations – also to remember the value of hybrid vigour and the awful sterile dangers of genetic standardisation.

As a campaign such as "Changing Minds: Every Family in the Land" strives to achieve this goal by opening up this inescapable agenda for public attention we shall still need to try to empower the mentally ill to test out the relevance, to their own potential self-interests, of the current Disability Discrimination act (DDA) and the soon to emerge UK human rights legislation. We may also need both to acknowledge our biologically driven behaviours before we can more effectively shape and curb them, and to become more knowledgeable about and comfortable about ourselves, before we become more at ease with mental illness in others. Apart from good protective legislation, greater public self-awareness is probably now essential for significant and enduring change. Meanwhile, Haghighat's contribution deserves recognition as an early building block and social prompt in our efforts to penetrate to and mute this unattractive and tenacious human trait of unfairly labelling and seriously disadvantaging others.

References

Allison-Bolger VY (1999) The Original sin of madness – or how psychiatrists can stigmatise their patients. *International Journal of Clinical Practice* **53**: 627–30.

Crisp AH, Gelder MG, Rix S et al. (2001) Stigmatisation of people with mental illnesses. *British Journal of Psychiatry* **177**: 4–7.

Department of Health (1999) General public attitudes to mental health/illness. Prepared for Central Office of Information CO1 Ref: RS4206.

Finzen A & Hoffmann-Richter U (1999) Chapter in: *The Image of Madness: The Public Facing Mental Illness and Psychiatric Treatment* (ed. J Guimón et al). Basel, Karger.

Gilbert P & McGuire M (1998) Shame; Social roles and status; the psychobiological continuum from monkey to human. In: Gilbert P & Andrews B (eds). *Shame; Interpersonal Behaviour, Psychopathology and Culture.* New York: Oxford University Press: 99–125.

Haghighat R (2001) A unitary theory of stigmatisation. *British Journal of Psychiatry* **178**: 207–15.

Kaminski P & Harty C (1999) From stigma to strategy. *Nursing Standard* **13**: 36–40.

Lewis CS (1943) *The Abolition of Man.* Oxford: Oxford University Press.

Littlewood R (1998) Cultural variation in the stigmatisation of mental illness. *Lancet* **352**: 1056–7.

Sontag S (1988) *AIDS and its Metaphors.* London: Penguin.

Wolff G, Pathare S, Craig T et al. (1996) Public education for community care: a new approach. *British Journal of Psychiatry* **168**: 441–7.

Acknowledgement

Copyright 2001 Royal College of Psychiatrists. Reproduced, with modifications, by kind permission of the Editor and the College from the *British Journal of Psychiatry* **178**: 197–9. http://bjp.rcpsych.org

Part 4

Self-inflictions, social adaptation or biological destiny? Models of psychopathology and their relationship to stigmatisation

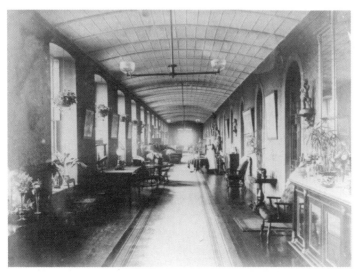

A women's ward in Bethlem, late 19th century

32 Models of the psychopathology of anxiety and their relationship to stigma

Michael Gelder

Throughout the world, ill people want to know the name of their illness and its cause. To name an illness gives a feeling of greater control over it, and to know the cause is a step towards effective treatment. Traditional healers know the importance of naming the illness and explaining the cause, and much of their popularity and their success stems from their ability to explain these things in ways that are readily understood by patients and others, and convincing because they fit well with these people's beliefs and with their culture. Traditional healers also understand the importance of stigma and their causal explanations are generally of a kind that removes blame from the patient and lessens stigma.

Doctors also name diseases and explain causes. However, the names they use and the explanations they employ are not always easily understood by patients or by other people, and they do not always fit well with their beliefs or with their culture. Misunderstandings of medical terms, and conflicts between medical concepts and cultural beliefs, can lead to an increase in stigma. For this and other reasons it is important to consider how the name "anxiety disorder" and the various theories of its aetiology may be understood by patients and by the people they know. Since there have been no satisfactory systematic studies of the public's understanding of the various models of the psychopathology of anxiety, the account which follows is necessarily based on clinical experience rather than on scientific evidence. Nevertheless it may serve to identify potential problems and suggest how they might be overcome.

There are five principal models of the psychopathology of anxiety: genetic, neurotransmitter, cognitive–behavioural, psychodynamic and social. Each will be considered, but before this we need to consider how the name anxiety disorder may affect public perceptions of the condition.

The term "anxiety disorder"

Doctors are sometimes criticised for using technical terms to describe conditions for which there are equally good everyday names which the public would understand better. Psychiatrists can be criticised for the opposite fault, that is for confusing the public by using everyday words to construct technical terms which have a different meaning. The term "anxiety disorder" is a case in point. Psychiatrists expect laymen to understand that the addition of the term "disorder" to the everyday word "anxiety", denotes an important change in meaning. Anxiety is a normal emotion familiar to everyone. Anxiety disorder is a serious pathological state, far removed from everyday experience. In Chapter 14 of this book, Nicky Lidbetter of the National Phobic Society reports that the name "anxiety disorder" suggests to patients and to the public that the condition is a minor one, akin to everyday anxiety. This misunderstanding leads to the idea that those affected are failing to deal with emotions that other people cope with every day. This idea leads directly to one of the common stigmatising opinions about mental illness: that the affected people could pull themselves together if they made sufficient effort. In this way, the condition is perceived as a weakness rather than a "real illness".

The problem does not stop with the general term "anxiety disorder". Several of the technical terms for specific kinds of anxiety disorder are open to similar misunderstanding since they too are constructed from words that are in common usage, namely "panic" and "phobia". (Although the word "phobia" may have started as a technical term it is now used in everyday speech to denote common fears.) Professionals combine these everyday words with the term "disorder" to denote conditions far more intense, prolonged and incapacitating than the states described by the everyday words "panic" and "phobia". It is noteworthy that among the various pathological states of anxiety, only post-traumatic stress disorder has a name that is clearly separate from the corresponding normal state, and this seems to be the term that is least stigmatising. Of course, technical terms such as schizophrenia and dementia are also stigmatising, but for other reasons and in the Royal College of Psychiatrists' opinion survey (see Chapter 3), few people expressed the opinion that people with these conditions could pull themselves together.

However unsatisfactory psychiatric nomenclature may be for laymen, it is now widely accepted by professionals and it is not likely to change. However, professionals need to be aware of these possible misunderstandings when they tell patients the name of their condition, and they need to consider how patients can best explain the name to the people who ask the inevitable question: What is wrong with you?

The genetic model

The genetic model supposes that people with anxiety disorders have an inherited predisposition to respond to stressful events with anxiety that is greater than that experienced by most people. The model has proved useful in research and it is supported by evidence. However, our interest here is not in the nature of this evidence but in the way in which the model may be understood by patients, and by other members of the public.

The genetic model is one of inherited vulnerability. Unfortunately the concept of vulnerability can be confused with the widespread idea that genetic disorders are evidence of inherited weakness. This misunderstanding leads to the idea that people with anxiety disorders lack courage and resilience, rather than the idea that they are overwhelmed by anxiety so severe that few people could endure it. There is a further potential for misunderstanding. Professionals recognize that genetic causes interact with environmental causes. Patients are likely to understand this idea, although they may have difficulty in explaining it to relatives, friends and people who ask what caused the condition.

Genetic explanations can be misunderstood in two other, potentially stigmatising, ways. First, they may seem to imply that the condition is lifelong and untreatable – though the idea that genetic disorders cannot be treated may become less prevalent as the public learns more about gene therapy. Second, genetic models of anxiety disorders may encourage the idea that the condition will be passed from parent to children. Of course, genetic models of anxiety disorders suppose a polygenic form of transmission which does not lead to this direct and inevitable inheritance.

Nevertheless laymen are likely to be more familiar with ideas about the dominant single gene inheritance.

The neurotransmitter model

This model proposes, essentially, that anxiety disorders are caused by an abnormality in one of the neurotransmitter systems of the brain. In these terms, anxiety disorders are similar to medical diseases and are clearly not the result of weakness. This might seem, therefore, to be among the least stigmatising of the aetiological models of the anxiety disorders. However, the model leads to a conclusion that can be misunderstood in a way that can increase stigma. The conclusion is that there is an overlap between the transmitter systems involved in anxiety disorders and those involved in depressive disorders. In keeping with this conclusion, anxiety disorders respond to drugs that are used to treat depressive disorders and are named after this action as antidepressants. In Chapter 14, Lidbetter reports that the prescription of antidepressants for anxiety disorders may lead relatives and friends to conclude that an anxiety disorder is "not an illness in its own right". This conclusion may either strengthen the opinion that there is nothing really wrong, or alternatively attach to the patient the stigmatising opinions associated with depressive disorders (described elsewhere in this volume).

The cognitive–behavioural model

In this model anxiety disorders are caused by irrational ways of thinking or by inappropriate ways of coping. An example of irrational thinking is the commonly encountered fear that palpitations, caused by emotional arousal, are signs of heart disease. This concern leads to a vicious circle in which palpitations cause anxiety which increases the palpitations, and leads thereby to even greater fear. An example of an inappropriate method of coping is the avoidance of situations that cause anxiety, an action which prevents the natural extinction that follows repeated exposure to these situations. The model contains no explicit statement about the origin of the irrational ways of thinking and inappropriate ways of coping. This lack of a clear reason for these ways of thinking or acting leaves the way open for the opinion that a more sensible person would not persist with them, he would pull himself together. Of course, cognitive behaviour therapists try hard to explain their model clearly since patients need to understand it before they can play their full part in treatment. However, patients may need additional help before they can explain the causes of their condition to other people in a way that avoids these potential misunderstandings.

The psychodynamic model

In this model anxiety disorders are viewed as the overt expression of more profound covert problems. Unlike the cognitive model, the psychodynamic model explains the origin of the problems and places it in events taking place during the patient's early life. In this way the cause is located outside the patient, who is not to blame and cannot be expected to overcome the problems by a simple effort of will – he cannot pull himself together. Nevertheless, the model could be stigmatising in three ways: the disorder is portrayed as more serious than it at first appears to be; recovery is likely to require complex and lengthy treatment; and blame may be attached to the parents. Despite these possibilities for stigmatisation, the model seems to be accepted sympathetically by most people. The first two implications of the model – that the disorder is more profound than it seems, and that treatment will be lengthy – may not in fact be stigmatising. We have seen already that people with anxiety disorders often feel stigmatised because their disorder is seen by others as trivial, and something they should be able to cope with on their own. By contradicting these assumptions the psychodynamic model may actually reduce stigma.

The third implication – that the disorder is caused in some way by failures of parenting – is a misunderstanding of the psychodynamic model but is nevertheless one that is commonly held. It seems likely that the idea has been reinforced by recent public statements about the long-term effects of sexual abuse in childhood. It is not a large step from this idea to the belief that other kinds of inappropriate parenting could give rise to conditions such as anxiety disorders. If this assumption is made, stigma may be attached to parents as well as to patients.

The social model

In this model, anxiety disorders are seen as the result of social stressors acting upon the patient. In its simplest form, the model does not assume that the patient is predisposed, though the model can incorporate the idea of an interaction between stressors and predisposition. The model also proposes that certain kinds of life experience can make people more vulnerable to stressors (for example the lack of a confidante, or the demands of caring for small children). The model should be easy to explain to the public, and it does not appear to be stigmatising because it places the causes of an anxiety disorder so clearly outside the patient.

The model used in family therapy can be viewed as a variant of the social model. In this model the patient's anxiety disorder is seen as an expression of current problems in the patient's family rather than a problem that originates within him. This model does not stigmatise the patient but it may divert stigma to the family. Family therapists see the causes of the identified patient's problems as lying within the functioning of the whole family, not within the individual members. However, it may be difficult for individual members of the family to explain the concept to the people who ask why they are all attending for treatment.

Multifactorial models

Nowadays few psychiatrists work within a single causal model, though some nonmedical psychotherapists still practise in this way. Multifactorial models reflect the complexity of aetiology with the interaction of genetic and environmental factors, the additional effects of early experience, and the involvement of underlying neurochemical mechanisms. Although it may not be difficult to explain this model to patients, they may have difficulty in explaining it to other people.

Conclusion

Models of psychopathology which are useful to professionals may be misunderstood by patients and by the wider public. Although much of the content of this chapter has necessarily been speculative, since there is no solid basis of research, the conclusions seem reasonably clear. There is good reason to suggest that professionals should bear in mind the importance to patients and to other people of naming a condition and explaining the cause. They need to remember also that other people will ask patients for this information. Technical terms carry special meanings that are understood by professionals but may be misunderstood by laymen in ways that can stigmatise patients. Therefore, not only should technical terms be explained to patients, but patients should also be helped to find everyday words to convey the true meaning of these terms to the other people who ask the inevitable questions – What is wrong and what caused it?

33 Is there a relationship between ideas about the origins/nature of depressive illness and its stigmatisation?

Arthur Crisp

Depression plays a central role in the human condition. It can be a negative consequence and then, by its impact, further crush the individual. Alternatively, when not overwhelming, it can sometimes ultimately enable a process of personal growth. In its straightforward expression alone, 10–20% of us can expect at least one episode in our lifetime. It alone can more or less justify the subtitle "Every Family in the Land" to the Royal College of Psychiatrists' campaign to combat stigmatisation of the mentally ill.

The 1998 campaign survey of public attitudes to seven mental illnesses (Crisp et al. 2000) showed that a variety of negative opinions were commonly held by the public concerning people with depression (Table 1). Roughly half of us report experiencing severely depressed people as *hard to communicate and empathise with*. This has the ring of truth about it. Mental illnesses can generate social handicaps and people with severe depression are withdrawn and unresponsive. Over half of us also report finding them *unpredictable*; an experience which may be related to our difficulties in communicating with them, leaving us unaware of how they may be thinking, feeling, and consequently behaving. Nearly a quarter of us report that people with severe depression are *dangerous to others* – surely a mistaken opinion fuelled by our view of them as unpredictable, also by our awareness that they may be dangerous to themselves and our feeling or suspicion that they might be a threat to our own mental stability. Nearly a fifth of us believe that such a person could *pull themselves together* if they chose, and 13% still think that they have *only themselves to blame*. Some of us may believe that it is easy for some people to shelter behind a diagnosis of depression for the purposes of secondary gain, as can happen with any illness.

Table 1. The British public's view of people with depression: the relationship it has to reality and its impact on the sufferer

Public perception	Percentage holding view	Reality	Outcome of negative public attitudes
Hard to talk to	62	*Often true*	*Distancing*
Feel differently	43	*Often true*	*Distancing*
Unpredictable	56	*? Consequence of distancing*	*Further distancing*
Dangerous	23	*Not dangerous*	*Distancing*
Could pull self together	19	*Hopeless / helpless*	*Further lowering of self-esteem and increased self-blame*
Only self to blame	13	*Hopeless / helpless*	*Further lowering of self-esteem and increased self-blame*

Within Table 1 there is also an attempt to represent the realities for the person who is depressed in the face of these negative views. The effects of such attitudes are severalfold. Depressed people become subject to avoidance/distancing by many of us. They may experience being shunned in all areas of life. It resonates with their lack of self-belief, and their self-esteem is further damaged. All of this can occur within the context of our own likelihood of developing depression at some stage in our own lives and despite our stated belief that they are likely to recover. Thus threequarters of the adult population surveyed considered that sufferers will recover and even more believed that *treatment could improve on that outcome.*

Of the six opinions expressed and outlined in Table 1, the first three appear to cluster together, the perception of them as dangerous may be relatively independent, whilst the last two may also cluster.

Some forces underwriting stigmatisation/distancing/discrimination

It has been suggested that there are biological, social and intrapsychic mechanisms at work in our present-day tendencies to regard as deviant and then to stigmatise and discriminate against people with mental illnesses (Figure 1).

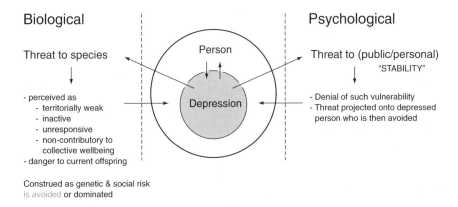

Figure 1. Possible factors leading to "distancing", operating against people with "depression".

In Chapter 30 of this book, Gilbert draws our attention to some of the alleged biological forces still at work within human nature. Apparent biological inadequacy is construed as a genetic threat to species survival and optimal evolution and similarly to personal survival, effective reproduction and the raising of offspring. Within nature, a member of the species perceived as territorially weak, inactive, unresponsive, noncontributory to collective wellbeing, a social burden and/or as a danger to current offspring would be rejected reproductively. Intimacy and social contact are dangerous and distancing/banishment the rule unless the impulse to dominate is invoked instead. Such biological imperatives can imaginatively be translated into present-day circumstances, for instance in terms of public reactions to the depressed person. Depressed people are not only inert and unresponsive but often territorially weak. As a consequence they may not naturally attract us. The workplace often rejects them and it has been suggested that, in our competitive Western society, we sometimes seize the opportunity to manipulate and dominate them socially and exploit them economically (Littlewood 1999; Haghighat 2001). Doctors sometimes advise people with manic-depressive illness not to reproduce. Such forces as these may have been at work disastrously in other arenas in the last century, for instance the Nazi attitude to and treatment of the mentally ill and those with learning disabilities. Biological and constitutional mechanisms also clearly underwrite the need for safety by over-inclusively categorising unfamiliar others who may pose a threat, and taking avoidant or confrontational action accordingly.

In Chapter 31 of this book, Hughes draws our attention to intrapsychic mechanisms allegedly generating the stigmatising process in relation to mentally ill people. We are conditioned to be in control of our impulses, thoughts and feelings. Such self-control is central to our personal and social identities and our self-esteem. Threats within ourselves to this adjustment generate panic. Splitting ourselves off from this threat and regaining a sense of security through denial of the personal problem can be essential. This is achieved by externalising it – in this instance attaching it to others who appear to have succumbed to/lost control of their impulses, thoughts or feelings. The apparent helplessness and hopelessness of people with depression may render us particularly uneasy and thus provoke this reaction. Such *projections* then reinforce our negative views of that person (rather than ourselves) and our consequent avoidance of them.

Into this arena also comes the belief in "choice". It is a tribute to the power of such projective mechanisms that our usual view on this matter – that we ourselves have the power to make choices whilst we believe we can predict the behaviour of others – is suspended. We now become judgmental and moral. They "could pull themselves together" and "have only themselves to blame".

In this sense it might seem that our tendency to stigmatise may have more to do with our own mental state than with any models we might have in our minds, medical or lay, as to how the disorder has arisen. But it may be that the two are related in terms of the model we adopt and apply to others and, more secretly, to ourselves.

Models of the (psycho)pathology of depression

Prior to the 20th century

Melancholia has been recognised as a major element in the human condition since antiquity. Gellert Lyons (1971) informs us that Shakespeare, Burton and other Renaissance writers on the subject drew upon this ancient tradition. It attracted medical, philosophical, spiritual and astrological attention. Many such schools developed aetiological models. The Hippocratic school of medicine generated a humeral model, rooted in alleged imbalances in body chemistry related to predisposing temperament and sometimes to external influences. Lyons reminds us that the word "melancholy" ("black bile") derives from this source and was defined as "fear or depression that is prolonged". It is noteworthy that Hippocrates recognised that anxiety and depression were linked.

Already there was a medical/non-medical divide. Hippocrates saw melancholia as an illness, labelled it and treated it. Aristotle was for respecting and cultivating it. "Why is it," he asked, "that all those who have been eminent in philosophy or politics or poetry or the arts are clearly melancholics, some of them to such an extent as to be affected by diseases caused by the black bile?" (Aristotle's Problems No. XXX; see Lyons 1971).

Such non-stigmatising thinking became the basis of theories of heroic melancholy held during the Renaissance, and of the later Puritan view that melancholy was the proper condition for mankind, one against which he should not protest but instead accept and recognise as a mainspring of self-improvement and faith, and which drove great poetry (Milton) and literature (Bunyan) as well as yielding great insights into its nature (Burton).

In our modern efforts to keep depression at bay are we ignoring its creative potential? It has been argued that it is the discomfort of unhappiness, the rage against the apparent pointlessness of death, that drives us to be artistically and scientifically creative. The fact remains that too severe a melancholy mind is no longer creative. It may become creative later or it may die. Death and the struggle to survive are traditionally medical matters. The overriding medical endeavour is still to identify biological and bodily physiochemical bases for "illness".

The 20th century

Biological models

In the late 19th century severe melancholy was again firmly labelled as a distinct medical condition. The word "depression" superseded it in common medical parlance once it had been adopted in translation from the German literature (Kraepelin 1921). Within decades there was great controversy in the world of psychiatry over whether or not depression was a disorder reflecting the continuum of disordered mood from mild to severe or whether there was a distinct category of so-called "endogenous" depression (with certain so-called "biological" hallmarks and wherein social precipitants were not readily revealed). Proponents of this latter view contrasted it with a category of "reactive" depression (generally milder and more often obviously related to social precipitants). This categorical dualistic thinking, though over-simplified and largely false (e.g. see Kendell 1968), generated a proper search for biological origins. Today this finds its most powerful expression in terms of identified genetic contributions. But whilst bipolar I mood disorder now stands up to some such scrutiny, the nature of the relevant genetic element remains unclear; it certainly does not account for all the expressions of the disorder, and the majority of depressive disorders relate less clearly to genetic factors. Of course it may be that polygenetic factors are at work, determining such contributory influences as temperament, vitality, self-esteem and cognitive organisation. These days, we are more convinced that the propensity for severe depression, as with other constitutional disorders such as anxiety, epilepsy, obesity, migraine, etc., exists within all of us. It is a balance between biological predisposition and the current social context.

Meanwhile, as mentioned earlier, this genetic approach may well also invoke stigmatisation unless the depression is interlaced with non-destructive and socially effective mild hypomania and/or valued creativity. But the labels "endogenous" or "genetic" do perhaps mute the condemnation that the individual could exercise "choice" and "pull themselves together". If anything is to blame it is the gene. Physical treatments for depression include the consumption of chemicals and the induction of epilepsy. They not only provide probes for chemical understanding of the brain but also, in the case of ECT, for revealing adaptive functions of the mind. Physiochemical treatments for depression are related to the notion that, within depression, brain neurotransmitter chemistry is disturbed. This approach may become attached in the sufferer's or the clinician's mind to a biological aetiological theory such as the genetic one and invoke the same reactions. It may otherwise be perceived simply as reflecting the brain condition under the current circumstances. Thus, physiochemical treatments may perhaps reinforce both the stigmatising and protective elements related to a label of biological illness whilst relieving the sufferer from a sense of responsibility for their state. At the same time, the individual may feel disempowered. Szasz (1973, 1999) is amongst those still passionately claiming that it is the medicalisation of depression in this last century that has generated its stigmatisation.

Social models
At the other extreme is the proposition (e.g. Brown and Harris 1978; Weissman and Paykel 1974; Littlewood 1999) that social factors are powerful in rendering people vulnerable to depression; for instance being female, tied to the tyranny and drudgery of home and children under impoverished circumstances, and without adequate personal and social support. The particular existential strains of manhood have been less comprehensively studied, though the French have never been in doubt that "woman is hope, man is despair".

Other less polarised models
Such exclusive biological and social models as these illuminate certain diagnostic problems. Le Fanu (1999) has dropped a hand grenade into the worlds of medical science and medical practice. The genetic and social models of disease have not generated the expected therapeutic mileage, he claims; nor will they.

On the one hand doctors are told, e.g. by psychiatrists and the pharmaceutical industry, that they are under-diagnosing depression. On the other hand they are considered sometimes to over-diagnose, e.g. as a label to conveniently adorn a sick note which the employer then distrusts. Depression of course, like many disorders, can be simulated. Moreover, although people with a whole range of apparently robust personalities can develop depression, those with avoidant or dependent personality disorders are more likely to do so. Such personality disorder may then loom large within a mild depression but the doctor is reluctant or ill-equipped to diagnose it. Moreover, once diagnosed, it would very likely attract even more stigmatisation. This grey area of diagnosis probably produces major "cross infection" so far as stigmatisation is concerned.

Moreover, pre-eminently amongst mental illnesses, depression has at its core a state of self-stigmatisation every bit as destructive as stigmatisation by others. The depressed person regards him/herself as helpless and hopeless, having failed and being to blame, and may be seriously intent upon self-destruction. Beset by shame and discrimination, if help is not forthcoming defences against such distress or alternative attempts at securing greater self-esteem may come

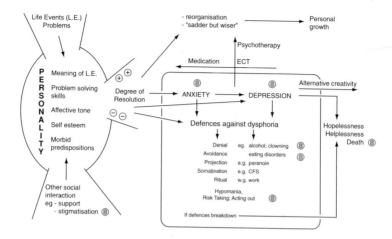

Figure 2. Depression (a working model) and defences against it.

into play. Figure 2 reflects a working model (which has best served me in my clinical practice) for the variety of expressions of depression and otherwise some defences that can be mobilised against it. These defences include avoidant responses e.g. resort to alcohol, eating disorders, preoccupation with the somatic expressions of dysphoria and search for relief from them, coupled with denial of primary mood disorder, clowning, hypomanic overdrive (presumably deriving genetically through its individual evolutionary survival value of re-engaging the retarded and inert depressed individual with life). Other behaviours driven by otherwise undefended dysphoria include excessive commitment to work, risk taking, anti-social behaviour, and the propulsion, previously mentioned, to artistic and scientific creativity. However, this still left the poet Philip Larkin with the awareness that "beneath it all, desire for oblivion runs". Schultz, creator of the immortal Peanuts cartoons, remarked that "All is the product of anxiety and melancholy"; and Einstein, partly in explanation of his creative drive, showed insight into his own solitary and depersonalised character. Some such expressions and defences invite their own forms of stigmatisation. In this chapter I will set out four instances that illustrate this ubiquity. The first, involving attempts to help someone with massive obesity, shows how a defence can protect an individual from the experience of underlying depression (Figure 3).

The patient's almost total inertia, stemming from her escalating massive obesity, was protecting her from confrontation with the experience and emotional consequences of her grandmother's death, for which the family had blamed her since it happened during her early teens. Her level of measured depression at the outset was 5 on a standardised scale. Dietary control, leading to weight loss, precipitated depression (score 8) which was tackled psychotherapeutically by entraining mourning. Weight loss enhanced her self-esteem and facilitated release of her underlying sociability (introversion/extroversion scores raising from 5 to 14). Further psychotherapy was associated with the development of new fulfilling relationships. More moderate residual obesity thereafter no longer dominated her life. In this case the patient was freed from excessive eating (which had been consonant with her late grandmother's

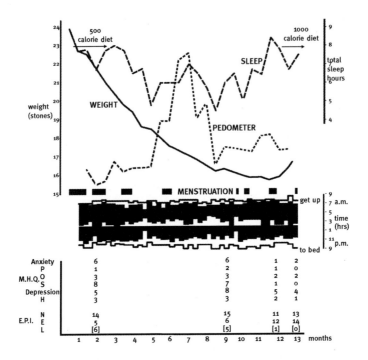

Figure 3. Massive obesity as a defence against depression. The record of body weight (1 stone = 14 lbs = 6.364 kg) of a patient being treated for massive obesity. Over the course of 10 months body weight fell by 51 kg and "depression" was exposed – see text. (The other data have to do with "biological" aspects of the case which were also the subject of study.) Reproduced from Crisp AH & Stonehill E (1970) treatment of obesity with special reference to seven severely obese patients. *Journal of Psychosomatic Research* **14**: 327–45. For further details, see this reference.

lifelong solution to all problems and whose wishes concerning her own teenage social behaviour she had flouted), and ultimate inertia and its protection for her from intolerable dysphoria. In the first instance she needed to confront and be allowed to deal with the sources of that dysphoria despite, in this case, resistance from her own family.

The second illustration shows how severe depression (and anxiety) can stand alongside antisocial behaviour (itself attracting the diagnostic label of "psychopath") probably driven by the associated dysphoria but which is so dominant as to swamp recognition by others of the underlying distress, but which, when social constraints on behaviour are applied without addressing the dysphoria, precipitates out self-destructively (Table 2).

The third example is of treatment of people with anorexia nervosa. Restoration of feared growth and physical maturation (through increased dietary intake), which is only acceptable if underlying problems are being addressed, often nevertheless precipitates out depression as stark awareness of the apparent hopelessness of the emotional challenge is rekindled. However, such depression can also significantly often provide the gateway to ultimate more satisfactory emotional adjustment, given appropriately targeted family therapy (Crisp 1980).

The contemporary controversy concerning the nature of chronic fatigue syndrome

(CFS) and also myalgic encephelopathy (ME) and their relationship to depression is the fourth example. In their excellent presentation of the current understanding of CFS, Wessely et al. (1998) emphasised its heterogeneity, especially in terms of aetiology. Somatisation of depression is one explanation, but is accompanied by angry denial by many of those afflicted. The matter remains sub judice but may follow in the footsteps of the once fashionable diagnosis of "neurasthenia".

Table 2. Undetected high levels of dysphoria in people diagnosed as "antisocial personality disorder/psychopathy"

Diagnosis	n	Anxiety	Phobic	Obsessional	Somatic	Depressed
Normals	1410	2.8	2.4	6.4	3.4	3.5
Anxiety state	84	10.0	4.2	8.0	6.3	6.0
Depressive illness	231	10.2	5.1	9.7	8.2	9.0
'Psychopathy'	137	8.1	3.1	7.1	7.0	7.9

Mean CCEI subscale scores for three clinically diagnosed groups of patients compared with those of a normal population. The mean score, on anxiety and depression scales, of those diagnosed as psychopaths, approximates to the mean score of those presenting with severe anxiety and depressive disorders.

Reproduced from Crown S & Crisp AH (1979) *Manual of the Crown–Crisp Experiential Index*. London: Hodder & Stoughton.

Classificatory problems; phenomenological and psychobiological

This arena, claiming to open up the true ubiquity of depressive illness, suggests a huge scale of problems concerning the continued stigmatisation of and consequent personal denials of such affliction, leading to the plethora of other medical presentations, social crises and personal distress that this generates.

Controversies over diagnostic boundaries have never been more intense, and have led, in recent times, to the search for international concensus on diagnostic criteria and aetiological factors relating to depression both within the *International Classification of Disease* (ICD-10) and the *Diagnostic and Statistical Manual* (DSM-IV). Dualistic thinking has largely gone out of fashion and the disorder has been seen more as a psychobiological reaction in the tradition of Meyer (1934). Genetic and social factors are recognised as interacting. However, both sets of classification are appropriately fairly skeletal and mainly descriptive in nature. There are also differences and conflict between the respective protagonists (see First and Pincus 1999). Moreover, they barely touch on the variety of affects (often not sadness but rather hopelessness, helplessness, anger, anxiety, envy, etc.) that the state can embody and which were elaborated on by Burton (1621) and Engel (1962). Further consideration of such complexities and also the potential for non-specific biological interactions within depression may take us towards a more complex model. For instance the affects just referred to are merely elements of psychobiological postures that can tangle and clash with each other, accounting for some of the wide variety of symptoms experienced by afflicted individuals. Non-specific biological mechanisms might include the tendency to react to any strain either with reduced appetite and consequent weight loss and disrupted sleep, or the converse. The complaint about early wakening might then be more accurately reframed as the depressed person's protest of "wakening too early". Figure 4 shows some aspects of such a model still operating within a social context of a provocative life event.

This leads us closer to a consideration of the individual with depression rather than just their genes or their social vulnerability. Might greater understanding of the individual help mute stigmatisation? One psychosomatic or psychobiological model that may allow this is suggested (Figure 5).

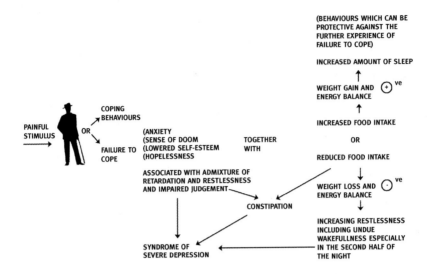

Figure 4. Depression and energy balance. Diagrammatic representation of one way in which a nutritional factor might sometimes contribute to the evolution of the typical syndrome of severe depression associated with weight loss and early morning waking, and also the less common syndrome of depression, weight gain and hypersomnia. Reproduced from Crisp AH & Stonehill E (1976) *Sleep, Nutrition and Mood*. London: Wiley.

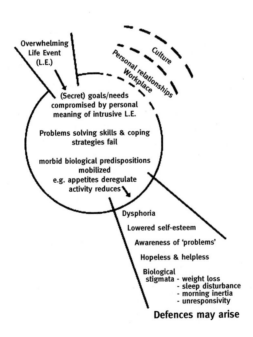

Figure 5. Psychobiological model for "depression".

Models incorporating individual uniqueness

The issues at stake here have to do with our degree of vulnerability expressed in terms of our basic and sometimes very secret and specifically human goals; our coping strategies, self-regard, interpersonal fulfilment and problem-solving skills set against our biological loading to react morbidly. Confronted by a problem/life event it becomes essential to understand its meaning to the individual before judge ment can be made about his or her resourcefulness or the morbid outcome. The aim in therapy becomes the challenge of muting or delaying the onset of illness rather than leaving the individual exposed to the risk of its "brought forward" time of expression (Brown et al. 1973).

Other models can fit within this process: for instance Seligman's model of "learned helplessness", Beck's (1976) cognitive model with its cognitive therapeutic consequences, and a model that places sleep and the failure to problem-solve at the centre of the process. It is argued that sleep is a principal forum for undistracted problem solving, and, in the potentially action-oriented human, failure to achieve this leads to and explains psychomotor retardation on wakening and bitter complaint about it (Crisp 1986). It is only within wakefulness that distractions begin to override the primary insoluble personal problems to which sleep remorselessly returns us.

Another model that emphasises the uniqueness of individuals and their circumstances stems from Freud's theory, elaborated upon by Bowlby (1980) and others, that depression is a personally meaningful response to loss (Freud 1917). This view also holds that loss itself is central to and inescapable in the human condition. Freud's view was that the infant's reaction to loss of the breast within its given social context could set the scene for subsequent responses to loss. Having often initially been "socialised" unconditionally in this way, the infant begins to experience constraints and more restricted conditional love. If these experiences are punitive then impotent anxiety and rage may precede a phase of unresponsivity. A propensity for severe depressive reaction is thus established. Losses in later life prompt it and lead to related processes of mourning that require the ultimate recognition of ambivalent feelings towards the lost object: "sadder but wiser" is the best possible outcome.

Such "depression" in relation to obvious loss is usually regarded sympathetically by the public (now they *do* know how the person feels). In some cultures it leads to great support, economic and emotional. Because of its acknowledged universal nature as a background phenomenon, it provides a setting within which others can get closer to a true understanding of the distressed person. Stigmatisation does not arise. But such a reaction, sometimes unrealistically, is expected to be time-limited. Moreover, many would insist that it does not provide a useful or accurate model for the majority of depressive illnesses. Sadness, rather than hopelessness, has been the central affect. However, we might serve the interests of destigmatisation well if we strove more to understand the extent to which the experience of loss in some form or other (e.g. meaningful objects and our own security and self-esteem and ultimately the prospect of our non-existence) is a trigger to "depression", and requires understanding of the person and his or her relationships. However, "loss" is both a human social and a biological challenge, and the fundamental mechanism culminating in hopelessness and inertia may still be rooted in the biological response to the overwhelming problem.

Conclusion

It is important to note that many members of the public do not report negative attitudes to people with depression. But sufficient numbers do for that person to feel stigmatised and to be discriminated against. Such stigmatisation and discrimination may reinforce their depression. Depression brings with it significant intrinsic social limitations. Nevertheless many people recover from depression with no residual handicaps.

Medical models and labels may invite and serve to focus some kinds of stigmatisation though that is not their intent. Furthermore, medical approaches are likely to persist and continue to contribute to unravelling the nature of the disorder. Within that context treatments need not always be biological in nature. The prospect that, one day, we shall be identifying the chemistry of every thought and feeling, the chemistry of memory and the chemistry of learning and unlearning will merely confront us with the moral challenge of whether to alter our thoughts and feelings by a direct chemical approach or through the ultimately chemical processes of learning and unlearning within a social context and with a sense of empowerment.

Powerful reinforcement of any negative views that observers hold concerning the depressed person can stem from their personal insecurities. Many of us are thereby likely to discriminate against those with depression, distancing ourselves or exploiting our advantage by domination. We need to acknowledge some of its potential strengths – the value of being "sadder but wiser" and the culturally rewarding creative forces that human dissatisfaction, dysphoria and the propensity to develop frank depressive illness can sometimes generate. This might liberate any caring side to our natures and allow us to recognise the need of the depressed person for our support, medical, social and moral (Kleinman and Kleinman 1996), rather than merely medical or social, and also the potential for our own personal growth that such support sometimes enables.

References

Beck AT (1976) *Cognitive Theory and the Emotional Disorders*. New York: International University Press.

Bowlby J (1980) *Attachment and Loss*. Vol. 3: *Loss, Sadness and Depression*. New York: Basic Books.

Brown GW, Sklair F, Harris TO & Riley JET (1973) Life events and psychiatric disorders. Part 1: Some methodological issues. *Psychological Medicine* **33**: 74–87.

Brown GW & Harris TO (1978) *Social Origins of Depression*. London: Tavistock.

Burton R (1621) *The Anatomy of Melancholy* (1621) (Dell F & Jordan-Smith P, eds). New York: Tudor.

Crisp AH (1980) *Anorexia Nervosa: Let Me Be*. London: Academic Press.

Crisp AH (1986) "Biological" depression: because sleep fails? *Postgraduate Medical Journal* **62**: 179–85.

Crisp AH, Gelder MG, Rix S, Meltzer HI & Rowlands OJ (2000) Stigmatisation of people with mental illnesses. *British Journal of Psychiatry* **177**: 4–7.

Engel GL (1962) *Psychological Development in Health and Disease*. Philadelphia: Saunders.

Wessely S, Hotopf M & Sharpe M (1998) *Chronic Fatigue and its Syndromes*. Oxford: Oxford University Press.

Freud S (1917) Mourning and melancholy. In: *Standard Edition of the Complete Psychological Works*. Vol. 14. London: Hogarth Press: 243–58.

First MB & Pincus HA (1999) Classification in psychiatry: ICD-10 v DSM-IV; a response. *British Journal of Psychiatry* **175**: 205–9.

Haghighat R. (2001) A unitary theory of stigmatisation. *British Journal of Psychiatry* **178**: 207–15.

Kendell RE (1968) *The Classification of Depressive Illnesses. Maudsley Monograph 18*. London: Oxford University Press.

Kleinman A & Kleinman J (1996) The appeal of experience; the dismay of images: cultural appropriations of suffering in our times. Daedalus. *Journal of the American Academy of Arts & Sciences*, Winter: 1–23.

Kraepelin E (1921) *Manic-Depressive Insanity and Paranoia*. Edinburgh: E & S Livingstone.

Le Fanu J (1999) *The Rise and Fall of Modern Medicine*. London: Little Brown.

Littlewood R (1999) In conversation with Rosalind Ramsay. *Psychiatric Bulletin* **23**: 733–9.

Lyons BG (1971) *Voices of Melancholy*. London: Routledge & Kegan Paul.

Meyer A (1934) The psychobiological point of view. In: Bentley M & Cowdry EV (eds). *The Problem of Mental Health*. New York: McGraw-Hill.

Seligman MEP (1975) *Helplessness: On Depression, Development and Death*. San Francisco: Freeman.

Szasz TS (1973) Mental illness as a metaphor. *Nature* **242**: 305–7.

Szasz TS (1999) Medical incapacity, legal incompetence and psychiatry. *Psychiatric Bulletin* **23**: 517–19.

Weissman MM & Paykel ES (1974) *The Depressed Woman: A study of Social Relationships*. Chicago: University of Chicago Press.

34 Malignant sadness: The evolutionary psychology of depression

Lewis Wolpert and Dylan Evans

There is a growing consensus that evolutionary theory can throw light on illness (Nesse and Williams 1994). For example, sickle cell anaemia has not been eliminated, because it can protect against malaria. The same approach can be applied to mental illness by drawing on the insights of evolutionary psychology, which tries to account for the adaptive basis of our various brain functions and behaviours (Evans and Zarante 1999). Many evolutionary psychologists are currently attempting to explain why depression is so common by looking at the evolutionary origins of this disorder. Could it be that schizophrenia is so common because there are associated genes that give individuals a reproductive advantage, and thus there is the possibility of mutations in these that then lead to the illness? Depression is a common illness found in most cultures, though often expressed in somatic form such as stomach pains. Why is this mental illness so common and how should it be looked at in evolutionary terms?

Social hierarchy

The best known evolutionary hypothesis about depression is the social competition hypothesis. This hypothesis sees depression as an adaptive response to finding oneself in a subordinate position in the social hierarchy. The idea was first stated explicitly by the British psychiatrist John Price (Stevens and Price 1996), and has since been developed by others. The hypothesis states that depression is an adaptation whose function is to inhibit aggressive behaviour to rivals and superiors when one's status is low. Depression is considered to preserve the stability of the group by preventing constant struggles for status in the social hierarchy. Many animals display submission cues to a conspecific aggressor who appears bigger and stronger. These submission cues usually prompt the aggressor to terminate the attack. The social competition hypothesis views depression in humans as homologous with these "involuntary yielding strategies".

Yielding prevents the aggressor from being more aggressive and promotes behaviour which encourages acceptance of a subordinate position and also enables the individual to conserve resources. According to the social competition hypothesis, depression will, in general, occur when the individual's perception of his/her status in the group falls below a critical threshold level. Possibly in the small primitive groups from which humans evolved such an individual might have been supported, but the almost universal stigma associated with mental illness could well outweigh the benefits obtained by such support. The main advantage to the individual is supposed to be that depression promotes adjustment to failure or defeat. According to the social competition hypothesis of depression, when the goals of the depressed person are given up they are not replaced by new personal goals, but rather by the goals of other more powerful group members. The depressed person tries to adopt these new goals, so that their goals become identical with the goals of the group or of its powerful members and this can lead to acceptance and reconciliation.

In these terms psychiatric disorders are not seen as a medical disaster but as an adaptive response that has become, in modern society, non-adaptive. Symptoms of depression can be thought of as growing pains. This evolutionary explanation of depression is unsatisfactory for a number of reasons. It is based on the assumption that depression is adaptive, but there are no grounds for believing that because it is widespread it serves a purpose any more than one would claim heart disease or cancer to be adaptive. Everything we know about severe depression in modern humans is that it is an illness, it is pathological and prevents an affected individual from functioning properly and so is not adaptive; there is no reason to believe that things would have been any different for depressed individuals in the environment of evolutionary adaptiveness. It is also well known that depression significantly increases the disability caused by physical illness and patients have shorter life expectancy as well as a much higher rate of suicide. There is also little evidence that humans are in a social hierarchy similar to those of the apes where it may be necessary to withdraw for safety – or even that such a withdrawal is similar to depression.

Emotions

If we are to understand depression then we need to understand the evolutionary significance of emotion, for depression is classified as an affective disorder. Emotion and cognition are best thought of as separate but interacting mental functions generated by different but interacting brain systems. Emotions have evolved through their adaptive value in dealing with social and environmental interactions. A possible common feature amongst these very different states is that they all represent some kind of response to potential benefit or harm. These responses may help the person gain a reward or avoid harm. For example, fear is one form of emotional reaction to the threat of physical damage. There are a number of basic emotions, which include happiness, fear, anger, sadness, disgust and surprise, and each is characterised by being initiated by a distinctive signal of rapid onset, short duration, and unbidden occurrence. Moods like contentment, feeling low, or anxiety are not considered basic emotions as they do not have distinctive signals and are much longer lasting.

There is good evidence for basic emotions that can be recognised by people in quite different cultures. Ekman showed photographs of people expressing emotions such as happiness, sadness, anger, fear and disgust to people of different cultures, including the isolated people of Papua, New Guinea, and all had no difficulty making up an appropriate story to fit the emotion in the photograph. That these emotions are so readily recognised supports the idea that they are human universals and that they provide social signals so others can readily know when someone is experiencing one of these basic emotions.

Sadness and grief

How do sadness and grief, which are the emotion and mood most similar to depression, as Freud so clearly pointed out, fit into this scheme (Wolpert 1999)? The answer seems to lie in attachment (Bowlby 1981). It is attachment that is adaptive, the need for a child to maintain a close bond with its mother, or carer, and for the mother to be attached to the child to help ensure the child's survival and thus that of her own genes. Attachment also promotes survival in a reproductive couple. For attachment to be effective the loss or removal of the mother from the child must necessarily cause distress for both and a search for the lost one. Sadness is thus the consequence of the loss of any desired person or object, the adaptive feature being the attempt to find it again so as to restore equilibrium. In a word, sadness is to attachment what hunger is to eating. The greater prevalence of negative as opposed to positive emotions may testify to their greater effectiveness in motivating action. The facial signal associated with sadness can signal to others the state of distress and so may result in help being given. The distress following separation has been well described in apes.

The feelings associated with bereavement are similar to those in depression, and unless we can understand bereavement we cannot understand depression. Sadness, like depression, is a very unsatisfactory term for it covers such a wide range of feelings and may give no sense of their terrible intensity, like the sadness associated with grief. Why should loss of a loved one be so devastating? Bereavement is the clearest example of depression-like symptoms where the cause is known and it is also a universal experience, though its expression is influenced by the local culture. What then is the adaptive nature of grief associated with bereavement, since it often leads to depression and ill health?

The answer lies in recognising that it is the result of the sadness associated with attachment and is the necessary trade-off of the commitment to attachment (Archer 1999; Parkes 1996). The negative aspects of bereavement, where the loss cannot be made good, are the inevitable consequence of the attempt to maintain the attachment. It is striking that loss of a limb or home can result in feelings similar to bereavement (Parkes 1996).

Malignant sadness

If one accepts that sadness is adaptive and a universal and normal emotion, as suggested above, then there is no difficulty in thinking of depression as pathological sadness. Something has gone wrong with the processes underlying the feeling of sadness so that the resulting depression is nonadaptive An analogy can be drawn with cancer, which is a normal growth process going out of control; depression is sadness out of control. Pursuing this analogy further, we may describe depression as "malignant sadness" (Wolpert 1999).

The evidence from animal studies is that depression is not linked to social hierarchy but rather to loss (Suomi 1997). About 20% of monkeys in a rhesus colony are more sensitive to novel stimuli from an early age and readily show fear and anxiety. If these monkeys experience poor maternal care, they have a high probability of showing depressive symptoms, becoming passive and anxious, and adopting a foetal posture away from the group.

A common feature of the depressed state is the negative attributions that, as Beck (1991) has proposed, maintain a depressed patient's self-defeating and pain-inducing attitudes even when objective evidence for positive factors are present. The assumptions in a depressed individual are dysfunctional because they are rigid and not necessarily related to reality. An essential feature of the theory is that all attributions are negative and such negative thoughts are automatic.

One model for depression would thus be the interaction between the biological basis of sadness, involving for example the amygdala, and negative cognitions. For a variety of reasons, usually involving a loss, a positive feedback loop may be set up. The negative thoughts may be driven by the emotion of extreme sadness and this in turn will reinforce the negativity. The adjective 'malignant' is appropriate in relation to sadness, as it can, just like malignant cancer cells, almost invade other mental processes, and so can affect in a profound way the thinking of the affected person. This is somewhat different from the conventional views on the relation between emotion and cognition in which primacy is usually given to cognition. On this model it is clear how both psychotherapy and antidepressants can cut the feedback loop.

Stigma

Are there studies on animals or ideas from evolutionary biology that could provide insights into the nature and origin of stigma associated with mental illness? As regards animal behaviour there do not seem to be any direct comparisons but there are, mainly anecdotal, cases of animals who are sick being picked on by their peers. Strangeness, it seems, elicits aggression from other animals. It has been suggested that this imposes uniformity of behaviour on the group, keeps down infection, and reduces the attention of predators.

Evolutionary theory might provide some insight. Animals and humans are selected with respect to reproductive success. In this process mate selection plays a key role. Animals go to great trouble to display how healthy they are and thus how desirable they are with respect to being a potential mate. This is particularly clear with the mating displays of birds. It is well established, for example among birds and other animals, that asymmetry in body form reduces the animal's chance of mating as it indicates unreliable embryonic development. Sick animals are in general avoided by others.

A mental illness which makes a person very different from the rest of the group will be stigmatised as it will be seen as internal – a genetic property of the individual – which will affect offspring. It may be that we were programmed during evolution to take such a stigmatised view of mental illness, in the same way that men are programmed to select as mates women with bodies that indicate good childbearing potential. Both men and women try to show how healthy and fit they are as potential mates. Illness clearly makes the individual a less attractive mate, particularly as the illness or disability may be genetic and thus passed on to the offspring, making them less likely to survive. The key here is that of the selfish genes – organisms work to promote the survival of their own genes. It is clear that some illnesses – colds for example – are transitory and will not affect reproduction. The important distinction is whether the illness has an external or internal origin. That is, is it due to external factors like bacteria or an accident, or is it an intrinsic feature of the individual, and thus genetic? In general, mental illness is seen as part of the affected individual's character and thus probably genetic, and so someone with whom mating would be undesirable. If this is correct then the perception of mental illness as not being due to external causes but being part of the individual's basic nature is fundamental.

A model for such thinking comes from an analysis of the incest taboo (Bateson 1995). Inbreeding has biological costs, but is this a product of Darwinian evolution? Is it possible that, like many other animals, humans choose as mates individuals who are a bit different to those whom they knew earlier in their lives? This might explain the widely found taboo on incest. The evidence is that people have actually learned the biological cost and thus the taboo.

Could the stigma of mental illness have a similar basis? People have come to realise that many mental illnesses have a genetic basis and so mating with such individuals should be avoided.

References

Archer J (1999) *The Nature of Grief. The Evolution and Psychology of Reactions to Loss.* London: Routledge.

Bateson P (1995) What about incest? In: Brockman J & Matson K (eds). *How Things Are.* New York: Morrow: 101–10.

Beck A (1991) Cognitive therapy: a 30 year retrospective. *American Psychology* **46**: 368–75.

Bowlby J (1981) *Attachment and Loss.* Vol. III. *Loss: Sadness and Depression.* London: Penguin.

Evans D & Zarante O (1999) *Introducing Evolutionary Psychology.* Cambridge: Icon.

Nesse RM & Williams GC (1994) *Why We get Sick The New Science of Darwinian Medicine.* New York: Vintage.

Parkes CM (1996) *Bereavement: Studies of Grief in Adult Life.* London: Routledge.

Stevens A & Price J (1996) *Evolutionary Psychiatry: A New Beginning.* London: Routledge.

Suomi SJ (1997) Early determinants of behaviour: evidence from primate studies. *British Medical Bulletin* **53**: 170–84.

Wolpert L (1999) *Malignant Sadness – The Anatomy of Depression.* London: Faber.

35 Drug and alcohol addiction

Andrew Johns

What does the public think?

A survey of public attitudes in Britain (Yamey 1999), conducted by the Royal College of Psychiatrists as part of its Changing Minds campaign against stigma, showed that drug and alcohol misuse was thought to be as dangerous a condition as schizophrenia. Between 65% and 75% of the population regard individuals with any of these conditions as dangerous and 11–15% of the population say of all three conditions that they would not improve. Important differences were that 60–67% of the sample thought that drug and alcohol misusers had "themselves to blame" compared with 8% for those with schizophrenia and, perhaps surprisingly, drug- and alcohol-related disorders were seen as having a better response to intervention, i.e. only 24% thought that drug or alcohol disorders would "never recover" compared with 51% for schizophrenia.

Table 1. Public perceptions of mental illness 1 (Yamey 1999); *N*=1737 subjects interviewed at home

	Schizophrenia	Alcohol misuse	Drug misuse
Dangerous	71	65	74
Self to blame	8	60	67
Will not improve	15	11	12
Never recover	51	24	23

In fact the same survey showed that taking the mean negative scores on eight attributes (dangerousness to others, unpredictability, hard to talk to, feel differently to us, self to blame, should pull themselves together, will not improve and will never recover) the score for drug misuse was 52, for alcohol misuse 47, and schizophrenia 43.

Table 2. Public perceptions of mental illness 2 (Yamey 1999)

Average negative score	
Drug misuse	52
Alcohol misuse	47
Schizophrenia	43
Dementia	42
Severe depression	32
Panic disorder	27
Eating disorder	27

This modest survey suggests that stigmatising views of addictive conditions are very common among the general population and not so different from the highly negative perception of schizophrenia.

Why are people who misuse drugs or alcohol stigmatised?

But what is stigma? Erving Goffman (1963) defined this as "an attribute that is deeply discrediting. Stigma can arise because of one possessing an attribute that makes that person different from others. . .and of a less desirable kind. She or he is thus reduced in our minds from a whole and useful person to a tainted, discounted one."

However, the effects of stigma are not wholly negative. For example the general awareness that misuse of some drugs is risky constitutes a protective effect. There can also be a form of secondary personal gain in which the person with the drug or alcohol problem may say something along the lines of "because I'm on methadone I can't work regularly" which has all the validity of the view "I have a wooden leg and therefore I can't play the piano"!

These issues aside, Goffman's definition remains generally applicable to the addictions, and anyone familiar with the problems of drug or alcohol misuse could suggest possible reasons for the imposition of negative stereotypes in these conditions. For example, drug or alcohol misusers are commonly perceived to be out of control, hard to treat and unrewarding. Substance misuse is seen as a self-inflicted behaviour, with a risk of self-harm and violence to others.

It has to be emphasised that stigma may not arise solely from the prejudices of others, but also from experience. Given that stigma arises from an interaction between the person with the problem and others around them, the factors that lead to the stigmatisation of drug and alcohol users may not be entirely invalid. Health care workers in particular are frequently exasperated by the attempts of drug users to obtain medications on prescriptions, and anyone working in a casualty department on a Friday or Saturday night will attest to the high levels of threatening and disagreeable behaviour consequent on intoxication.

These issues are also complicated by the marked ambivalence of society towards the addictive substance. Opiates for example were considered chic by the lakeside poets, more generally accepted as a panacea in 19th century East Anglia, and as something rather exotic in the opium dens in the East End towards the end of the 20th century. The mid-1980s saw the appearance of young adolescents using heroin, who were termed "scag-heads" as a general term of disapproval. More recently we have seen ultra-thin female models described as "heroin waifs". Cocaine was initially described by Freud as non-addictive, used by Sherlock Holmes in a form of a 7% solution as an antidote to boredom, and more recently has been regarded as a yuppie drug or "God's way of telling you that you are making too much money". Cannabis was widely portrayed in the 1940s and 1950s as a mind-damaging drug and yet nowadays even a president of the USA can admit to some earlier familiarity with the drug.

It would appear that the general perceptions of drug and alcohol misusers are complex. How can we reconcile such apparently conflicting views? Take a reasonably common scenario. A young man shows disturbed and threatening behaviour. If his behaviour is attributed to schizophrenia then it is regarded as "not his fault" and even if he is not "liked" as a patient, he is regarded as "deserving" of care. If, however, the young man's behaviour is attributed to drugs or alcohol misuse then it would often be regarded as "his fault" and even if he is "not liked" he is regarded as less deserving and less likely to receive appropriate medical care. It is a tangible consequence of addiction that some drug or alcohol misusers with the highest level of need are rejected by health care systems.

It may reasonably be suggested that it is the extent to which drug or alcohol misuse is regarded as chosen or not chosen which is perhaps the main determinant of stigma.

Therefore the psychopathology of action versus inaction, i.e. of taking or of not taking a particular drug is important in shaping the stigmatic response.

However, our understanding of the psychopathology of substance misuse has changed very considerably over the years (Johns 1990). To take Elizabethan England as a starting point, habitual drunkenness was well recognised and described frequently in Shakespeare. The contemporaneous paradigm would be that the drunkard "chose" to get drunk because men always act according to rational self-interest. This is the philosophical notion of rationalism. It is therefore appropriate for drunken misbehaviour to attract sanctions or punishment from society, as would any other offending behaviour. By the end of the 18th century a great change of outlook had occurred. The scientific method had yielded startling results from a study of the material world, i.e. Newton's laws of motion. The same approach was then applied to an explanation of human drives and actions. Human behaviour was seen as determined by forces outside the individual's control and yet susceptible to scientific explanation, with the result that habitual drunkenness was explained by the disease of addiction. Dr Benjamin Rush of Philadelphia (1745–1813) and his counterpart in Edinburgh, Dr Thomas Trotter (1760–1832), each wrote highly influential tracts in which addiction to alcohol was described as "a disease of the will". It was argued that once a "craving" for ardent or distilled spirits had developed, the addict could not then resist the impulse to drink. Drunkenness was not seen as a vice or a personal weakness, since the sufferer had lost control over his drinking. The only remedy was complete abstinence from drink and so the Temperance movement was born. By the end of the 19th century, the diseases of alcoholism and morphinisim had been described, with, however, an important shift in aetiological concepts. These addictive conditions were regarded as the product of "diseased cravings and paralysed control" and the product of "moral bankruptcy or insanity". Addicts and alcoholics were then regarded as morally reprehensible, partly to blame for this misfortune and undeserving of medical attention. These are considerable results of stigma.

Matters did not change much until the 1940s when Dr Jellenek established the Yale Centre for Alcohol Studies and re-emphasised the disease concept of alcoholism. The function of this approach was to legitimise drug and alcohol misusers and the actions of those who help them.

By the 1950s it was apparent that the use of the terms "addiction" and "disease" not only meant that drug- or alcohol-related problems were regarded as a stigma but also failed to acknowledge the contributions of the social sciences and hindered the proper development of services. This re-evaluation led to the seminal paper by Edwards and Gross (1976). The key features, such as compulsion to drink, prominence of drink-seeking behaviour, tolerance, withdrawal symptoms etc., were adapted and incorporated in earlier editions of the International Disease Classifications. However, the most recent DSM-IV (American Psychiatric Association 1994) does not include the term "compulsion", and ICD-10 (World Health Organization 1992) makes reference to "strong desire or a sense of compulsion to use" without further defining the compulsion. Elsewhere in the same volume, obsessive compulsive disorder compulsion is described as "stereotyped repeated behaviour not inherently enjoyable" so this does not immediately relate to drug or alcohol consumption.

It is then necessary to review findings from the social learning literature in order to make more sense of the concept of compulsion and its contribution to stigma. It has been a long established principle of operant conditioning that behaviour may be controlled by its consequences, and those consequences which increase the rate or frequency of behaviour are known as "reinforcers".

As to the nature of reinforcers, there has now been isolated a whole family of opiate receptors interacting with exogenous and endogenous opiates to mediate brain reward mechanisms. Mu opiate receptors act to reinforce in that they produce euphoria, but stimulation of kappa opiate receptors is not reinforcing. As a further example, genetic variation in the alcohol catabolising enzymes can confer an effect protective of alcoholism (Johns 1990).

There are also environmental factors which may act as reinforcers, and perhaps availability is the predominant one. The availability of any drug and in some countries any form of alcohol is dependent upon its legal status. Laws may also determine access and, if illicit, lead to a complicated system of dealers, networks and social proscription. Among personal factors relating to compulsion must be included expectancy effects and craving, the reinforcement schedule of misuse of drugs or alcohol, and perhaps predominantly, the extent to which the individual is able to balance short-term versus long-term effects of the substance of misuse.

There are clearly interactions between stigma as a final attitude and elements of compulsion. With regard to expectancy effects, a stigma may shape the "desirability" of the drug and its effects. In relation to the reinforcement schedule, stigma may effect the availability and pattern of use. In relation to an individual's ability to balance the short-term versus long-term effects of any drug, it is probable that the individual who overvalues short-term gain against long-term problems receives the greater disapprobation or stigma.

So much for the addictive sciences, but there are other perspectives on the issue of compulsion to use drugs or alcohol. The law has something to say on this issue. In 1998, a Mrs Tandy strangled her daughter. Mrs Tandy generally drank a bottle of vodka a day and was clearly an alcoholic in the medical sense. The question arose in court as to whether her alcoholism was a "disease" which then met criteria for a plea of diminished responsibility and hence not guilty of murder. After protracted arguments between experts had failed to resolve the issue, the judge ruled that if Mrs Tandy was unable to resist the first drink of the day then her alcohol-related problems could be regarded as a disease (Rex v Tandy 1967). This "first drink of the day test" introduced a concept of addiction hitherto unappreciated by medicine.

The law has also generated the concept of capacity, i.e. to decide in particular as to whether an individual accepts or rejects health interventions. This has led to the notion of lack of capacity defined as follows: by reason of a mental disability a person is unable to make a decision because he or she is (i) unable to understand or retain the information necessary to that decision, or (ii) unable to make a decision based on that information.

The obvious question becomes: does a capacity-based test help in understanding addictive behaviour? Based on clinical experience it is reasonable to conclude that the majority of drug or alcohol using individuals retain, at point of use, a capacity to decide whether to use that substance or not but give greater priority to short-term gain over long-term loss. However, all clinicians have encountered a minority of drug- or alcohol-misusing individuals who, at the point of use, also clearly lack capacity to decide whether that substance misusage is in their interests or not.

There are considerable implications to this argument. From the point of view of research, it should be feasible to develop tests of capacity at point of use of drugs or alcohol. In terms of policy, it is reasonable to conclude that the majority of drug or alcohol misusing individuals retain capacity, and it is therefore appropriate for them to be held responsible for the consequences of their actions.

It is also reasonable to conclude that Mental Health Act disposals are not appropriate for the majority of drug or alcohol users who retain capacity, and in any event these conditions are explicit exclusion criteria from Section 1 of the 1983 Act, a situation likely to be unchanged in any imminent revision of the Mental Health Act.

It may also be concluded that drug or alcohol misusers have a responsibility for themselves and for their carers. It follows that the duty of care to drug- or alcohol-misusing patients is not absolute but conditional.

Conclusions

As part of the stigma campaign, health carers should be saying to drug or alcohol misusers "you should not be disadvantaged by any misinformed view about your condition, but you may be disadvantaged by unacceptable behaviour". It may be appropriate to suggest a revision of the Patients' Charter for drug or alcohol misusers, emphasising their general right of access to good quality services and their onus to behave appropriately. For the carers, such an explicit charter could remind them of the need to offer treatment, but not unconditionally. No doctor or nurse should expect to be assaulted by a drug or alcohol misuser who has been judged to retain capacity.

The College campaign is aimed at reducing the stigma associated with various mental disorders. In relation to addiction, much use may be made of appropriate websites, as the American experience shows. But perhaps our main target for this campaign are our fellow health professionals to whom we need to emphasise the legitimacy of health care interventions balanced by a reframed duty of care.

References

American Psychiatric Association (1994) *Diagnostic and Statistical Manual of Mental Disorders,* 4th edn (DSM-IV). Washington, DC: American Psychiatric Press.

Edwards G & Gross M (1976) Alcohol dependence: provisional description of a clinical syndrome. *British Medical Journal* i: 1058–61.

Goffman E (1963) *Stigma: Notes on the Management of Spoiled Identity.* Englewood Cliffs, NJ: Prentice-Hall: 2–3.

Johns A (1990) What is dependence? In: Ghodse AH & Maxwell D (eds) *Substance Abuse and Dependence: An Introduction for the Caring Professions.* London: Macmillan: 5–29.

World Health Organization (1992) *The ICD-10 Classification of Mental and Behavioural Disorders.* Geneva: WHO.

Rex v Tandy (1967) 87 Court of Appeal Report 45.

Yamey G (1999) Young less tolerant of mentally ill than old – BMJ news item. *British Medical Journal* **319**: 1092.

36 The stigmatisation of eating disorders

Gerald Russell

The subject of this chapter is the stigmatisation of patients suffering from obesity, anorexia nervosa, and related eating disorders. Curiously, obesity is sometimes omitted from the grouping of eating disorders. It is essential not to repeat this error in this context for two reasons: first, a great deal is known about the stigmatisation of obesity, in contrast with the paucity of knowledge on stigmatisation in anorexia nervosa; secondly, at least in the anorexic patient's mind, the justification for her behaviour is her immense dread of fatness. It may be said that the anorexic patient has incorporated society's contempt for fat persons.

The word *stigma* is generally taken to be derogatory. In its original meaning from the Greek it refers to the brand with which slaves and criminals were marked. The word may also have a positive connotation when *stigmata* refers to the marks of Christ's wounds impressed on the bodies of saintly persons. The claim was first made in the case of St Francis of Assisi, who received his stigmata in a state of ecstasy on Mount La Vema in 1224. The impressions on the body of Saint Francis corresponded to the wounds received by Christ during his crucifixion. Later on, other saints have been credited with these marks of holiness, and especially important for the present subject is Saint Catherine of Sienna, a Christian mystic who lived in the 14th Century, and whose strictly ascetic life led her to a state of emaciation diagnosed retrospectively as anorexia nervosa (Bell 1985; Rampling 1985).

I should return to the commoner derogatory meaning of the term of stigma and consider the principal features of this concept. In Chapter 30 of this volume Paul Gilbert clarifies various related terms describing the components of stigmatisation. He accepts Goffman's (1963) argument that stigma is a mark of social devaluation. It is associated with shame which may be internal or external, and when extreme felt as humiliation. For the purpose of the present chapter the external stigmatisation due to prejudice will be termed "*discrimination*". *Shame* will be taken to mean self-devaluation which may indeed result from external discrimination. The distinction between internal shame and external discrimination is important because they do not necessarily go hand in hand, as will be seen later in patients with anorexia nervosa.

In this chapter, the stigmatisation of obese persons and patients with anorexia nervosa will be discussed in turn. Stigmatisation in anorexia nervosa will be examined in relation to the prevailing views on the nature of the disorder. Prejudice, on the part of the media, official bodies, and medical professionals will be examined in turn so as to identify sources of stigmatisation and attempts to destigmatise patients with anorexia nervosa.

The Stigma Campaign by the Royal College of Psychiatrists

In 1998 the Royal College of Psychiatrists began a five-year campaign on "Changing Minds: Every Family in the Land". The title was specially chosen to emphasise the fact that every family is affected by mental illness because one of its members will probably suffer from it at some stage in his or her life. The Royal College commissioned a survey to assess the prevalence of stigmatising attitudes towards people with mental illness. In this survey 1,737 adults were questioned about their views regarding seven different mental disorders: severe depression, panic attacks, schizophrenia, dementia, alcohol addiction, drug addiction and finally eating disorders. Unfortunately, the term "eating disorders" was not defined in this survey and one has to guess it referred to anorexia and/or bulimia but not obesity.

The survey was carried out on behalf of the College by the Office for National Statistics: 2,679 adults were chosen from households in a national sample, stratified by region, economic and social status. The questions asked from the interviewees were selected according to the views put forward by Hayward and Bright (1997). These workers had concluded that stigmatisation was associated with enduring themes of people with mental illness being perceived as dangerous, unpredictable, difficult to talk with, feeling different to the way we do, having only continuously themselves to blame, able to pull themselves together, unlikely to improve if treated, and incapable of recovery.

Table 1. Survey by the Royal College of Psychiatrists

	Perceptions of British Adults (n = 1,737) (percentages show negative opinions)		
	Severe depression	Panic attacks	Eating disorders
Dangerous to others	23%	26%	7%
Unpredictable	56%	50%	29%
Hard to talk to	62%	33%	38%
They are to blame	13%	11%	35%
Could pull themselves together	19%	22%	38%
Would not improve with treatment	16%	14%	9%
Would never recover	23%	22%	11%
They feel differently	43%	39%	49%

Table 1 summarises some of the results and is derived from the Royal College of Psychiatrists' survey (Crisp et al. 2000). For example, people with depression were often viewed as unpredictable, difficult to talk with and feeling different from the way we do. Similar negative opinions were obtained about people with panic attacks, although these opinions were somewhat less frequent. Patients with eating disorders were viewed somewhat differently. On the whole they attracted fewer negative opinions. Nevertheless, more than one-third of the respondents thought that these patients "could pull themselves together", "have only themselves to blame", and "are difficult to talk with". On the other hand, almost 90% of the respondents thought that patients with eating disorders would recover eventually – a surprisingly optimistic view. These patients were not thought to be dangerous or unpredictable. Two of these opinions stand out: these patients were judged to be blameworthy and capable of solving their own problems, which is tantamount to saying that their illness is self-inflicted. The authors of the Royal College publication rightly concluded that this opinion is stigmatising.

For the reasons I have already given, the stigmatisation of patients with eating disorders will be taken to cover obese subjects and patients with anorexia nervosa and related disorders. They will be discussed in turn.

Obesity

There is a much greater awareness of the stigmatisation of obesity in comparison with anorexia nervosa and related eating disorders. A Medline search showed that the number of articles listed on stigmatisation was in the ratio of about 30 on obesity to 1 on other eating disorders. The psychological reactions to obesity are multiple. They were gathered together under the umbrella of "psychologic burden" when the health implications of obesity were considered by a consensus conference on obesity organised by the National Institute of Health in 1985. They concluded that "obesity creates an enormous psychological burden ... in terms of suffering, this burden may be the greatest adverse effect of obesity" (NIH 1985). This conclusion applied to all obese persons, but particularly to the minority who suffer from severe obesity (100% overweight). This is an arresting statement given that the physical burden borne by obese persons is well recognised in terms of the numerous complications that may afflict them.

The "psychological burden" of obesity has to be analysed in terms of its different components. It does not mean, for example, that the obese show increased psychological disturbances. Stunkard and Wadden (1992) observed that epidemiological and clinical studies refute the popular notion that overweight persons as a group are emotionally disturbed. Although obese people are subjected to intense prejudice and discrimination, they show a tremendous resilience of the human spirit (Stunkard and Wadden 1992).

On the other hand, when the obese person's sense of "shame" is considered along the lines proposed by Gilbert, it has been shown that they are extremely disparaging of their own bodies and see themselves as disabled. The first of these components of shame has been documented in the severely obese; their feelings of body disparagement improved remarkably after surgical treatment which led to loss of weight (Halmi et al. 1980).

The degree of shame and disability perceived by severely obese subjects was also disclosed when they were asked a series of forced-choice questions in a study by Rand and Macgregor (1991). The method has been called "owning one's disability". In a series of 47 severely obese persons who had maintained an average weight loss of 45 kg after surgical treatment, they were asked to say whether they preferred their previous obesity to being deaf, dyslexic, diabetic, or having heart disease. Not a single patient preferred the former obesity to one of these hypothetical handicaps. Only leg amputation or legal blindness was considered worse than the obesity.

The evidence of widespread prejudice and discrimination against the obese in most areas of social functioning has been reviewed by Stunkard and Wadden (1992):

1. Obese high school students are less often accepted than normal weight students by prestigious colleges in the USA.
2. When seeking employment the obese face marked discrimination, e.g. 16% of employers said that they would not hire obese women under any condition.
3. Prospects for marriage are more limited for obese women. They are twice as likely to descend rather than ascend in their social class.
4. More than 80% of obese patients perceived themselves as physically unattractive, expressing the view that others make disparaging comments about their weight.
5. Most worrying is the finding that 78% of severely obese patients said they had been treated disrespectfully by the medical profession because of their weight (Rand and Macgregor, 1990). This disparagement of the obese is long-standing, having been detected in 1969 in a survey of physicians who described their obese patients as "weak willed, ugly and awkward".

In conclusion, discrimination against the obese is widespread among different social institutions. It is not surprising that many obese persons are ashamed of their bodies and consider their size as a disability. It is remarkable that they appear not to react with frank psychiatric disturbance. On the other hand, society's condemnation of the obese has been incorporated in the thinking of patients with anorexia nervosa and related eating disorders, as will be discussed now.

Anorexia and related disorders

Psychological disturbances in anorexia nervosa

An important diagnostic feature of anorexia nervosa is the patient's dread of fatness. It has already been said that the anorexic patient has therefore incorporated society's contempt of fat persons. But she has done this to such an extreme degree that her dread of fatness amounts to an over-valued idea, or even, occasionally, a frank delusion. On the other hand anorexic patients often take pride in their thinness. This observation led German psychiatrists to name the illness *Magersucht*, meaning "seeking after thinness". In part the pride is derived from the patient's sense of achievement that she has lost weight through dieting, something that the majority of women fail to do when they attempt to lose weight. This pride in thinness is illustrated in a case vignette.

Patient 1

A young student decided to reduce her weight from 54 kg and began to diet. Her menstrual periods soon stopped. Within a few months her weight had fallen to 46.2 kg (BMI 17.6). After two years of out-patient treatment her weight had risen to only 49.5 kg and amenorrhoea persisted. She said she regretted that she could no longer feel the bony points of her body. She asserted that for her anorexia nervosa was not a stigma. "Anorexia" was attractive because it carried a romantic and glamorous image, as shown by ballet dancers and models. Moreover, looking "anorexic" gave the impression of being sensitive and serious. By being thin she elicited concern from other people who showed that they cared about her.

In anorexia nervosa, therefore, the patient may not experience shame of her illness, in contrast with the obese person. The wish to look frail and vulnerable is consistent with anorexia nervosa as an expression of asceticism. This has been stressed in the literature on the mediaeval saints, among whom St Catherine of Sienna stands out as the best documented example (Bell 1985). It is recorded that St Catherine "was compelled to let a fine straw or some such thing be pushed far down her throat to make her vomit" (Rampling 1986). This account suggests that extreme forms of Christian asceticism might lead to anorexia nervosa.

Discrimination against patients with anorexia nervosa

The role of the media

Eating disorders are probably discussed more frequently in the media than any other mental illness. For example, British newspapers became interested in the Kendall sisters, identical twins who suffered from anorexia nervosa. After the first twin died there was much publicity surrounding the second twin, especially when she decided to attend a special treatment clinic in Canada. Sadly the second twin also died a few years later (*Guardian* 1994). Another tragic victim of anorexia nervosa was Lena Zavaroni, who had been a child singing star. She died from the illness in October 1999 at the age of 35, and her story appeared in daily newspapers (*The Times* 1999). These newspaper articles regularly express compassion for these patients. At other times they may convey helpful advice. Victoria Beckham, one of the "Spice Girls", attracted widespread attention when newspaper photographers showed her as having lost a great deal of weight. The article quoted a medical expert who said that "women's ideal body shape is too unhealthy", "Trying to look like Posh Spice can damage your health" (*Daily Express* 1999).

Stigmatisation by officialdom

In 1991 a tragic series of deaths on the children's ward at the Grantham and Kesteven General Hospital was found to have been caused by a nurse, Beverly Allitt, who had murdered them while they were under her care. An independent inquiry rightly concluded that this nurse had a major personality disorder (Allitt Inquiry 1994). Unfortunately the committee gave erroneous advice on how to diagnose a serious personality disorder, and this led to discrimination against applicants for nurse training. It was rightly said that it is difficult to diagnose a serious personality disorder, but it was wrongly suggested that consideration should be given to "excessive absence through sickness, excessive use of counselling or medical facilities, or self-harming behaviour such as attempted suicide, self-laceration, or *eating disorder*". The Royal College of Psychiatrists recognised that this part of the report was discriminatory and the President of the College persuaded the NHS Executive to produce new advice as follows: "Individual factors may not be significant if taken in isolation: for example, young people in particular may make extensive use of counselling, or may suffer from short-term eating disorders, without this indicating any serious underlying pathology" (NHS Executive 1994).

Prejudice among healthcare professionals

In an Australian study, testing a wide range of healthcare professionals, the respondents were asked to express their attitude to patients with the following diagnoses: schizophrenia, recurrent drug overdoses, and an eating disorder (Fleming and Szmukler 1992). The healthcare professionals were asked to estimate (in percentages) the degree to which patients were "responsible for their own condition". The patients with anorexia nervosa were held to be almost as "responsible" as patients who took drug overdoses (59% for anorexia nervosa, 71% for recurrent overdoses, and 18% for schizophrenia). The respondents were also asked to express their liking for patients in each diagnostic category. It transpired that none of the patient groups was particularly liked by the healthcare professionals, but schizophrenic patients were preferred to patients with anorexia nervosa, who were in turn preferred to those who took drug overdoses.

Another example of discrimination against anorexic patients by healthcare professionals is the harsh rationing of treatment under various schemes of "managed care". In the USA the duration of in-patient treatment is severely limited. In Britain the scarcity of beds in specialised eating disorder units has led to a dependence on extra-contractual referrals to outside health authorities or private hospitals, leading to a close scrutiny of the costs incurred. This author has come across medical reports written by psychiatrists suggesting that certain patients had already cost the National Health Service a great deal of money and that further expenditure was not justified, even though they were still extremely ill. Such reaction indicates the trivialisation of anorexia nervosa, even by psychiatrists who fail to appreciate the danger of the illness and the extreme suffering it causes.

Discrimination against patients with bulimia nervosa

There is little information about discrimination specifically directed against bulimic patients. However, it is well recognised that these patients, in contrast with anorexic patients, express a great deal of shame about their bulimic behaviour and self-induced vomiting, which they often keep secret. It is noteworthy that when Princess Diana declared at a conference on eating disorders in London in 1993 that she too had experienced bulimia nervosa, the disorder became somewhat more acceptable. This may be an example of gentrification, as discussed by Porter in Chapter 1 of this volume.

Stigmatisation depends on the public's view of the nature of the disorder

It is possible that the level of stigmatisation varies according to a person's model of the disorder. In the case of healthcare professionals this means their perception of the causes and pathogenesis of the disorder. In Chapter 1 Porter shows how stigmatisation may be enhanced or reduced according to the public, and especially the medical, conceptualisation of an illness. For example, explaining it in terms of an underlying physical disturbance tends to remove blame from the patient and restore her dignity. A number of aetiological models will be examined.

Aetiological models

Anorexia nervosa as a disease
Some experts have been struck by the intractable course of anorexia nervosa and consider it to be a disease. In recent years it has become clear that genetic factors contribute to its causation. Such a model of the illness may help to reduce discrimination against anorexic patients.

Anorexia nervosa results from a cult of thinness in Westernised societies
There is a widespread view that the cult of thinness, with its tyrannical pressures on young women, leads many to experiment with weight-reducing diets, and the most vulnerable among them succumb to an eating disorder. This model blames society and therefore absolves the patient.

Psychological explanations for anorexia nervosa
One of the most beguiling explanatory models is that anorexia nervosa is a "flight from growth" (Crisp 1980). On entering adolescence the youngster may find the biological and psychological effects of puberty overwhelming. She experiences unwanted and frightening pubertal "fatness" rather than simple obesity per se as the source of her problem, and automatically seeks relief by limiting her food intake, thereby switching off her own pubertal development. An acceptance of this persuasive model may also help reduce negative feelings towards anorexic patients.

Fleming and Szmukler's (1992) model indicated that a common view is that the family is a causal influence. This is a two-edged sword. Patients are regarded as less responsible for their illness as it is attributed to faulty family interactions. The unfortunate consequence, however, is the blaming of the parents.

Conclusions on different aetiological models

Any of the above explanatory models may go some way towards reducing the prejudice felt for patients with anorexia nervosa, but none of them may overcome the widespread view that anorexia nervosa is a relatively trivial problem which is self-inflicted. It is indeed difficult for health professionals to ignore the fact that most of these patients do their utmost to avoid treatment and sabotage programmes of refeeding. This was summed up by Samuel-Lajeunesse (1994) who suggested: "Denial of the illness, lies, cheating, manipulation, are characteristic of the behaviour of anorectics".

Anorexia nervosa is a dangerous disorder which causes immense suffering

Perhaps the most powerful counter to the stigmatisation of anorexia nervosa is the clinician's experience of witnessing the severity and persistence of a patient's suffering. A case history will make the point.

Patient 2

An adolescent girl had already begun to lose weight when she injured her hip while running. A fracture was identified which was thought to be pathological and due to osteoporosis. Operative pinning of the femur was at first unsuccessful and she needed a second operation, which still left her with a painful limp. She was twice admitted to eating disorder units and was able to achieve a gain in weight from 38 to 52 kg. She remained depressed, however, and was plagued by obsessional rituals. Family therapy for one year sustained her weight, but only temporarily. With the recurrence of weight loss she required another admission, this time to a medical unit. Subsequently she lost weight again. Hypoglycaemia led to an emergency admission when she was fed through a nasogastric tube. She developed a gastric perforation, followed by acute peritonitis and renal failure. She was then treated on an intensive care unit, but the gastric perforation led to a fistula. In spite of naso-jejunal tube feeding, her emaciation became worse. She required ventilation through a tracheostomy. She improved temporarily when renal function returned but she had become severely anaemic, weighed only 26 kg and had bed sores. When the tracheostomy tube was removed pulmonary infection ensued with consequent respiratory failure and death.

This unfortunate young woman had been ill for four years. For much of this time she suffered enormously, as did her family. Her last few weeks were painful in the extreme. Such a case history should remind us that anorexia nervosa can often be a serious illness which should give rise to appropriate professional concern and therapeutic endeavour.

Mortality rate

An important reason for heeding the plight of sufferers from eating disorders is their high mortality rate. A comparison of standardised mortality ratios for patients with "all eating disorders" was made with other psychiatric illnesses (Harris and Baraclough 1998). The mortality for patients with eating disorders exceeded that of other psychiatric disorders including schizophrenia, alcohol abuse, bipolar disorder and even suicidal attempts.

Conclusions

1. Society's contempt for the obese is universal.
2. In anorexia nervosa the patient is likely to take pride in her ability to lose weight and maintain her thinness.
3. Serious stigmatisation has arisen in the past from confusing eating disorders with major personality disorders.

4. Discrimination by medical professionals against patients with anorexia nervosa carries the risk of poor standards of care.

5. Important factors in the stigmatisation of anorexia nervosa are the trivialisation of the disorder and the perception that it is self-inflicted.

6. Stigmatisation is best combated by recognising that anorexia nervosa causes much suffering and carries a high mortality rate.

References

Allitt Inquiry (1994) *Independent Inquiry relating to Deaths and Injuries on the Children's Ward at Grantham and Kesteven General Hospital during the period February to April 1991 (The Cecil Clothier Report)*. London: HMSO.

Bell RM (1985) *Holy Anorexia*. Chicago: University of Chicago Press.

Crisp AH (1980) *Anorexia Nervosa: Let Me Be*. London: Academic Press.

Crisp AH, Gelder MG, Rix S et al. (2000). Stigmatisation of people with mental illness. *British Journal of Psychiatry* **177**: 4–7.

Daily Express (1999). Thin may be ideal but we should all plump for the fuller figure. 8 December.

Fleming J & Szmukler GI (1992) Attitudes of medical professionals towards patients with eating disorders. *Australian and New Zealand Journal of Psychiatry* **26**: 436–43.

Guardian (1994) Anorexic's mother pins hopes on Canada. 10 May.

Goffman E (1963) *Stigma: Notes on the Management of Spoiled Identity*. Englewood Cliffs, NJ: Prentice Hall.

Halmi KA, Long M, Stunkard AJ et al. (1980) Psychiatric diagnosis of morbidly obese gastric bypass patients. *American Journal of Psychiatry* **137**: 470–2.

Harris EC & Barraclough B (1998) Excess mortality of mental disorder. *British Journal of Psychiatry* **173**: 11–53.

Hayward P & Bright JA (1997) Stigma and mental illness: a review and critique. *Journal of Mental Health* **6**: 345–54.

NIH (1985) National Institute of Health Consensus Development Panel on the Health Implications of Obesity. Health complications of obesity. *Annals of Internal Medicine* **103**: 1073–7.

NHS Executive (1994) Occupational Health Services for NHS Staff. HSG (94) 51, para. 15.

Rampling D (1985) Ascetic ideals and anorexia nervosa. *Journal of Psychiatric Research* **19**: 89–94.

Rand CSW & Macgregor AMC (1990) Morbidly obese patients' perceptions of social discrimination before and after surgery for obesity. *Southern Medical Journal* **83**: 1390–5.

Samuel-Lajeunesse B (1994) Troubles du comportement alimentaire: aspects sémiologiques. In: Samuel-Lajeunesse B & Foulon Ch (eds). *Les Conduites Alimentaires*. Paris: Masson: 91.

Stunkard AH & Wadden TA (1992) Psychological aspects of severe obesity. *American Journal of Clinical Nutrition* **55**: 524S–32S.

The Times (1999) Zavaroni "made suicide threat" to get surgery. 9 December.

37 Mad *and* bad? Models of psychopathology and the stigmatisation of people with schizophrenia

VY Allison-Bolger

It is a fact that people with schizophrenia are stigmatised. They are stigmatised by people in a society which has particular views about madness. These views shape the interpretation of psychopathological models. To understand the impact of such models on stigmatisation we must understand the social context in which they are applied.

Folk psychology and attitudes to madness

Folk psychology is the name given to commonsense theories about why people think, feel and act as they do. We use these theories in everyday life to explain why people say and do the things they do. These explanations are based on the assumption that we are all more or less the same.

Madness marks the limits of folk psychology. It is by definition irrational, unreasonable. The mad are beyond ordinary understanding. They are bizarre and unpredictable.

This is one source of unease with madness and mad people. Another is their behaviour. It is not only difficult to understand and predict – it is also socially deviant. They do not do what is expected of them. As Szasz (1970) wrote 30 years ago, they "violate ethical, political and social norms". This violation marks them out as bad citizens (Allison-Bolger 1999).

As bad citizens they are open to blame. Being blameworthy means both acting in a reprehensible manner and being deserving of blame. Certain groups are excused from this on the grounds that they are not responsible for their actions – principally young children and the mad, who are believed to be unable to form proper intentions.

The difficulty comes in distinguishing bad citizens who are, and bad citizens who are not, responsible for their actions. In England we make a distinction between psychopaths and people with mental illness. The latter group are excused because they are deemed ill.

The concept of illness

Most psychopathological models of schizophrenia are underpinned by the idea that schizophrenia is an illness. Illness and disease are hard to define (Fulford 1989) because they encompass a complex set of relationships between the body, the person, his behaviour and society. This is hard to capture in a single sentence!

One aspect of the concept of illness, of great relevance to psychopathological models, is given in this definition:

"Illness is a cause [of failure of function] which is revealed indirectly as symptoms".

The key feature of the definition is that it describes a causal relationship. The essence of illness is that observable events (or states) are attributed to hidden forces (or agents).

We are usually blinded to this simple formulation by our concern with defining what it is that is bad about illness. In this definition the "wrongness" is contained in the phrase "failure of function", but it could be replaced equally well by another criterion of illness, such as "arousal of therapeutic concern", or "social and biological disadvantage". In focusing on these phrases we have missed something very important. That is, our account of abnormal mental states has the same underlying basis as our account of normal mental states. Both are attributed to hidden forces – be they beliefs, desires, the unconscious, demons or chemicals.

But, when we seek to explain why people with schizophrenia think, feel and act as they do we use a causal model which is subtly different from the one we use to explain ordinary human action. We use the illness model, which, as we have seen, emphasises the wrongness, rather than the cause. In so doing we magnify the distinction between the mad and the sane.

There are three routes to the idea that there is something wrong with mad people. Firstly, we don't understand them; secondly, they are bad citizens; thirdly, they are ill. The first of these is a source of fear and mistrust, the second is a source of blame, the third is a reason for forgiveness.

Psychopathology

Psychopathology is the study of symptoms which are to do with the mind. Mental symptoms are abnormalities of thinking, feeling and acting which are attributed to mental illness. Psychopathological models are used to explain the causes of mental illness.

The term "psychopathology" presupposes a medical conception of conditions such as schizophrenia. Within this medical paradigm the experiences of people with schizophrenia are regarded as signs of illness.

Schizophrenia

Schizophrenia is a term used to refer to a particular set of symptoms. A person with a number of these symptoms may be diagnosed as having schizophrenia. They include hearing voices when no one else is there, having other people's thoughts put inside your head, seeing signs or receiving messages, having experiences of telepathy or mind reading.

People with schizophrenia can have bizarre or impossible beliefs about the world or their place in it. They may have trouble thinking straight or getting themselves motivated to do things. They may say or do odd things. Psychopathologists describe and name these symptoms and create theories to explain how they come about.

Three psychopathological models of schizophrenia
Biological models

In the 19th century the prevailing view was that mental illness was brain disease. The popularity of this view has waxed and waned, but now most psychiatrists agree that schizophrenia is caused by abnormalities of brain function.

There are many sophisticated theories about how the brain might cause symptoms.

They may result from faulty connections, probably between frontal and temporal lobes (Weinberger 1997). Genetic and environmental factors can affect the formation of these connections. Subsequently their function can be influenced by neurotransmitters and neuromodulators (Johnstone 1996).

Psychological models

Supporters of psychological models may say that brain processes alone are not sufficient to explain schizophrenic symptoms. Jung (1944) certainly took this view as did Laing, who described the person with psychosis as ontologically insecure and so unable to take the realness, aliveness, autonomy, and identity of himself and others for granted (Laing 1965).

Psychoanalytic theories hold that schizophrenia is a disorder of ego boundaries (Federn 1953). This means that the individual is unable to distinguish between self and not-self. This is seen in passivity phenomena, for example, when the patient believes that others control his actions or know what he is thinking.

Cognitive neuropsychology is a refinement in which cognitive mechanisms are proposed as the hidden forces. For example, passivity phenomena are explained as a failure of internal monitoring of action. That is, the mechanism by which we are aware of what we are doing as we are doing it. Recently this has been attributed to "an inability to represent our own mental states" (Frith 1994).

Social approaches to madness

Social models are concerned with the nature and function of an individual's relationships with significant others and with society in general. Some theories concentrate on the nature of mental illness and whether it is a real disease entity or a social construct (e.g. Hacking 1998). Others are concerned with the external factors that influence the course of that disorder or the effects of illness on a person's social conditions – employment, wealth, housing and so on. Social historians tend to focus on the experiences of the individual patients (e.g. Porter 1987).

Social models are rarely causal accounts in the way that biological and psychological models try to be. Exceptions to this are the family dynamic and expressed emotion theories – the former are concerned with factors which can cause psychosis, the latter with those which exacerbate it. Family dynamic theories such as the double bind in which a parent communicates two contradictory messages simultaneously have not been proven to cause schizophrenia (Arieti 1974).

However, exposure to high expressed emotion (emotional over-involvement, intense critical and/or hostile comments) can cause the person with schizophrenia to relapse (Leff and Vaughan 1985).

Both these theories are interesting in emphasising the role of stressful communication in bringing about psychotic symptoms. These interactions may reflect the ambivalent beliefs that people have about mental illness, which must be compounded if the patient is a loved one.

Models of psychopathology as augmentors of stigmatisation

The biological model and stigmatisation

The core belief of the biological model is that the person with schizophrenia is ill, and therefore, a suitable case for treatment. If the patient is not compliant then the profession's tolerance is eroded – he is seen as a difficult customer and is resented.

This may have more to do with how doctors see their role than with anything to do with the patient. The imperative to heal the sick is so strong that any obstacle is resented – be it lack of resources (organ transplants), absence of effective treatments (many cancers) or denial of consent (refusal of blood transfusion on religious grounds).

The case of the person with schizophrenia is even more entangled, because people with mental disorder are the only group subject to compulsory treatment under the law. This puts them in the unique position of being the objects of both compassion and social control. The person with cancer doesn't need controlling, because he poses no threat to society. Unlike the control exerted over criminals, detention in a hospital is seen as being in the individual's best interests.

This can be argued convincingly for particular individuals in particular situations. But it is profoundly stigmatising for the group of people with schizophrenia. In folk terms, they are seen as "wild mad people" who need locking up for their own good and for the good of society. Subtly, they are seen as people who are not capable of acting in their own best interests. This perception can persist even when the person is no longer disturbed.

The biological model is not directly stigmatising. Many would claim that in banishing myths it paves the way to treating the person with schizophrenia with the respect he deserves. Its alliance with medical venues may also be seen as a good thing, evoking the need for compassionate treatment.

The biological model is the cornerstone of physical treatment. Drugs are arguably the most effective therapy we have. But, in being wedded to the perceived need for treatment, and in enforcing it against the patient's will, we create a class of people who receive not only the benefits of treatment but also condemnation.

Psychological models and stigmatisation

Psychological models seek to explain the causes of symptoms. They may focus on symptoms rather than syndromes but they are still subject to the pitfalls of categorisation, because as causal accounts they are concerned with general theories rather than particular cases.

Their general theories are to do with how individuals make sense of, and respond to, things and events in the world. Particular ways of responding are then linked to particular symptoms. So there is a shift from the person to the personality, and to personality types.

Categorisation is seen as a problem for individuals because it appears to deny that which they most highly prize – their individuality. But we are all members of groups. Membership of certain groups is seen as desirable. The insult is not in being labelled personally, but in the implications of the label that one is given. Changing the name of the group doesn't change the criteria for membership of it. If these criteria mean having symptoms which are regarded as "bad", then it doesn't matter whether one is called "schizophrenic" or "cognitively biased".

Social approaches and the process of stigmatisation

Social approaches can reveal the paradoxes at the heart of the process of stigmatisation. Firstly, they highlight the uniqueness of mad people; secondly, their marginalisation; thirdly, the efforts made by society to assimilate them.

So, uniqueness is social deviance, or a sane response to an insane world. The individual is blamed for behaving badly or a society is condemned for expecting conformity. The mad person is marginal because he refuses to participate, or because participation is denied. Treatment is a form of annihilation of the individual, or a release from suffering.

Conclusions

Stigmatisation is a complex phenomenon to which all three psychopathological models contribute in different ways. Their contribution is best understood within the broader context of social attitudes to madness. Much turns on the identification of madness with deviance – specifically with actions which contravene the social order. The person who is silently and inactively mad does not come to our attention. The person with schizophrenia who does come to our attention is the one who kills a person or an animal, or who shouts, or strips, or knocks the hats off policemen. Society may probably resent these acts and that may spill over into resentment of the person. Such a person is one of the most likely to be detained. This generates a significant confluence of judgments and acts – deviance, resentment and compulsory treatment. In this light professional intervention can be seen as punitive or controlling. Introduce the notion of illness and there is an entirely different spin – professional intervention is both necessary and compassionate.

Illness explains the deviance and provides the grounds for forgiveness. Strawson (1974) says that to forgive is "to accept the repudiation and forswear the resentment". Forgiving is easier if the person does repudiate his resented acts and attitudes – in this case, if he abandons his madness. But he might not see it as something which should be resented. He was just doing what he had to do – whether it was killing a witch's familiar or passing a message to the Freemasons. This clash of world views lies at the heart of the confrontation that characterises so many psychiatric consultations. The doctor says that the patient is mad. The patient says that he is not. It is from this opposition, and its repetition in the waiting room, the home, the street, the work place and the social club, that stigmatisation springs.

References

Allison-Bolger V (1999) The original sin of madness – or how doctors can stigmatise their patients. *International Journal of Clinical Practice* 53: 627–630.

Arieti S (1974) *Interpretation of Schizophrenia*. London: Crosby, Lockwood & Staples.

Federn P (1953) Ego psychology and the psychoses. In: Weiss E (ed.). *Maresfield Reprints*, London: 229.

Frith C (1994) Theory of mind in schizophrenia. In: David AS & Cutting JC (eds). *The Neuropsychology of Schizophrenia*. Hove: Psychology Press: 154.

Fulford KWM (1989) *Moral Theory and Medical Practice*. Cambridge: Cambridge University Press.

Hacking I (1998) *Mad Travellers: Reflections on the Reality of Transient Mental Illnesses*. Charlottesville: University Press of Virginia.

Johnstone EC (ed) (1996) Biological psychiatry. *British Medical Bulletin* 52(3): Royal Society of Medicine Special Issue.

Jung CG (1944) *The Psychology of Dementia Praecox* (translated by AA Brill). Nervous & Mental Diseases Monograph Press.

Laing RD (1965) *The Divided Self: An Existential Study in Sanity and Madness*. London: Penguin Books.

Leff JP & Vaughn C (1985) *Expressed Emotion in Families*. New York: Guilford Press.

Porter R (1987) *A Social History of Madness: stories of the insane*. London: Phoenix Giants.

Strawson PF (1974) *Freedom and Resentment and other essays*. London: Methuen: 1–25.

Szasz T (1970) The myth of mental illness. In: *Ideology and Insanity*. London: Penguin.

Weinberger DR (1997) On the plausibility of "the neurodevelopmental hypothesis" of schizophrenia. *Neuropsychopharmacology* 14: 1S–11S.

38 Stigma in dementia

John Kellett

Introduction

Although the madness of George III may have made mental illness more respectable (Macalpine and Hunter 1966), the suggestion that it was due to porphyria, a metabolic defect, might have removed this benefit. It suggests that mental illness caused by a known metabolic defect is less stigmatised than one whose cause is unknown, so-called functional psychosis. One should not therefore be surprised by the finding of the Royal College of Psychiatrists' survey (Crisp et al. 2000) that subjects with dementia harbour the least blame of all mental conditions though they also suffer the worst prognosis. Taking dementia as a whole, these public attitudes are correct.

Blame

However, it was not always so. Dementia paralytica, the dementia of cerebral syphilis, was attributed to excessive masturbation (Hare 1962), and even when its cause, a venereal infection, was established the patient was open to criticism. The same applies to AIDS dementia today, though the dementia is only apparent in the terminal stages of the disease. Unlike other mental conditions, some dementias are catching, if only through cannibalism like Kuru, or blood contamination. This leads to serious problems of stigma for the neuropathologist with the corpse of a patient with a prior dementia even if health workers are more relaxed when caring for the living. It is clear that stigmatisation of dementia relates as much to the cause of the dementia as it does to the condition itself. Neuroses gain opprobrium through the notion that the sufferer could have overcome the deficit. Psychogenic dementia does not exist, though some may feign the condition. The idea that atrophy follows disuse has been applied to the brain – a concept which is difficult to disprove since the first sign of dementia, apathy, may precede dysmnesia by several years. However dementia is no respecter of class or premorbid intellect, and it is most unlikely that a demented subject can be held responsible for their condition, unless this extends to a failure to take hormone replacement therapy, or arises from a head injury.

Different dementias

Some dementias affect frontal lobe function either exclusively (as in normal pressure hydrocephalus (NPH) and Pick's) or at least dominate the early stages of the condition (e.g. Huntington's). These poor people earn their stigma by their sociopathic behaviour. Without showing cognitive defects they allow their standards of hygiene, and ethical standards, to fall until they become pariahs. No longer bothering to answer letters or pay bills, they are evicted from their homes and may face civil or even criminal prosecution (e.g. for sexual abuse). They lose insight early and may even regard their plight with amusement. The patient with NPH falls to the ground when standing up giggling at their weakness. Not surprisingly, busy nurses think them silly. Of all mental patients they benefit most from expert medical attention which can sanction their need for care and even cure the condition (NPH by inserting a ventriculo-peritoneal shunt.) Rarely Alzheimer's disease can present with such symptoms, though questioning will quickly reveal the accompanying loss of short-term memory.

However, the vast majority of the dementias are forms of Alzheimer's disease, vascular damage, or mixtures of the two, and largely are confined to the elderly. This has enabled medicine to neglect the area to the extent that care is shared between those in the least glamorous parts of medicine: psychiatrists and geriatricians. There are plenty of examples of medical discrimination against the elderly, and indeed if one has to choose between giving life-saving treatment to the old or young one naturally chooses the one whose life is largely ahead of them.

Giving the diagnosis

Another measure of stigma is the willingness of doctors to impart the diagnosis to the patient. The same problems arise with cancer, but by avoiding the term and using words like lymphoma and oat cell neoplasia, the oncologist can soften the blow and the patient may learn about their condition and obtain an accurate prognosis. At least, however, the patient can understand the implications, and retain hope through miracle cures. With dementia that hope is difficult to sustain in that its very presence indicates denial. A patient in the early stages of the condition has every right to prepare for it by drawing up an enduring power of attorney, arranging their estate and future care, and leaving instructions about resuscitation in the later stages. However, the grim tidings may well exacerbate a depression which often occurs at the start of the dementia, and creating hope is not easy. The slow progress gives the patient and their family months of relative normality which can be destroyed by depression and irritability. As the dementia progresses, insight may not be so painful but equally may not be retained. The husband of a lady with a profound dementia died when she was in hospital. She was informed, and taken to the funeral. She wept and all assumed that mourning was progressing until a week later she asked the whereabouts of her husband. She was reminded that he had died and she wept bitterly. After the third occasion it was clear that she was re-experiencing the loss each time and it was more humane to tell her the lie that he would be visiting later. In the same way a rigid belief in the right to a diagnosis can be nothing more than a self-justification for a morally correct but rigid doctor. If a patient can take the diagnosis with equanimity, he can hardly have understood the implications, but if it causes distress at every telling, ignorance is merciful.

On the other hand a patient can hardly be criticised for the absence of insight if no one has told them of the diagnosis. Like so many decisions in medicine there is no universal rule. Even if it is felt damaging to force information about the diagnosis on the patient, this is no reason to ignore their wishes. "Does he take sugar?" is more often asked of the carer of the dement than of the child with learning disability. Patients are infantilised "for their own good", and a doctor who instructed his nurses not to force fluids on his reluctant demented patient was recently struck off by the GMC for 6 months.

Paying for treatment

Another measure of stigma is the value society places on treatment. Just as many schizophrenic patients have to endure the apathy induced by dopamine antagonists rather than the benefits of the newer but much more expensive neuroleptics, so the introduction of cholinergic drugs was greeted with unpardonable apathy by doctors and by some of the Alzheimer's Disease Society. Many health authorities placed a ban on their use under the NHS or imposed severe rationing. An example was the refusal by the Wandsworth Ethical Committee to allow patients who had completed a six-month double-blind study of medication to continue the medication in an open label study. They felt it unlikely that any medication could help a dementia, and any such proposals should be restricted to the most scientifically valid procedure. On the other hand, patients who felt they had benefited were bitterly upset, and were referred to another centre, rather than give up hope. The results of the trial showed that the committee was too pessimistic – a lesson that ethical purity may lead to human misery.

One reason for such an attitude is that ageing should be respected and not treated. Certainly 20% of 80-year-olds are dementing, as are 50% of those over 90. It is easy to see how the stigma of dementia is not so much the result of the stigma of ageing as the cause. Healthy ageing may involve some loss of interest in current events and a willingness to see a pattern in human events which repeats itself generation by generation, thus creating an apparent sang froid. Prompt recall of the name of the Prime Minister or the date is no marker for psychological health and yet a patient of mine was nearly denied the opportunity to marry his sexual partner of many years for that reason. The ability to weigh the merits of a decision to marry is regarded as a waning power of the ageing, which can be readily removed by legal action, whilst the foolish impulses of the young are regarded with equanimity. The cynic might feel this has something to do with the financial consequences of such a decision for the younger generation.

Premorbid states

Unlike schizophrenia most dementias present in the senium after a successful life. The very fact that one has reached such an age is an indication of psychological health (Sims 1987). There should be no surprise that such subjects should have become Presidents of the USA (Rooseveldt, Reagan) and British Prime Ministers (Churchill, Wilson). The willingness of President Reagan, in particular, to acknowledge his condition has helped to reduce the stigma of Alzheimer's disease. Even though his prosopagnosia (difficulty recognising faces) caused difficulty during his presidency, the dementia did not prevent him being an outstandingly successful holder of that office. Alzheimer's dementia does not arrive on a clean slate. The dementia and disinhibition interact with the premorbid personality such that the dominating irrascible dement is just as much if not more intolerable, as the triggering of such outbursts become increasingly meaningless. Maybe it is for this reason that the public see dements as unpredictable and even dangerous. A patient did indeed murder her sister by pushing her downstairs, but acts of deliberate and sustained aggression are rare, especially in the later stages. When they do occur they are usually the result of cognitive defect, as for example when a demented lady threw her husband out of bed in the morning thinking that the elderly man in her bed had little resemblance to the young man she thought was her spouse. The degree to which patients reduce their age does not help. In mild dementia the patient may exhibit marked irritability not unlike the experience of premenstrual tension, and cause despair in the carer. As the condition progresses, however, apathy becomes the predominant emotion and sleep the predominant state. The carer has to come to terms with the loss and can only successfully nurse their patient through the final stages when the bereavement process is complete (see below). There are few more tragic interactions than a despised daughter trying to extract an expression of love from a demented mother who only has memories of her absent son.

Stigma is imposed on the sufferer not only from assumed blame but also because the disorder makes them unpredictable, irresponsible and incurable. For all these reasons a diagnosis of dementia disadvantages the subject, often with good reason. Certainly one would not want someone suffering from dementia to be driving, running dangerous machinery, or indeed making decisions for the population at large by holding the nuclear key. The failure of some cervical smear programmes has been because of a tendency to redeploy those doctors with brain damage into this area, where the loss of vigilance is critical. The progressive removal of the privileges of citizenship must cause pain for the carer if not for the subject. The supposed irreversibilty leaves the exceptional subject who does recover in difficulties to prove the extent of their recovery.

Medicalisation

Whilst the stigma of the functionally ill may be increased by medicalisation, knowledge of the brain damage of the dement is essential if the patient is to escape censure from her healthy peers. Such an attitude must not lead to therapeutic nihilism, but a determination to enjoy and exploit declining powers. For example many people with Alzheimer's disease continue to appreciate music and retain the ability to play their instrument. Becoming less critical of their peers, their personality may change for the better, such that the care of these patients may be unusually rewarding, provided the carer has indeed passed through the process of bereavement, and is prepared to enjoys the skills which remain. The occasional response reminding one of previous skills is no longer seized on with hope for full recovery but seen as a marker of the past. The efforts of the patient to cope with the simple demands of a social programme can be rewarded as an indication that all is not lost.

Self help

The carer has to cope not only with the increasing demands of their patient but also the withdrawal of those who do not know how to relate to the person who was once their colleague and friend. This reaction is not so much due to stigma but the response of many to change and hurt. This emphasises the value of the Alzheimer's Society, which can keep carers in contact with one another, and lessen the impact of death. Cognitive loss is likely to be a necessary part of ageing, but the current advances in knowledge of the chemistry of Alzheimer's dementia suggests that this mental illness will be less stigmatised in the future.

References

Crisp AH, Gelder MG, Rix S, Meltzer HI & Rowlands OJ (2000) Stigmatisation of people with mental illness. *British Journal of Psychiatry* **177**: 4–7.

Hare E (1962) Masturbatory insanity; the history of an idea. *Journal of Mental Science* **108**: 1–25.

Macalpine I & Hunter R (1966) The insanity of King George III: a classic case of porphyria. *British Medical Journal* **i**: 65–71.

Sims A (1987) Why the excess mortality from mental illness? *British Medical Journal* **294**: 956–7.

Commentary on Part 4

Sally Mitchison

This commentary considers points raised in the preceding chapters and also during the subsequent discussion at the RSM Psychiatry Section meeting on 11 January 2000 (references to contributions made during the discussion at the London meeting are attributed to the individual speakers).

Stigmatisation within psychiatry

The contributors to this section consider different aspects of stigmatisation. They discuss stigmatisation of the mentally disordered, differential stigmatisation of different mental disorders, self-stigmatisation and failure to perceive disorder in the self contributing to a lack of insight. While these are all interesting and relevant to the Changing Minds Campaign, I am particularly concerned with stigmatising perceptions of mental disorders in doctors and nurses. Only if we put our own house in order can we criticise others. The spring-cleaning entailed will include much rearranging of mental furniture and some throwing out of comfortable but old-fashioned and now somewhat threadbare assumptions. Unfortunately there is little recent evidence on the extent to which doctors and nurses stigmatise mental disorders. Much more is known about the models suggested – usually by psychiatrists – to account for such disorders. In Chapters 33, 35 and 37 Crisp, Johns and Allison-Bolger give historical accounts of different models of mental disorders.

Different models

Models that focus on agency – that a patient's behaviour is responsible for the disorder – are stigmatising if we assume that we are all equally able to chose how we live and behave. We need to avoid the trap of blaming victims. A social adaptation model, as Gelder and Russell point out in Chapters 32 and 36, may simply shift the stigma from the patient to the patient's family (or occupation, social group or ethnic group). A biological model risks the stigma of tainted genes. Genetic difference may be considered socially adaptive (though not necessarily more acceptable) as Wolpert and Evans point out in Chapter 34. But a biological model may also foster a eugenic view and paternalistic legislation rationalised as necessary and compassionate (Chapter 37).

Non-understandable behaviour

Stigma does not just arise out of the model. Allison-Bolger argues that stigmatisation of the mad arises partly as a result of madness being construed as the result of illness (a biological model) but also because madness is beyond common understanding and the behaviour of the mad deviates from social norms. In Chapter 38 Kellett makes a strong plea for medical diagnosis – frontal lobe dementia – of some deviant behaviour.

Behaviour is a key issue for the Changing Minds Campaign. It is what the most negative attributions in the Royal College of Psychiatrists' survey of public attitudes are concerned with: "unpredictable" and "dangerous to others". Some functional disorders such as migraine and irritable bowel syndrome carry little stigma. This is because they do not normally result in behaviour that is non-understandable or non-acceptable.

I would challenge Russell's equation of prejudiced stigmatisation with discrimination. Kellett makes the point that it can be dangerous to have patients with some disorders in charge of machinery. In some situations it is right to discriminate. But Russell is right to point to the risk of prejudice replacing careful discrimination in determining when someone is fit to train as a nurse. Or, I would suggest, in deciding who is fit to drive a car.

At the London meeting, Dr Sandy Robertson suggested that in tackling stigmatisation we need to think carefully how to respond to judgemental views about people with mental disorders. An illness model may explain behaviour and make it more understandable. But it does not necessarily excuse it. Crisp acknowledges the part personality and particularly personality pathology has to play in the stigmatisation of depression. But for "cross infection" from personality pathology one might expect to find more compassion and tolerance for depression. Depression is a relatively understandable disorder even though we project onto the depressed our own fear of giving in to despair. Yet, one in five of the public surveyed think that patients with a severe depression "could pull themselves together".

Johns addresses the problem of behaviour directly. He suggests that whether or not some difficult behaviour should be tolerated depends on capacity. If the patient can understand and believe what the doctor says and retain it for long enough to weigh it in the balance before making a decision then that patient has capacity.

A psychiatric diagnosis

There are different views about whether a psychiatric diagnosis increases or reduces stigmatisation. It can help to have frightening or despairing personal experience confirmed as a feature of a known illness. It can also be destigmatising. Russell argues strongly for the inclusion of obesity in our thinking about eating disorders. We resist seeing serious obesity as the disorder it really is; we won't allow that it is an illness. This leads not just to personal distress but to under-treatment of a disorder that has high costs for the health service as well as for the patient.

Yet Allison-Bolger emphasises the limiting and alienating assumptions behind using an explanatory illness model for mental disorder. And Crisp finds it necessary to point out that in our polarisation of depressed as opposed to normal feeling we deal with our own insecurities at the cost of reifying the experience of others. He also reminds us of the potential for depressive experience to generate wisdom. There is no mention of this in most psychiatric textbooks.

The naming of a disorder is important. Gelder would wish for more distinctive names to be given to anxiety disorders.The changes from "mental handicap" to "learning disability" and from "mental illness" to "mental health disorder" were prompted by a wish to destigmatise. But changing the signifier – a name – does not in itself change the perception of what is signified – the disorder. It is difficult to open one's mind to really think about mental disorders without stigmatisation. Allison-Bolger suggests we consider the individual and society in a way that Gestalt psychotherapy might construe as "figure and (back)ground".

Holding other possibilities in mind

Allison-Bolger invites us to hold in mind the possibility that the patient is the sane person in an insane world. This may be difficult to achieve in clinical situations structured by psychiatric institutions – even in day hospitals or assertive outreach projects. But it may be possible to hold an open mind on models of mental disorder. Ordinary psychiatric care could benefit from adopting routinely the multifactorial approach described by Crisp.

Professor Martin has studied changes in brain activity demonstrated by neuroimagery in depressed patients treated either by an antidepressant or by interpersonal psychotherapy (Martin 1995). Each group improved substantially and showed different but consistent changes in brain activity. This is one of only two studies that have assessed the effect on the brain of medication compared with therapy. It is a measure of unifactorial thinking there has not been more interest in this field and that this remarkable finding, first reported in 1995, has yet to be replicated. I would suggest that belief in a sole model of psychopathology, while comfortingly straightforward, contributes to the view that mental disorders happen to unfortunates other than ourselves. The slogan "Every Family in the Land" is intended to remind us that our families and ourselves also suffer mental disorders. We see the patients we care for as different from ourselves and our families. It becomes all too easy to judge and stigmatise.

Differences

Difference is hard to accept. Claire Rayner made this point at the London meeting. Dr Mike Shooter followed on to suggest that our current government has stirred up strong feeling by trying to deny that there are differences: between those who are ill and those who are not, between different disorders and between different experiences of disorder. Melba Wilson from Mind suggested that tackling social exclusion means that differences have to be addressed. If we are going to acknowledge that differences exist we could start with differences in psychiatric provision within the National Health Service. At the London meeting Cliff Prior from the National Schizophrenia Fellowship (now Rethink) urged that "the best should be(come) routine". This will require more resources for basic clinical services and training than we currently have. But I suggest that training and treatment geared around any single model of psychopathology will not deliver a good, all-round clinical service. Some disorders and some patients will be seen as different and viewed as not really ill, not treatable or not appropriate for psychological interventions. This is stigmatising. What is lacking is a greater acceptance of difference – an open mind.

Reference

Martin SD, Rais S, Martin E, Richardson M et al. (1999) SPECT changes with interpersonal therapy versus venlafaxine for depression. *Syllabus and Proceedings of the American Psychiatric Association 1999 Annual Meeting.* Washington, DC: APA: 45–46.

Acknowledgement

I am grateful to Dr Sandy Robertson for the assistance and support he has provided in helping me develop the ideas expressed in this discussion.

Part 5

Personality disorder, its nature, stigmatisation, relationship to mental illness and its treatment possibilities

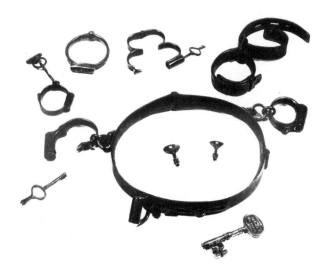

"Instruments of restraint" used in Bethlem Hospital up to the early 19th century

39 Personality disorder: The origins of the concept. Nature and nurture

Michael Shooter

Introduction

The concept of personality disorder has run into rough waters. Storms have raged around the report of Judge Fallon's Committee of Inquiry into the Personality Disorder Unit, Ashworth Special Hospital, and the proposals of the then Home Secretary, Jack Straw, for managing dangerous people with severe personality disorder. Politicians and practitioners have been swept into very public debate over treatability issues and civil rights on a tide swelled by press accounts of lurid, criminal cases.

In the process, use of the terminology for the basic subgroups of personality disorder (PD) has become confused. Concepts like severe personality disorder (SPD) and dangerous severe personality disorder (DSPD) have been used as if they were bona fide psychiatric disorders in their own right with some sort of inevitable progression between them.

This has obscured the deeper, underlying issue of whether there is any such thing as a "normal" personality, integrated, stable and pervasive, against which any personality disorder might be judged (Dowson and Grounds 1995). This presentation sets out to trace the history of the issue and its consequences for modern psychiatric practice.

General historical overview

Not surprisingly, the river that runs down to these current debates is difficult to navigate. Its source lies somewhere in the classical masks of Greek theatre and the concept of bodily humours, laid down by Hippocrates, developed by later writers into a first theory of personality types, and transformed by Aquinas into the medieval "condition of a person".

Thereafter, it meanders through a semantic swampland over half a millennium with rival schools of philosophy on either bank. On the one hand, personality is seen as a surface representation and its disorder as a disturbance of physical functions. On the other, personality is part of the inner character and its disorder a disruption of the continuity of "self".

Not until the nineteenth century does "science" attempt some rationalisation of the problem – albeit with a continuing debate overlaid, for the first time, with moral overtones. The school of "automatism" saw personality disorder as a lower form of existence escaping from higher controls. The schools of faculty psychology and associationism attempted rival theories of mind that would pave the way for both psychoanalytic concepts of the early twentieth century and the later twentieth-century packaging of taxonomy, statistics and rating scales.

The modern concern has been to define more clearly the trait components of personality, their clustering into types, and the diagnosis of disorders based upon those types. Beneath that concern, however, the murkier historical waters run deep and surface occasionally around debates on the relationship between personality disorder in general and the body of mental illness, whether it is or is not the proper concern of psychiatrists, and the particular arguments about "psychopaths" or their DSPD equivalent.

The remainder of this presentation looks in more detail at those historical phases and the delicately balanced questions with which we are left.

Classical background

The Latin *persona* is borrowed from the masks of Greek theatre in which the actor held a megaphone to the mouthpiece, through (*per*) which the sound (*sona*) was amplified. It was therefore a device by which the actor projected a role to the outside world (Casey 1998). The persona was part of a drama on stage or in life; it was the semblance of things that the actor wished us to see. It was not the actor himself.

Hippocrates thought that all disease arose from imbalances between the four bodily humours: yellow bile from the liver, black bile from the spleen, blood and phlegm. A disordered person could therefore be described as choleric, melancholic, sanguine or phlegmatic, and Hippocrates' pupil Theophrastus subdivided these into 30 or more personality types. Empedocles linked these to the four elements (earth, air, fire and water) which worked in harmony or discord through the intervention of Love or Strife. Galen, who thought Empedocles the founder of the Italian School of Medicine, associated these with more modern sounding concepts of temperamental style that are still rooted in the "forms" of disease. St Thomas Aquinas, in his description of personality as the "condition or mode of appearance of a person", harped back to the masks of Greek theatre once more.

Through all these classical writings runs the search for recognisable forms of human behaviour, but the personality remains a very bodily function. It is a concept that would be part of the debate for the next eight hundred years.

The semantic swamp

During succeeding centuries, words like "personality", "type", "constitution", "temperament" and "character" float in and out of usage in what is a taxonomist's nightmare. Without becoming bogged down too deeply in the nuances of meaning, perhaps two broad trends can be identified.

In one view, the "self", insofar as it exists as an integrated and personalised set of characteristics that would be recognised by someone as different from another, is reflected in physical aspects. Disorder is a disturbance of bodily functions or of self-awareness in an almost organic sense – like sleep-walking or hysterical anaesthesia or disintegration of consciousness. This physical interpretation can be traced through Gall's phrenology (in which the shape of the skull gave clues not only to the underlying shape of the brain but also to a person's character itself) to Kretschmer's personality types (in which the stocky, pyknic type was linked with manic depression and the thin, asthenic to schizophrenia) and Sheldon's endomorphs (the viscerotonic, social, relaxed pain avoiders of life), mesomorphs (the somatotonic, assertive, energetic but often callous disregarders of other people's feelings), and ectomorphs (cerebrotonic, often awkward, social isolates) (Casey 1998).

In the other view, the "self" is a more metaphysical sense of personal identity – the unchangeable "core character" of Kant and John Stuart Mill, the self-awareness of

Descartes, Hume's series of perceptual moments linked by memory, and the more interactionist theories of Royce and Baldwin, in which continuity relies on feedback from others and the way we are seen (Berrios 1993).

Nineteenth-century rationalisation

The argument escapes from this through typical nineteenth-century rationalisation – but only at the expense of dispute between individual schools of psychology, based, it has to be said, on historical fashion rather than true empirical evidence.

The concept of the hierarchical nervous system, as championed by Hughlings Jackson, was paralleled by automatism in which personality disorder was a lower form of behaviour escaping from higher controls. It would live on in modern English criminal law as "involuntary conduct" in which a person could commit an act that would be an offence if under normal control of bodily movements. Even where the offence was one of strict liability, the accused would not be criminally responsible for the consequences unless the loss of control arose from his own failure to take reasonable precautions.

Faculty psychology, drawing on the writings of Kant and Thomas Reid, saw the world as a set of functions (intellectual/cognitive; emotional/orectic; volitional/cognative) in which experience alone could not explain all knowledge. Personality disorder was a failure of mental faculty – of the "will".

Associationism, grounded in the work of British philosophers like Locke, and Maine de Biran's concept of "habitude", saw the mind as an empty slate with knowledge coming in from the external world by combinations under the rules of association. Personality disorder was therefore a loss of coherence between cognitive, emotional and volitional information rather than the faculties themselves (Berrios 1993).

The Faculty psychology school would contribute to later personality profiling and ideas of brain localisation and mapping. Associationism would contribute to psychophysics and psychological quantification. Both paved the way for the new twentieth century psychiatric taxonomy.

Psychoanalytic concepts

It is a moot point as to whether Freud was really interested in the "character" of a person as opposed to the interpretation of his individual symptoms; but personality is linked to his developmental phases and colours the defence mechanisms arising from them. Thus, being "stuck" in the oral phase, in its sucking and biting sub-phases, leads to the oral dependent type (gullible, swallowing anything he is told) and the oral sadistic type (distrustful, sarcastic and cantankerous). The anal phase and battles over sphincter control may lead to the obsessional, anankastic type. The phallic phase may lead to the narcissistic type, the hysterical type and the masochistic type.

Reich's "character disorder" was based on psychosexual conflict, the neurotic solution to which encouraged the formation of a rigid "armour" against perceived threats in the world. Vaillant classified personality disorder according to defence mechanisms in general. Millon regarded personality as a sort of psychological "immune system" that protected its thin- or thick-skinned host against both external and internal stresses but created symptoms in the process (Casey 1998). Stone revived echoes of the past in his idea of a circular process in which the personality was the true "face" of an individual, as opposed to a mask-like protective "façade", which could become a new, true "face" if it was worn for long enough and its defences pervaded and overwhelmed the individual's original character. It is no surprise that DSM-IV talks of a "defence functioning scale" as a measurement of coping styles.

The ego psychologists set the personality in the context of relationships both within the self (between ego reality and id unconscious) and between the self and others. Sullivan's anxious need for security can lead, paradoxically, to the exploitative, ambitious character. Adler's inadequate character strives to repair his deficits and over-compensates in the process. Horney identified three responses: the "move towards people" of the dependent (compliant) personality; the "move against people" of the sociopathic (aggressive) personality; and the "move away from people" of the schizoid (detached) personality. Kernberg delved deeper into the specific "basic fault" of the borderline psychotic.

Twentieth-century packaging

From these historical waters, by a path never less than tortuous, the river emerges into the delta of modern measurement techniques. Monolithic (molar) descriptions of human behaviour are broken down into trait (molecular) components (Berrios 1993). Traits themselves are defined as those clusters of enduring and pervasive patterns of perception, thinking and relationships of mixed constitutional and social origin, that influence a person's behaviour from early childhood on. By the new science of correlation, statistics and probability theory, the elusive traits are measurable in rating scales. Attempts are made to localise them on maps of cerebral function. Clusters are seen to go together to make up broader descriptions of personality types. The traits are at once what marks out the individual as unique from his neighbour and as similar to all those of the same disposition (Oldham 1994).

The personality disorder can be distinguished from the several norms as clusters of traits that are inflexible and maladaptive, that cause significant functional impairment or subjective distress, and one exhibited in a wide range of important social and personal contexts. The personality disorders finally take their place in the twentieth century psychiatric taxonomy of the International Classification of Diseases (ICD-10) and the Diagnostic and Statistical Manual (DSM-IV).

And yet the central question remains. Is this the final reduction of a rambling, psychophilosophical debate to scientific reality – the long sought after specific personality disorders that adequately describe the disturbance of an individual's functioning? Or is it a specious validity superimposed on what is a hotchpotch of overlapping traits, vague symptoms of distress, variable patterns of behaviour, loose psychodynamic concepts, moral judgements, gender discrimination and legal conveniences?

Relationships with mental illness

Nowhere is this question more insistent than in the relationship of personality disorder to the main body of mental illness – and its corollary: Is personality disorder part of the remit of mainstream psychiatry?

Personality disorders in general were once seen as "formes frustres" of nineteenth-century insanity (Berrios 1993). But could there be true insanity without intellectual delusion? Pinel ("manie sans delire"), Esquirol ("monomanias"), Trélat ("folie lucide") and Pritchard ("moral insanity") offered their own affirmative resolutions to this question and laid the path for acceptance of affective disorders without psychosis, for the removal of its sufferers from criminal responsibility, and for the recognition, perhaps, of personality disorder as part of mental illness. Thereafter, the argument could shift to the relationship of personality disorder to other disorders. Were the neuroses the periodic manifestation of underlying personality disorder? Were personality disorders separate illnesses in their own right? Since, according to the French "theory of constitutions", the personality was the total synthesis of an individual's existence, were its disorders the very stuff of all mental illnesses whether of minor or major degree?

The strange and unique case of the "psychopath" raised even more debate. It began as a description of all mental disorders that were simply "psychopathological" in its broadest sense. Koch's concept of "psychopathic inferiority" introduced an element of moral judgement. Schneider saw the "psychopathic personality" as a form of being rather than an illness. Kahn plotted an imbalance of impulse, temperament and character in what was, for him, a sort of three-legged semi-illness (Berrios 1993). Only with Henderson does psychopathy become a true illness "state" but one which is difficult to treat and the existence of which makes everything else about an individual difficult to help too. Thus does the concept of treatability, whatever the status of psychopathy as a mental disorder, become all-important – and the foundation of the modern political debate become entrenched.

Conclusions

And so, finally, we are left with a number of delicately balanced issues for debate. Can the categories of personality and their disorders be seen as discrete entities or are they a loose and overlapping amalgam of different concepts? Can eleven clusters of traits ever be enough to pin down the huge range of human morbidity? What is the relationship between "traits" (useful but more arbitrary) to "dimensions" (less arbitrary but of questionable clinical use)? Are personality disorders really stable over time and context or are they a product of their circumstances? Do the differences between the taxonomy of ICD-10 and DSM-IV reflect a lack of true scientific validity? Are personality disorders really part of mental illness at all or part of the general spectrum of social behaviour (Kendell 2002)?

Those who would deny that they were a bona fide mental illness would point to difficulties of definition, vagueness of symptomatology, obscurity of aetiology and a lack of clearly worked-out treatments – the very antithesis of the disease concept. To include them within the psychiatrist's remit would be to make him the arbiter of social behaviour and land him, paradoxically, in a position of responsibility without power. The very terminology used – "psychopath" and "hysteric" – is a vehicle for stigma and abuse.

The opposite camp would affirm their place among the mental illnesses as serious conditions that cause psychological damage to the individual and those around them, and increased morbidity and mortality. To deny their existence as illnesses leads to legal nonsenses such as the "irresistible impulse". More importantly, if the individual with a personality disorder is "not ill" he is responsible for his own suffering, is regarded as "bad" and consigned to the dustbin of therapeutic neglect (Casey 1998).

There is no clear resolution to this debate and it will go on, for it is the product of a history which is as much to do with philosophical fashion as empirical, scientific evidence. The question of "nature" versus "nurture" is not primarily about aetiology; rather, it is about whether the idea of personality, and therefore its disorders, really exists as a natural entity or a figment of the literary imagination of famous protagonists and the faith of their followers. If the latter, can we grumble if modern politicians add their own labels to the taxonomy in the interests of political convenience?

References

Berrios GE (1993) European views on personality disorders. *Comprehensive Psychiatry* **34**: 14–30.

Casey P (1998). In: Stein G & Wilkinson G (eds). *Seminars in General Adult Psychiatry.* London: Gaskell: 753–814.

Dowson JH & Grounds AT (1995) *Personality Disorders: Recognition and Clinical Management.* Cambridge: Cambridge University Press.

Kendell RE (2002) The distinction between personality disorder and mental illness. *British Journal of Psychiatry* **180**: 110–115.

Oldham JM (1994) Personality disorders: current perspectives. *Journal of the American Medical Association* **272**: 1770–6.

40 Co-morbidity: Personality disorder and mental illness – the nature of their relationship

Jeremy W Coid

Introduction

Co-morbidity is generally taken to imply the occurrence of independent psychiatric disorders in an individual patient. This is of considerable clinical and theoretical importance as the presence of one disorder can markedly affect the treatment, course, and phenomenology of another. Furthermore, the extent and pattern of co-morbidity will also indicate areas of overlap and redundancy among diagnoses. The study of co-morbidity is therefore of major importance in the refinement of psychiatric diagnosis. However, the process of separating personality disorders from major mental disorders into different axes of a multi-axial system is not without problems. The introduction of the DSM-III-R Manual pointed out that "there is no assumption that each mental disorder is a discrete entity with sharp boundaries (discontinuity) between it and other mental disorders". Vize and Tyrer (1994) were critical of this system, concluding that considerable confusion remains and that many studies show a continuum between mental state and personality disorders for certain categories. Nevertheless, both the DSM and ICD glossaries persist with the categorical rather than the dimensional approach, as does most published research on personality disorders.

Epidemiology of Axis I co-morbidity

Considerably more is known about the co-morbidity of Axis I than Axis II conditions, with the exception of antisocial personality disorder (ASPD). The epidemiologic catchment area (ECA) study was the first to document that co-morbidity is widespread, not only amongst patients but also in the general population (Robins et al. 1991). Over 54% of ECA respondents with a lifetime history of at least one DSM-III psychiatric disorder were found to have a second diagnosis. Similar results were found in the more recent National Co-morbidity survey in the USA (Kessler 1995) where 56% also had one or more disorders. Associations were found between almost all disorders, especially between major depression and dysthymia and mania. Disorders of a single type, e.g. affective disorders, tended to be more strongly related to each other than another type, e.g. substance-use disorders. Only 21% of all lifetime disorders occurred in a sub-sample of respondents who had no additional lifetime co-morbidity. Thus 79% of disorders occurred with lifetime co-morbidity. Furthermore, over 50% of lifetime disorders occurred in 14% of the population who had a history of three or more disorders. Overall, co-morbidity was associated with both severity and chronicity.

Axis I–Axis II co-morbidity

Excessive co-morbidity within Axis II can result from a series of diagnostic arte-facts. Caron and Rutter (1991) pointed out that the DSM and ICD follow quite dif-ferent approaches. Problems can occur with the DSM system where diagnoses are made on algorithms based on specified constellations but without regard to the presence or absence of accompanying symptomatology of a different kind, apart from a few exceptions. Consequently, when a patient has one diagnosis there is usually at least one other diagnosis. The ICD-10 system allows multiple diagnoses, but tends to discourage them by adoption of a pattern approach. Caron and Rutter argue that the underlying concept of the WHO approach is probably correct because it is more likely that a patient would have a single disease rather than sev-eral.

Loranger (1992) reviewed the literature on research diagnostic instruments and concluded that self-reporting inventories are not suitable for making personality disorder diagnoses, although they may have potential use as screening devices. Self-report instruments produce considerably more Axis II categories than research diagnostic interviews, indicating a high level of false positives and inevitably lead-ing to excessive co-morbidity. Earlier versions of interviews also experienced prob-lems. Artificial co-morbidity could arise when the same criterion appeared in more than one diagnostic category. This problem is largely eliminated from recent inter-view schedules. But subtle differences between superficially similar criteria in two or more different categories does require considerable sophistication in interview-ing skills.

Additional problems can arise when disorders defined in terms of one main symptom complex are sub-divided into various sub-categories, particularly in the DSM system. In some cases, one disorder may represent an early manifestation of another, or could be part of, or a secondary manifestation of, another. However, studying artefactual co-morbidity may be helpful in throwing further light on the nature of the disorders involved.

Caron and Rutter (1991) proposed four potential processes which can lead to true co-morbidity:

1. *Shared risk factors:* Overlap may occur when two disorders share the same risk factor or factors. Many psychiatric disorders are multi-factorial in origin and many aetiological factors are not diagnosis-specific.
2. *Overlap between risk factors:* Even when the risk factors for two disorders are distinct and different, there may still be co-morbidity because the risk factors themselves are associated. In this case, the individual may be at risk for two separate conditions.
3. *The co-morbid pattern constitutes a meaningful syndrome:* A constellation with a co-morbid set of symptoms which shows relatively poor response to treatment compared to a "pure" constellation of symptoms would tend to suggest that there are indeed two separate conditions present.
4. *One disorder creates an increased risk for the other:* Life stressors can be risk factors for psychiatric disorder. Evidence suggests that individuals shape and select their own environments and that various psychiatric disorders play a part in generating stress and adversity. For example, stress induced by one dis-order, such as ASPD, could lead to a higher risk of other disorders, e.g. depression.

Clinical difficulties in differential diagnosis

In the UK, undergraduate and post-graduate training schemes do not routinely teach how to diagnose personality disorder. In the USA, residents training in psychiatry are taught to consider both Axis I and Axis II disorders when carrying out a diagnostic formulation. But even with training in the multi-axial approach, it can still be difficult to make a satisfactory differential diagnosis. For example, it can be exceptionally difficult to make an Axis II diagnosis in the presence of pervasive Axis I disorder, especially severe psychotic illness. Furthermore, personality psychopathology may complicate both the diagnosis and the treatment of Axis I disorder. Even in the absence of Axis I disorder, personality disorder psychopathology may not be initially apparent and some features of Axis II disorder may not be diagnosed until the clinician knows the patient well. The theoretical orientation of the clinician may also influence whether an Axis I or Axis II diagnosis is made. Nevertheless, it is essential that an adequate differential diagnosis is made because Axis II disorders can be as severe and disabling as Axis I disorders.

Clinical difficulties are influenced by several theoretical difficulties. It remains unclear whether personality disorders should always be separated from clinical syndromes in a multi-axial system. Is there a continuum between mental state and personality disorders? For example, it has been argued that borderline personality disorder (BPD) may be a variant of affective disorder (Coid 1993). Similarly, there is increasing consensus that there is no clear dividing line between avoidant personality disorder and social phobia. A study of the aetiology of personality disorders further supported the argument that not all should be contained in a separate Axis (Coid 1999). Preliminary findings suggest that avoidant personality disorder and BPD fail to maintain diagnostic stability over time in a significant percentage of patients, undermining the criterion of temporal stability within the definition of personality disorder.

Studies of inter-Axis co-morbidity

A literature search was carried out of studies of inter-axis co-occurrence using Medline and Psychlit. This was supplemented by a hand search of references from available publications. Only studies which employed a standardised assessment procedure to establish both Axis I and Axis II diagnoses were included. Studies which used self-report data to establish Axis II diagnoses were excluded. Only two previous studies were found which examined the full range of disorders from both Axes and then carried out a statistical examination of co-morbidity between the individual categories (Alnaes and Torgerson 1988; Zimmerman and Coryell 1989). Four other studies carried out statistical analyses after combining personality disorders into clusters or clinical syndromes into broad groupings (Oldham et al. 1995; Maier et al. 1991; Nestadt et al. 1992), or else limited the number of conditions studied (Jackson et al, 1991).

An alternative and less satisfactory method of examining Axis I/Axis II co-morbidity is to include studies which selected a single Axis I category but examined the full range of Axis II disorders. This method is limited in that few Axis II disorders occur in isolation over the lifespan in a single subject, as has been discussed above. Differences between studies may have emerged due to the presence of additional but unreported Axis I conditions which confound the findings. The differences between samples and research diagnostic instruments will also contribute to the variability between studies. However, bearing these limitations in mind, the main findings from this review are summarised in Table 1.

Table 1. Summary of Axis I/Axis II co-morbidity from review of literature

Axis I disorders	Co-morbid Axis II disorders
Mood disorders	Borderline Avoidant Dependent
Schizophrenia, delusional	Schizotypal Paranoid
Substance use	Antisocial Borderline
Phobias	Avoidant Dependent
Anxiety / Panic	Borderline Avoidant Dependent
Obsessive–compulsive	Obsessive–compulsive Dependent
Eating disorders	Borderline Avoidant Dependent
Post-traumatic stress	Borderline Obsessive–compulsive Avoidant Paranoid

Mood disorders

The suggestion that mood disorders correlate with Cluster B disorders (Siever and Davis 1991), particularly BPD, received moderate support from the review of literature. There was greater co-morbidity with avoidant and dependant personality disorders from Cluster C. There was a strong association between dysthymia and BPD, but this was not always the case for depressive disorder. The relationship between BPD and mood disorders is not entirely resolved (Kroll and Ogata 1987; Gunderson and Phillips 1991). The defining features of BPD include affect dysregulation, physically self-damaging acts, chronic feelings of emptiness and intense relationships. BPD may represent a variant of mood (and impulse) pathology in the same way that schizotypal personality disorder is a characterologic variant of schizophrenic pathology. It has been argued that BPD represents a diagnosis that is literally on the boundary of mood disorders and may thereby represent both a personality and a mood disorder (Widiger 1989).

Psychotic disorders

Several studies demonstrate high levels of co-morbidity between schizophrenia and related psychotic disorders and schizotypal personality disorder and, in certain studies, with BPD and paranoid personality disorders. The latter demonstrate moderate consistency across studies (Zimmerman and Coryell 1989; Oldham et al. 1995; Jackson et al. 1991). Cluster A (schizotypal, paranoid, schizoid) disorders are more prevalent in subjects with lifetime schizophrenia and schizoaffective disorders compared to other categories. Schizotypal personality disorder was a new addition to the DSM-III and intended to describe certain psychopathological characteristics which are usually stable and assumed to be genetically related to a spectrum of disorders, including chronic schizophrenia (Spitzer et al. 1979). However, the ICD-10 now includes this condition in the section with schizophrenia and not as a personality disorder.

Substance use disorder

Co-morbidity between substance use disorders and Axis II is complex. There is strong evidence that personality disorder may act as a risk factor for the development of substance abuse. Axis II disorders also modify the course of dependence on alcohol and drugs. Subjects with co-morbidity tend to have earlier onset of substance abuse, more additional psychiatric symptoms and higher rates of polysubstance abuse. Similarly, features of Axis II psychopathology may emerge as a consequence of substance abuse, although there is less evidence of this phenomenon.

Drug dependency has been found to have a high level of co-morbidity with ASPD followed by BPD. However, the internal consistency of this research is compromised by the questionable independence of ASPD and substance use disorders (Gerstling et al. 1990). Several criteria are similar in each condition. When early onset of drug abuse occurs, it can be difficult to decide whether the criteria for ASPD are the result of drug-seeking behaviour, including a criminal lifestyle.

Phobic disorders

Studies are consistent in demonstrating co-morbidity between avoidant and phobic disorders, especially social phobia, followed by dependent personality disorder. BPD also appeared moderately prevalent and was somewhat more so in the context of lifetime studies of Axis I diagnostic data. However, as has already been noted, there no longer appears to be strong evidence for retaining avoidant personality disorder within a separate Axis from social phobia (Herbert et al. 1992; Turner et al. 1993).

Anxiety and panic disorder

Anxiety and panic disorders demonstrate a similar pattern of Axis II co-morbidity with Axis II studies to the phobic disorders, although the overall prevalence of personality disorders tends to be somewhat lower and with less consistency observed between studies. Overall, these tend to show moderately elevated associations with borderline, avoidant, and dependent personality disorders.

Obsessive–compulsive disorder

The review demonstrated a moderate degree of consistency across five studies, demonstrating, as expected, that the highest level of co-morbidity was between obsessive–compulsive disorder, compulsive (now obsessive–compulsive) person-ality disorder and dependent personality disorder. The relationship between obsessivecompulsive disorder and compulsive personality disorder continues to be a matter of debate between those who traditionally view the two conditions along a continuum and those who strongly support separation between the two elements.

Eating disorders

There was a relatively high degree of consistency for association between eating disorders and BPD, followed by avoidant and dependant personality disorders. Binge-eating can be a sign of generalised impulsivity and is included among the criteria for impulsivity in the diagnosis of BPD, indicating a strong potential for overlap. Lacey and Evans (1986) suggest that a "multi-impulsive" subgroup of bulimics exists with many features of BPD and a poor response to treatment.

Post-traumatic stress disorder

Post-traumatic stress disorder is associated with high levels of co-morbidity with several other Axis I conditions. There have been few studies of association with Axis II disorders. The evidence suggests that BPD is most prevalent, followed by compulsive, avoidant and paranoid personality disorders. This could reflect an overlap between diagnostic criteria within two Axes. Several criteria for avoidant personality disorder are similar to symptoms of withdrawal and emotional numbing within PTSD. Similarly, hypervigilance and diminished trust overlap with features of paranoid personality disorder.

There are two views of character pathology within PTSD. Firstly, that personality disorder traits were present in these patients before the trauma occurred and have thereby contributed to the actual development of PTSD. Secondly, severe trauma may be sufficient to cause secondary change in character in individuals who have normal pre-morbid functioning. Thus, the high prevalence of BPD could be partly explained by trauma.

The influence of personality disorders on the outcome of Axis I disorder

It is generally thought that personality disorders have a negative effect on the outcome of major mental disorder. The presence of personality disorder tends to impair the response to treatment of the common neurotic disorders (Greer and Cawley 1966), anxiety disorders (Kass et al. 1985), depression (Shea et al. 1992; Mulder et al. 1994), eating disorders (Skodol et al. 1993), schizophrenia (Smith et al. 1993), adolescent, emotional and conduct disorders (Rey et al. 1995), alcohol (Helzer and Pryzbeck 1988) and substance use disorders (Links et al. 1995), and patients treated with crisis intervention (Andreoli et al. 1993). Despite this strong body of evidence, a review by Tyrer et al. (1997) concluded that the view that personality disorder always has a negative effect on the outcome of Axis I order should no longer be held universally.

Tyrer and colleagues argued that previous studies may have measured personality disorder but did not make any allowances for this when planning treatment programmes. Where a worse outcome has been reported, this tends to have been overstated. Many studies demonstrated important baseline differences, and subjects with Axis I–Axis II co-morbidity tend to have higher baseline ratings. But because co-morbid patients have higher baseline ratings, they can improve to exactly the same extent as those with Axis I disorders alone, even though they still have higher levels of pathology at the end of the treatment study. Furthermore, the evidence is not always consistent. For example, several studies suggest that co-morbidity, such as ASPD and substance abuse, may not always have poor outcome. This could be a consequence of planning treatment programmes appropriately in these studies.

There are some limited indications that co-morbidity may result in different outcomes with specific treatments compared to patients with Axis I disorder alone. Tyrer et al. (1997) argued that co-mobidity needs to be considered in the larger context of psychiatric services. The general idea that patients with personality disorders should be excluded from inpatient care because of poor response should be investigated more closely in future. Patients with Axis I/Axis II co-morbidity tend to have more severe conditions. But one study demonstrated that they may have a better outcome, particularly in terms of social function, and when treated as inpatients rather than in the community (Tyrer et al. 1994). The opposite finding was shown with similar patients who had no personality disorder.

Conclusion

Many of these findings are preliminary, but demonstrate the importance of further research and that clinicians should not always assume poor outcome for mental disorders with co-morbid personality disorder. However, there remain a series of problems to be overcome. These include artefactual co-morbidity resulting from poor diagnostic validity and reliability, and diagnostic practices that lead to the misclassification of both Axis I and Axis II disorders. Future studies should include epidemiologically representative samples, particularly samples drawn from the community. Many previous studies have examined a single mental disorder then measured the prevalence of personality disorders in highly selected clinic samples, increasing the risk of Berkson's bias. Statistical error as a result of confounding is rarely addressed within these studies, and analysis may require logistic regression for categorical data or multiple regression when using dimensional scores. It will also be necessary to incorporate aetiological measures in an attempt to examine whether apparently separate diagnostic categories have similar risk factors.

The majority of studies suggest that co-morbid personality disorder leads to a poorer outcome for major mental disorder. But it is time to re-evaluate this evidence as this may have been overstated for certain conditions, and plan for co-morbid Axis II psychopathology in future treatment programmes. In the past, patients have sometimes been excluded from inpatient services in the UK on the basis of a diagnosis of personality disorder, even when suffering from severe mental illness, but where difficult and uncooperative behaviour has been anticipated. The development of new treatments for personality disorder remains in the early stages. But, in future, it will be increasingly important and necessary to make accurate clinical diagnoses of personality disorder when co-morbid with major mental disorder, devise suitable treatment programmes, and evaluate their effectiveness.

References

Alnaes R & Torgersen S (1988) The relationship between DSM-III symptom disorders (Axis I) and personality disorders (Axis II) in an outpatient population. *Acta Psychiatrica Scandinavica* **78**: 348–55.

Andreoli A, Frances A, Gex-Fabry M, Aapro N, Gerin P & Dazord A (1993) Crisis intervention in depressed patients with and without DSM-III-R personality disorders. *Journal of Nervous and Mental Disease* **181**: 732–7.

Caron C & Rutter M (1991) Comorbidity in child psychopathology: concepts, issues and research strategies. *Journal of Child Psychology and Psychiatry* **32**: 1063–80.

Coid JW (1993) An affective syndrome in psychopaths with borderline personality disorder? *British Journal of Psychiatry* **162**: 641–50.

Coid JW (1999) Aetiological risk factors for personality disorders. *British Journal of Psychiatry* **175**: 530–8.

Gerstling LJ, Alterman AI, McClellan AT & Woody GE (1990) Antisocial personality disorder in patients with substance abuse disorders: a problematic diagnosis? *American Journal of Psychiatry* **147**: 173–8.

Greer HS & Cawley RH (1966) Some observations on the natural history of neurotic illness. In: *Australian Medical Association, Mervyn Archdall Medical Monograph* No. 3. Glebe: Australasian Medical Publishing Company.

Gunderson JG & Phillips KA (1991) A current view on the interface between borderline personality disorder and depression. *American Journal of Psychiatry* **148**: 967–75.

Helzer JE & Pryzbeck TR (1988) The co-occurrence of alcoholism with other psychiatric disorders in the general population and its impact on treatment. *Journal of Studies on Alcohol* **49**: 219–24.

Herbert JD, Hope DA & Bellack AS (1992) Validity of the distinction between generalised social phobia and avoidant personality disorder. *Journal of Abnormal Psychology* **101**: 332–9.

Jackson HJ, Whiteside HL, Bates GW et al. (1991) Diagnosing personality disorders in psychiatric inpatients. *Acta Psychiatrica Scandinavica* **83**: 206–13.

Kass F, Skodol AE, Charles E, Spitzer RL & Williams JB (1985) Scaled ratings of DSM-III personality disorders. *American Journal of Psychiatry* **143**: 627–30.

Kessler RC (1995) The national comorbidity survey: Preliminary results and future directions. *International Journal of Methods in Psychiatric Research* **5**: 139–51.

Kroll J & Ogata S (1987) The relationship of borderline personality disorder to affective disorders. *Psychiatric Developments* **2**: 105–28.

Lacey JH & Evans CDH (1986) The impulsivist: a multi-impulsive personality disorder. *British Journal of Addiction* **81**: 641–9.

Links PS, Heslegrave RJ, Mitton JE, van Reekum R & Patrick J (1995) Borderline personality disorder and substance abuse: consequences of co-morbidity. *Canadian Journal of Psychiatry* **40**: 9–14.

Loranger AW (1992) Are current self-report and interview measures adequate for epidemiological studies of personality disorders? *Journal of Personality Disorders* **6**: 313–25.

Maier W, Lichtermann D, Klinger T et al. (1991) Prevalences of personality disorders (DSM-III-R) in the community. *Journal of Personality Disorders* **6**: 187–96.

Mulder RT, Joyce PR & Cloninger CR (1994) Temperament and early environment influence comorbidity and personality disorders in major depression. *Comprehensive Psychiatry* **35**: 225–33.

Nestadt G, Romanoski AJ, Samuels JF et al. (1992) The relationship between personality and DSM-III Axis I disorders in the population: results from an epidemiological survey. *American Journal of Psychiatry* **149**: 1228–33.

Oldham JM, Scodol AE, Kellman HD et al. (1995) Comorbidity of Axis I and Axis II disorders. *American Journal of Psychiatry* **152**: 571–8.

Rey JM, Morris Yates A, Singh M, Andrews G & Stewart GW (1995) Continuities between psychiatric disorders in adolescents and personality disorders in young adults. *American Journal of Psychiatry* **152**: 895–900.

Robins LN, Locke BZ & Regier DA (1991) An overview of psychiatric disorders in America. In: Robins CN & Regier DA (eds). *Psychiatric Disorders in America: the Epidemiologic Catchment Study*. New York: Free Press.

Shea MT, Widiger TA & Klein MH (1992) Comorbidity of personality disorders and depression: implications for treatment. *Journal of Consulting and Clinical Psychology* **60**: 857–68.

Siever LJ & Davis KL (1991) A psychobiologic perspective on the personality disorders. *American Journal of Psychiatry* **148**: 1647–58.

Skodol AE, Oldham JM, Hyler SE, Kellman HD, Doidge N & Davies M (1993) Comorbidity of DSMIII- R eating disorders and personality disorders. *International Journal of Eating Disorders* **14**: 403–16.

Smith TE, Deutsch A, Schwartz F & Terkelsen KG (1993) The role of personality in the treatment of schizophrenic and schizoaffective disorder inpatients: a pilot study. *Bulletin of the Menninger Clinic* **57**: 88–99.

Turner SM, Biedel DC & Townsley RM (1992) Social phobia: a comparison of specific and generalized subtypes and avoidant personality disorder. *Journal of Abnormal Psychology* **101**: 326–31.

Tyrer P, Merso S, Onyet S & Johnson T (1994) The effect of personality disorder on clinical outcome, social networks and adjustment: a controlled clinical trial of psychiatric emergencies. *Psychological Medicine* **24**: 731–40.

Tyrer P, Gunderson J, Lyons M & Tohen M (1997) Extent of comorbidity between mental state and personality disorders. *Journal of Personality Disorders* **11**: 242–59.

Vize C & Tyrer P (1994) The relationship between personality and other psychiatric disorders. *Current Opinion in Psychiatry* **7**: 123–8.

Widiger TA (1989) The categorical distinction between personality and affective disorders. *Journal of Personality Disorders* **3**: 77–91.

Zimmerman MT, Coryell W (1989) DSM-III personality disorder diagnoses in a non-patient sample. *Archives of General Psychiatry* **46**: 682–9.

41 The stigma of dangerousness

John Gunn

Introduction

Dangerousness has long been associated with mental disorder. Headlines such as "maniac runs amok and stabs three nurses" are all too common. The association between violence and mental disorder in popular imagination goes back thousands of years. When Socrates was told that there were many mentally disordered people in Athens he retorted "how could we live in safety with so many crazy people? Should we not long ago have paid the penalty at their hands, and have been struck and beaten and endured every other form of ill usage which madmen are wont to inflict?" In the middle of the 19th century Benjamin Franklin wished to set up a mental hospital in his new state of Pennsylvania, and he failed to persuade anyone of this virtue until he hit upon the notion of telling the people that they were at risk from dangerous mentally disordered people and they should build a hospital for their own protection (Monahan 1992). It opened in 1751.

Words matter

Although it's amusing to criticise political correctness in language, everybody is at some level sensitive to the impact which words can have on stigma and prejudice. To call a black man a "coon" or a "nigger" is totally unacceptable and may even transgress the law because of the stigmatising effect of these terms. The word "dangerous" is a stigmatising word in its own right. When she was very angry with him, Lady Caroline Lamb called Lord Byron "mad, bad and dangerous to know". She was probably using the three worst expletives that she could think of in polite society, and it's worth noting how related the concepts of badness, madness and dangerousness are juxtaposed even in the early nineteenth century.

Psychiatric patients have been stigmatised by a whole range of words for a long time. "Lunatic" is now out of use but "schizophrenic" is extremely common and almost passed as acceptable by the medical profession. Worse are words such as "psychopath", "sectioned", "untreatable" and "personality disordered". Personality disordered can be made more stigmatising by describing an individual as *severely* personality disordered, or, if you really want to produce a monster, along the lines of the "psychopath", you can do as the current Government does and say individuals are "dangerous severe personality disordered".

A study by Gerbner et al. (1981) showed that mental illness played a role in 17% of all American TV dramas in the early 1980s, 73% of the mentally disordered were portrayed as violent, and 23% of the violent were homicidal. Paradoxically, although the press and general prejudice can associate mental disorder with violence in one direction, there is a reluctance to do it the other way round. When the chief executive of Broadmoor Hospital complained to a newspaper about the stigmatising terminology used in respect of one of his patients he received this reply. "Truly the world is going mad where we have to refer to a murderous criminal like Ronnie Kray as a patient" (Kaye 1998). To be a patient is to have acceptability.

The word "dangerous" has many synonyms according to *Roget's Thesaurus*. These include deadly, desperate and destructive, but prominent among them are *bad*, *menacing* and *nasty*. The concept of dangerousness probably includes three important elements: destructiveness, predictability and an element of fear. These elements being rolled into one broad concept are then reified so that an individual is said to have "dangerousness" or worse to suffer from "dangerousness" as though this complex concept which is largely in the eye of the beholder were in fact a real thing which could be found somewhere in the monstrous individual who is said to have it, and as if it were an immutable characterisation like eye colour.

The medical profession has made some attempt to get away from this and to switch the concept of dangerousness into one of risk. It is possible to consider risk in relation to circumstances and time so it is easier to conceptualise risks that change as circumstances change and as individuals change. The statement "he poses a risk" prompts discussion. When, where, how can it be reduced? "He is dangerous" has an air of finality and rejection.

Violence and mental illness

For much of the twentieth century it was believed in psychiatric circles that the mentally disordered were less likely to commit violence than other people in the general community. We now know that this is not true and that there is a weak but important association between mental disorder and violence (e.g. Taylor and Gunn 1984). We looked at a consecutive sample of male prisoners who had been remanded in custody in London and who were awaiting trial. We interviewed the more serious offenders. All men charged with homicide in London during our study period fell into the sample. Five out of these 46 men (that's almost 11%) suffered from schizophrenia. This relationship between schizophrenia and violence has now been replicated in a number of other important studies. Perhaps the best known is the study in the community in the USA, the ECA Study, which Swanson revisited in 1990 and showed that patients with a diagnosis of schizophrenia were four times more likely to be violent than those who had no diagnosis. The more important part of his study was to show that as the number of diagnoses for an individual increased so the likelihood of violence for that individual also increased, and there was a particularly strong association between having a dual diagnosis of schizophrenia and substance abuse.

These findings have been further replicated in a new study by Mullen and his colleagues in Australia (2000). They were concerned not only to investigate the relationship between violence and mental disorder but also to see whether there was a change in the relationship between violence and mental disorder between 1975 and 1985. The significance of these years is that during that decade mental hospitals were largely closed down and community care came into operation. The authors found the same association as has been found elsewhere between schizophrenia and violence. Patients with schizophrenia were five to six times more likely to have been violent during the course of their life than other members of the population. This liability to violence did not change during the period studied but it was possible to show in the 1985 sample the additive effect of substance abuse as Swanson had shown (Swanson et al. 1990).

Summarising a lot of studies, some from the Institute of Psychiatry in London, it's now fairly clear that the increased risk of violence in psychiatric patients is associated with schizophrenia to some extent but particularly with drug and alcohol abuse. Patients with schizophrenia who do eventually become violent are not usually violent in the early part of their illness. The violence seems to be related in part to the presence of delusions, particularly passivity delusions and particularly to the emotional impact that those delusions have upon them.

It is important to get all this in perspective, and Taylor and I showed that the number of people in England and Wales who are convicted of homicide and are found to be of diminished responsibility because of a mental disorder has not really changed over almost 40 years (Taylor and Gunn 1999). However, the murder rate in England and Wales has risen sharply during that period and so the proportion of cases who are now deemed to be mentally disordered has fallen sharply because, whilst the numbers of mentally disordered cases remain much the same, the overall homicide rate has climbed.

Let's get serious about dangerousness

It's clear that in spite of the falling proportion of homicide cases who are deemed to be mentally disordered there is an increasing public awareness, possibly panic, about the relationships between mental disorder and violence. Indeed, following a notorious case which was subject to a public inquiry – when Christopher Clunis killed Jonathan Zito, who was standing waiting for a train on an underground platform – the then secretary of state made it a mandatory requirement that all homicides that occur involving a patient in treatment should be subject to a public inquiry. Many such public inquiries have now been published. They tend to arrive at similar conclusions, and they tend to cause much damage to the professionals involved – sometimes damage to their health, sometimes just to their morale. Some psychiatrists have given up work after such an event.

Nevertheless, inquiries do tend to highlight serious problems in the individual cases they study. I just picked two old cases, the one just mentioned, in respect of the Clunis case (Ritchie et al. 1994) and an earlier one when a young woman called Sharon Campbell killed her social worker who was working late at night in the hospital (DHSS 1988). Simple comparisons between these two cases suggest some interesting hypotheses (Gunn 1996). In both cases there was a change of diagnosis as time went by from psychosis and schizophrenia into personality disorder or "social difficulties". Further, in both cases there was a steady escalation of violence from the possession of sharp weapons to damaged property, to threats, to small knife attacks, punching, and then finally very serious violence. Christopher Clunis was passed like a parcel between various professionals and different types of accommodation. He had, in the six years between 1986 and 1992, 13 admissions to 8 different hospitals, lived in 4 hostels, had 4 periods of living in bed and breakfasts, once had a flat of his own, and twice was in prison. During this time he was attended to by no less than 35 mental health and social work professionals. Moving house just once is a life event which may precipitate psychiatric symptoms!!

The Ritchie Report made a list of the usual recommendations such as "better communication" and "do not allow geographical boundaries to interfere with care". It also made a series of recommendations for Her Majesty's Government, and they are perhaps worth spelling out in view of the Government's recent policy priorities, to lock up in special Home Office institutions patients with so-called "dangerous severe personality disorder" (Home Office/Department of Health 1999):

1. Provide more medium security beds
2. Provide more general psychiatric beds
3. Provide a range of health service accommodation
4. Provide more approved doctors (i.e. psychiatrists)
5. Provide more social workers

Successive governments have made some progress towards implementing these unarguable recommendations, but not very much. The policy for this new class of dangerous people has been floated without reference to evidence, and is to be implemented, so it is implied, whether evidence supports it or not. We don't know who this new, highly stigmatised, category of people really are. Noting the politics behind the proposal, they are probably individuals who threaten or commit sadistic crimes and who molest children. Such a heterogeneous group of people will undoubtedly contain a lot of mental disorder but of a wide variety of types, including psychosis (like Christopher Clunis and Sharon Campbell). The proposed new "treatment" has not been subjected to a cost-effectiveness analysis, and it has not been sent to the National Institute for Clinical Excellence (as all expensive new medical treatment should). Above all, no attention has been paid to the allimportant question of staffing these new institutions. Some of us believe that the new policy may already be deterring appropriate staff such as psychiatrists.

Treatability

One of the most stigmatising things that is said within psychiatry is that certain patients are "untreatable". This remarkable epithet which is not used in any other branch of medicine is normally reserved for patients who are said to have "a personality disorder", a stigma which is applied to difficult patients as they become more chronic and more difficult whatever their basic psychopathology. It is easy to see how "untreatable patients" can be transformed into "dangerous people". It is important therefore to demonstrate more effectively than we have done hitherto how much treatment can be given and how effective it is. Certainly this is reinforced by an interesting paper from Israel which suggests that the concepts of dangerousness and treatability are negatively correlated (Arikan et al. 1999).

Conclusion

Whilst it's clear that there is an association between some violent behaviour and some mental disorder, this association does not fit the mad axeman stereotype nor is it reasonable to regard large numbers of patients as dangerous. The important policy initiatives which can be used to reduce risk are to tackle more vigorously the problems of substance abuse, and to provide more services for patients who have chronic disorders and are shown to have increasing risks. It's also extremely important for psychiatrists to modify their language so that patients are not stigmatised by the things that are said about them, and I would recommend in the context of this discussion that the word "dangerousness" is dropped entirely from the psychiatric lexicon. If dangers are to be thought about they should be in the rubric of risk. It's quite possible for professionals to undertake risk assessments and then to go on to manage any risks discovered. Stigma will also only really begin to melt away when treatment is applied with more enthusiasm by psychiatrists and with more research to demonstrate what aspects of treatment work and what do not. It is highly unlikely that stigmatising a group of patients with the label "dangerous severe personality disorder" and building a whole new range of expensive institutions to be run by the Home Office will provide a solution for anything. It's likely to compound the problem and may increase the risk to the public.

References

Arikan K, Uysal O, and Catin G (1999) Public awareness of the effectiveness of psychiatric treatment may reduce stigma. *Israel Journal of Psychiatry and Related Sciences* **36**: 95–9.

DHSS (1988) *Report of the Committee of Inquiry into the Care and Aftercare of Miss Sharon Campbell.* Cmd.440. London: HMSO.

Gerbner G, Gross L, Morgan M & Signorielli N (1981) Health and medicine on television. *New England Journal of Medicine* **305**: 901–4.

Gunn J (1996) Let's get serious about dangerousness. *Criminal Behaviour and Mental Health* Supp: 51–64.

Kaye C (1998) "Press and public relations". In: Kaye C, Franey A (eds). *Managing High Security Psychiatric Care.* London: Jessica Kingsley.

Home Office/Department of Health (1999) *Managing Dangerous People with Severe Personality Disorder: Proposals for Policy Development.*

Monahan J (1992) Mental disorders and violent behaviour. *American Psychologist* **47**: 511–21.

Mullen PE, Burgess P, Wallace C, Ruschena D (2000) Community care and criminal offending in schizophrenia. *Lancet* **355**: 614–17.

Ritchie JH, Dick D & Lingham R (1994) *The report of the Inquiry into the Care and Treatment of Christopher Clunis.* London: HMSO.

Swanson JW, Holzer CE, Ganju VK & Jono RT (1990) Violence and psychiatric disorder in the community: evidence from the Epidemiologic Catchment Area Surveys. *Hospital and Community Psychiatry* **41**: 761–70.

Taylor PJ & Gunn J (1984) Violence and psychosis I. Risk of violence among psychotic men. *British Medical Journal* **288**: 1945–9.

Taylor PJ & Gunn J (1999) Homicides by people with mental illness: myth and reality. *British Journal of Psychiatry* **174**: 9–14.

42 Stigma and quality of life in personality disorder: The Cassel/North Devon study

Jeremy Holmes, Anna Harrison-Hall, Charles Montgomery, Marco Chiesa and Carla Drahorad

Many patients suffering from personality disorder – especially those in contact with general psychiatric services – are, literally, stigmatised. Etymologically, a stigma is a mark made with a pointed stick or a brand. Self-mutilation is a frequent feature of patients suffering from borderline personality disorder, many of whom cut or scratch themselves with razor blades, knives, broken glass, drawing pins or other sharp implements. Burning one's flesh with lighted cigarettes or the infliction of pressure burns with the hands is also common. The most frequent sites for such assaults are the hands, forearms, abdomen, legs, and occasionally genitals. The significance of such actions is not entirely clear, but patients often report temporary feelings of psychological relief at the time of self-injury, a phenomenon some have speculated to be associated with endogenous opiate release. Other possible meanings include a switch from passive to active mastery of pain and rejection inflicted on a body which in childhood was physically or sexually assaulted; a way of distancing potential further abusers; a non- verbal attempt to communicate mental pain – a "ventilation" of feelings which also connects with the botanical use of the term stigma to denote a respiratory vent in a leaf; and an attempt to signal a sense of shame and unworthiness.

In everyday speech a stigma is an unwelcome distinguishing feature, often associated with social exclusion. Ambivalence about the distinctiveness of their disorder is common among those suffering from mental illness. On the one hand people may wish that their disability were visible –"if only I had a broken leg then the neighbours would understand why I can`t go to work and stop accusing me a of being a scrounger"; on the other, there is a fear of being singled out as "a personality disorder" – with all the negative connotations of that term – and a wish to merge into the background. In the West the cultural significance of stigma is inescapably linked with the Christian image of the suffering and rejected Godhead – here social exclusion is reversed: stigmata become a mark of holiness, a contemporary echo of which can be found in the reverence afforded in some circles to those who have been sexually abused.

Stigmatisation is all pervasive and self-perpetuating. Themselves often the victims of stigmatisation ("psychiatrists are all mad", "don't you find it depressing working with those sort of people all day?"), mental health workers are not immune to its perpetration, a phenomenon described by Anna Freud as identification with the aggressor. Patients with personality disorder are a common target, as anyone who has tried to persuade ward staff to admit someone suffering from PD to a ward on a Friday evening will testify.

As Lewis and Appleby (1988) put it, people with personality disorders are "patients psychiatrists dislike" – and not without good reason. Fear, ignorance and helplessness, based on a two-way process of projection, fuel stigma. All three feelings can easily be aroused by the presentation of such patients in general psychiatric settings. By definition they make unpredictable, abrasive, or overdependent relationships with others, including mental health workers. They seek out attachments, but are unable to profit from them. Their psychic life is dominated by projective identification in which those with whom they come in close contact are unconsciously assigned humiliated or humiliating roles. Similarly, feelings of anger or hopelessness that originate in the patient`s psyche but chime in with the recipient's own uncertainties may come to lodge uncomfortably in the psyche of the mental health worker. Above all, outside a few specialist centres, there is a lack of good, evidence-based, structured treatments for these people (but beware the construction "these people…" a sure sign of a stigmatised discourse). The result is a vicious circle in which the more incompetently the patients are managed, the more problematic they become – until at worst their handling in psychiatric settings becomes a species of "retraumatisation" which repeats the rejection or abuse they suffered in childhood.

In an attempt to describe and help tackle this problem – and, stigmatisation aside, these patients are highly problematic and resource-consuming – we initiated a research project, first in North Devon (Study 1), and then in collaboration with the Cassel Hospital (Study 2). The presentation of our findings to date forms the main part of this chapter. Our long-term aim is to establish a viable personality disorder service within the limitations of a district mental health unit. Research and audit is an essential part of that service, and the clinical implications will be spelt out at the end of the chapter. Before presenting our findings, some comments on quality of life and psychiatric disorder are needed.

Social medicine, stigma and quality of life

Our starting point is that patients with personality disorder suffer from disadvantage and social exclusion. There are complex associations between psychiatric illness, stigma, and social disadvantage. As with physical illness, psychiatric illness is both a cause and a consequence of poverty. However it seems that relative poverty – i.e. inequality – may be a more important promoter of ill health than absolute levels of income (Wilkinson 1996). Inequality in turn is linked with stigma – in unequal societies the "haves" tend to stigmatise the "have nots", presumably as a social protection mechanism that attempts to justify their unequal (and from an ethical perspective unfair) share of resources. The impoverishment of the psychiatrically ill can thus be traced partly to the type of society – equal or unequal – in which the sufferer lives, partly to the secondary consequences of the illness itself, and partly to stigmatisation consequent upon the illness and the social context.

Psychiatry is thus inescapably an aspect of social medicine; psychiatrists have to make difficult decisions about where, as doctors, their role in the treatment of illness ends and society`s responsibility for tackling disadvantage begins. Different practitioners place the divide differently – but stigma always lurks on the far side of the Rubicon. Nowhere is this more true than in personality disorder, in which an extreme position holds that patients with Axis II disorders are not "ill" and therefore represent a social rather than a medical responsibility. Given the disruption to health settings which such patients are capable of causing, and the lack of clear treatment models, this position is understandable.

It is also, however, untenable. As we shall show, patients with personality disorders have a high incidence of Axis I pathology; conversely, the difficult Axis I cases that tend to be referred to psychiatric services are often complicated by Axis II disorders

(Alnaes and Torgerson 1997). Patients with personality disorders cannot be defined out of existence – they will continue to present to and cause difficulty for psychiatric services.

In schizophrenia social disadvantage and poor quality of life are seen as legitimate targets of psychiatric involvement. The HoNOS scales, which were developed mainly with schizophrenia in mind, take poor quality of life as a major mark of severity and target for treatment. In schizophrenia poor quality of life is a consequence of the illness. We suggest that in personality disorder the reverse is true: developmental difficulty leads to poor quality of life, which in turn is a vulnerability factor leading to the depression and anxiety, transient psychotic symptoms, and substance abuse that are the Axis I accompaniments of the disorder. The origins of poor quality of life in personality disorder are inextricably bound up with the developmental nature of the disorder and the social responses to it.

In an attempt to counteract the process of stigmatisation within psychiatry, in which schizophrenia is viewed as a legitimate focus for medical work, whereas personality disorder is seen as problematic or beyond the pale, we decided to try to delineate the extent of social disadvantage, dependency on medical services and impoverishment of quality of life experienced by patents suffering from personality disorders. Our working hypothesis was that these would be roughly comparable to those found in schizophrenia.

Defining quality of life is not easy (Atkinson et al. 1997). A useful concept is that of the discrepancy between a person`s expectations and hopes and their actual experience. Influenced by the HoNOS scales, we identified a number of distinct domains relevant to quality of life in which we felt that personality disorder would be likely to have an impact. These include:

- the presence or absence of mental pain, as revealed in Axis I psychiatric disorders.
- the ability to work, either in a voluntary or paid capacity
- feeling part of a community
- the presence or absence of intimate relationships
- having a sense of purpose and meaning in life
- having a sense of autonomy – the capacity to make choices and to feel in control of one's destiny

Clearly there are many routes by which an individual might be disadvantaged in one or other of these domains, of which personality disorder would only be one. The most obvious example is unemployment. If feeling economically productive is a key component to a good quality of life then clearly the state of the economy will play a part in an individual's quality of life, independent of psychiatric disorder. Indeed the sense of a good or compromised quality of life is a complex mixture of personal and social factors, objectively identifiable disadvantage and an individual`s subjective reactions to that disadvantage.

The North Devon Personality Disorder Study

Method

In the first instance consultant psychiatrists and frontline mental health workers in the area were asked to identify those patients aged between 18 and 45 on their caseload to whom they would apply a primary diagnosis of personality disorder on clinical grounds. These were then screened using the Personality Disorder Questionnaire 4 to confirm the presence of at least one Axis II diagnosis. Those patients who agreed to participate in the study were then given a battery of tests, which included the SCID-I

& II diagnostic interviews, the General Health Questionnaire, the Beck Depression Inventory, the Symptom Check List 90, the Global Assessment Scale, the Social Adjustment Scale, the Adult Attachment Interview, and measures designed to identify and quantify service utilisation and total cost of disability. These were repeated at one and two years. Patients who were found to be suffering from schizophrenia, paranoid psychosis or organic mental illness, and those who were in psychotherapy at a frequency of once a week or more, were excluded from the study sample. A total of 80 patients were therefore selected.

In addition, in Study 1 the patients' keyworkers were interviewed in an attempt to estimate the stress or "burden" which the patients represented, using a Lickert scale. In Study 2 a case control method was used to compare the North Devon cohort with two samples of patients attending the Cassel Hospital. Here the aim was to compare the impact of two patterns of delivery of intensive psychotherapy with the "standard care" available to the North Devon sample.

Results

Study 1 (Montgomery et al. 2000)

The mean GHQ for the 80 patients was 14.58 and the mean BDI 28.22, indicating high levels of morbidity. The mean number of personality disorders as measured by the PDQ-4 was 4.2, a figure roughly similar to that found in an in-patient psychiatric population (Dowson 1992). One quarter of patients (21/80) had been admitted at least once to a psychiatric ward in the previous year, and 17% (13/80) had presented to the casualty department in the previous two months. Tables 1 and 2 show the relationship between keyworker stress and GHQ and BDI scores, the main finding of this phase of the study being that the number of personality disorders was not in itself associated with admission to hospital, whereas levels of BDI were.

Table 1 Relationship between keyworker stress and GHQ and BDI scores

CPN stress	GHQ score, mean and 95% CI	BDI score, mean and 95% CI
Yes	16.29 (13.71–18.87)	30.75 (26.85–34.65)
No	10.91 (8.01–13.81)	23.91 (21.90–25.92)
t-value	2.72	2.42
p	0.008	0.018

Table 2 Relationship between the hospital admission and BDI and PDQ scores

	n	BDI	Age	PDQ
Admitted	20	34.14	35.7	39.95
Not admitted	53	25.52 (1)	42.3 (2)	36.10

(1) $t = -2.86$; $p = 0.0005$; (2) $t = 2.60$; $p = 0.011$

The number of personality disorder diagnostic criteria met by each patient was not in itself associated with subjective "burden" in keyworkers, or with level of psychiatric service utilization such as in-patient admission. Rather, it seems that the combination of a personality disorder and the presence of major psychiatric symptomatology and clinical levels of mental health as assessed by the BDI and GHQ is what determines the impact of such patients on a district psychiatric service.

Study 2

Here 70 patients drawn from Study 1 were available for interview as possible participants in an extended and more detailed study. Once those failing to meet inclusion criteria and unwilling to participate in the study had been excluded, together with those who dropped out at the baseline stage, a group of 50 active participants in the study was achieved. Remarkably, only one had dropped out of the study at 2 years. Table 3 indicates the general demographic and background characteristics of the 50 patients who met inclusion criteria and agreed to participate in this phase of the study. The mean age of the sample was 34, and two thirds of the sample were female. As expected, difficult and unhappy backgrounds were common. There was a high incidence of early maternal deprivation (44%), early loss (36%), reported severe sexual abuse (26%), and moderate to severe reported parental brutality (36%). Common too were involvement in violence (58%), drugs and alcohol abuse (42%).

Table 3. Cassel baseline questionnaire data for North Devon sample ($n = 49$)

Age	34 years (mean)
Sex	66% female
Marital status	62% single
Early maternal deprivation	44%
Early loss	36%
Severe sexual abuse	26%
Severe parental brutality	36%
Education beyond GCSE	22%
Currently employed	12%
No close contact with friends or family	58%
No sexual contact	49%
DSH at least once in previous year	36%
At least one hospital admission	58%

A bleak picture of quality of life in personality disorder emerges from the study. The majority was educationally disadvantaged; one third had either taken no school-leaving exams or 78% had achieved no more than GCSEs. They were similarly disadvantaged in the area of work. Only 12% were currently employed, and 76% had had no employment in the previous year. One third had little or no social contact with friends, and two thirds reported an absence of close relationships in their life. 42% had no sexual relationship.

As far as psychiatric status was concerned one third self-harmed in the previous year; 58% had had hospital admissions at some point. The mean length of previous hospitalisation was 40 days. Only 6% had never been on psychotropic medication, and 70% had been on medication for at least 12 months. With regard to psychiatric diagnosis, 56% were suffering from current major depression. Half had current panic disorder and/or agoraphobia, 10% had an eating disorder and 20% a current alcohol or drug dependence. The SCID-II findings showed that 70% had a cluster B disorder, and 66% of these had borderline personality disorder. Ninety percent had Cluster C disorders, of which avoidant (68%) and dependent (34%) were the most common. Forty-four percent had a Cluster A paranoid personality disorder. The low incidence (8%) of antisocial personality disorder was noteworthy, and shows how different are this group of patients with personality disorder compared with a forensic sample.

Our basic hypothesis in the case control study was that only patients undertaking psychotherapy at the Cassel Hospital would show significant change over time. Table 4 shows the three main measures – the GAS, SAS and SCL-90 at intake and at one year – and Figure 1 shows individual GAS scores over two years. In general the results confirm that social adjustment and satisfaction in life changed little over the period of the study, although there was a non-significant improvement in the SCL-90. By contrast, the GAS did show significant improvement over the two-year period, with a move to a higher band in which the patients were less psychiatrically ill and dependent than at the start of the study.

Table 4. Means of main measures at baseline and one year (n = 49)

	Baseline	1 year
SCL-90	1.87	1.74
SAS	2.7	2.7
GAS	45	49*

* $p = 0.02$
Note: 1. Nithsdale SAS for schizophrenia: 2.19
        2. In-patient SCL-90: 1.4

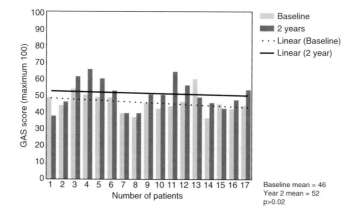

Figure 1. GAS scores at baseline and 2 years.

Implications

Stability and quality of life

By almost any standards this group of patients would be judged to experience a poor quality of life. Virtually none were employed, few had close relationships, many had spent long periods in hospital, almost all took psychotropic medication, more than half were currently severely depressed and a significant proportion suffered from eating disorders and alcohol or drug dependence. The level of symptomatology as measured on the SCL-90 was worse than in a typical psychiatric in-patient population.

Study 1 reveals the important finding that it is not personality disorder as such which leads to intense involvement with psychiatric services, but the associated Axis I disorders, for which, presumably, personality disorder is a major vulnerability factor (Figure 2). Compared with the Cassel patients the general impression was of a slightly older group who had to some extent adjusted to their very restricted situation. The very low drop-out rate from the study (only 1/50 in two years) is a mark of this stability. It

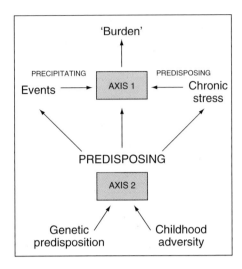

Figure 2. Co-morbidity in SPD.

seems that those patients in whom Axis I disorders are contained can lead a reasonably stable life, albeit one that is very restricted – with no employment, few friends or social contacts and often an avoidant or quasi-agoraphobic lifestyle.

Impact of general psychiatric services

These patients consume a large amount of medical and social resources. Given our finding of the general lack of improvement in these patients, is this amount of investment justified? If not, how should it be better deployed? In answer to these questions, a number of relevant points emerge from our study.

First, there is no doubt that much unproductive psychiatric work is done with these patients. Many spend long periods in general psychiatric wards, with doubtful benefit, or have intensive but fruitless contact with community keyworkers. However, it is also true that GAS levels improved significantly over time, and it seems likely that psychiatric input played some part in achieving this modest change. This has to be contrasted with the non-significant improvement on the SCL-90, a subjective measure of satisfaction, and no change at all on the SAS, a measure of social adjustment. The methodology of our study means that we cannot be sure that this improvement is due to medical intervention rather than natural remission, but the difference between the measures at least suggests that it may well be a treatment effect. If this is a robust finding then it seems likely that general psychiatric services are able to make a small but significant impact on the 'illness' component of personality disorder – the Axis I aspect, or mental distress – but not on the social disadvantage and relationship difficulties. This is not surprising since, by and large, general psychiatric services concentrate on symptoms, whereas psychotherapy services target relationship difficulties, and, by definition, this group of patients did not receive psychotherapy. Although outside the scope of this chapter, the comparison with the Cassel group, in whom significant improvement in SCL-90 and SAS did occur (Chiesa and Fonagy 2000), is consistent with this conclusion.

How to improve services for patients with personality disorder

Our study suggests that psychiatric services may not be sufficiently equipped to meet the needs of patients with personality disorders. There is a lack of relevant psychotherapy input and excessive investment in standard care, which has only a small impact on the overall disability characteristic of this condition. A three-stage model is required, with the possibility of movement between the levels. First, there is a group of patients for whom standard care is sufficient to maintain a restricted but relatively untroubled quality of life. At the second level there is a group of patients who have frequent contact with services, are experienced as a "burden", and who are highly distressed. Here there are two key requirements: firstly, active, intensive individual therapeutic engagement with the patient that can withstand the tendency in personality disorder to undermine intimate relationships; secondly, to engage the patient with others in a group or community setting that is likewise able to maintain psychic health. In other words to offer the patient a secure base that is proof against the fears and insecurity and destructiveness inherent in the condition (Holmes 1999). These require intensive psychotherapeutic management by skilled workers, based around individual and group work at a frequency of no less than twice a week and a therapeutic environment in which social and relationship skills can be acquired. General psychiatric hospital admissions for this group should be planned and brief. All this is potentially achievable within a district service by diversion of existing resources currently unproductively deployed with these patients. Thirdly there is a sub-group for whom intensive specialist therapeutic community facilities are required, which may need to be provided on a supra-district basis, for example through partial hospitalisation (Bateman 1995) or Specialist Outreach Services. Further clinical and empirical research is needed for a clearer identification of these three sub-groups of PDs with their different indications for treatment and prognosis.

Quality of life in personality disorder and schizophrenia

The literature is equivocal about quality of life in schizophrenia compared with personality disorder. Gunderson et al. (1975) found no significant differences between the two groups when followed up for two years post-hospitalization. MacEwan and Athawes (1997) in their Scottish schizophrenia sample found SAS levels of 2.19: indicating better adjustment than our sample with 2.7. By contrast, McGlashan's study of the Chestnut Lodge cohort (1986) – all of whom had undergone intensive psychotherapy – with a much longer follow-up period extending to decades, found a better prognosis in the personality disorder group, especially in the second decade after discharge. A French study of schizophrenia (Huguelet et al. 1995) found GAS scores above 50 in 30% of patients at 4-year follow up, which can be compared with 50% over 50 after 2 years in our study. We are planning further work in this area, in collaboration with the University of Bristol. A tentative view that patients with personality disorder are comparable in symptomatology and quality of life to the "upper" end of patients suffering from schizophrenia seems reasonable at this stage.

Conclusion

The concepts of stigma and personality disorder are both social constructs. Both emerge from the intersection of psychological and social forces on groups and individuals. What we call "personality disorder" is a final common pathway for factors which include inherited temperament, adverse developmental pathways, negative psychological meanings, and restricted social contexts. The notion of personality disorder highlights the extent to which "medical" concepts can be used both to transcend and to perpetuate implicit ethical and social values. A diagnosis of personality disorder implicitly rescues the sufferer from connotations of blame and moral turpitude, but also labels the patient and so opens the door to stigmatisation and rejection.

If we are to extend the notion of medical responsibility to include attempts to improve people's quality of life, then there needs to be a concomitant widening of the scope of medical skill and technology. We continue to tackle the social aspects of psychiatry with outmoded tools and concepts. The discomfort created by patients with personality disorders for both sufferers and carers exposes this discrepancy. One way to deal with the discomfort is by projection and stigmatisation – we stigmatise these patients because we just do not know what else to do with them. The other is to update our medical repertoire to include psychotherapeutic skills, and group understanding. Only then – to take an evidence-based perspective – will the SAS and SCL-90 scores in our personality disorder patients keep pace with improvements in the GAS. That in turn – to move to an ethical perspective – will enhance mental health workers` sense of mastery and effectiveness, and thereby reduce their need for stigmatisation of personality disorder sufferers.

References

Alneas R & Torgeson S (1997) Personality and personality disorders predict development and relapse of major depression. *Acta Psychiatrica Scandinavica* **95**: 336–42.

Atkinson M, Zibin S & Chuang H (1997) Characterizing quality of life among patients with chronic mental illness: a critical examination of the self-report methodology. *American Journal of Psychiatry* **154**: 99–105.

Bateman A W (1995) The treatment of borderline patients in a day hospital setting. *Psychoanalytic Psychotherapy* **9**: 3–16.

Chiesa M & Fonagy P (2000) Cassel Personality Disorder Study: Methodology and treatment effects. *British Journal of Psychiatry* **176**: 485–91.

Dowson J (1992) The assessment of DSM-III-R personality disorders by self-report questionnaire: the role of informants and a screening test for co-morbid personality disorders (STCPD). *British Journal of Psychiatry* **161**: 344–52.

Gunderson J, Carpenter W & Strauss J (1975) Borderline and schizophrenic patients: a comparative study. *American Journal of Psychiatry* **132**: 1257–64.

Holmes J (1999) Psychotherapeutic approaches to the management of severe personality disorder in general psychiatric settings. *CPD Bulletin Psychiatry* **1**: 35–41.

Huguelet P, Zabala I, Cruciania G et al (1995) Evolution durant quatre ans de l'adaptation psychosociale d'une cohorte de patients schizophrenes. *L'Encephale* **XXI**: 93–8.

Lewis G & Appleby L (1988) Personality disorder: the patients psychiatrists dislike. *British Journal of Psychiatry* **153**: 44–9.

MacEwan T & Athawes W (1997) The Nithsdale schizophrenia surveys: XV. Social adjustment in schizophrenia. *Acta Psychiatrica Scandinavica* **95**: 254–8.

McGlashan T (1986) The Chestnut Lodge follow-up study. *Archives of General Psychiatry* **43**: 20–30.

Montgomery C, Holmes J & Lloyd K (2000) The burden of personality disorder – a district-based survey. *International Journal of Social Psychiatry* **46**: 164–9.

Wilkinson R (1996) *Unhealthy Societies – The Afflictions of Inequality*. London: Routledge.

Commentary and discussion on Section 5A

Commentary

Oscar Hill

In Mike Shooter's contribution (Chapter 39), what occurred to me was that while there are very strong philosophical arguments for determinism of behaviour, unfortunately there are equally strong philosophical arguments for free will. Between the two lots of philosophical arguments, what we finally decide in the practical world is often more to do with personal prejudice, sometimes dressed up as science. If we take Gilles de la Tourette syndrome, self-damaging behaviour is extremely common. We take the view in Gilles that it is disease-determined, quite another in personality disorder, where we usually conclude that it is willful.

The cultures in which our patients grow up are so very diverse. I recently looked into variations in homicide, suicide and violence in the London boroughs, with Harry Kennedy and Rachel Iveson (1999), and the variation is quite remarkable. In the worst parts of London, rates of homicide are 16 times greater than in the least affected areas. If you want a quiet life go to Sutton. If you would prefer to be surrounded by violence, go to Camden, Islington, Lambeth or Southwark. Violence against the person is 6 times as high in the worst boroughs as it is in the best. In the worst boroughs, 1 in 100 of the total population commit crimes of violence against the person. These are only the offences that are identified by the police, and average figures. Within a borough there are enclaves where matters are much worse than the average. Most criminals and most victims are involved with parents, brothers, sisters, children, friends, so that a substantial part of the local community is affected by violence in these enclaves. We can only conjecture at what this does to the people who live and grow up there. Further, if you live in gentle Sutton, your perspective on violent behaviour is likely to be very different from the natives of the more disturbed boroughs. It is sufficient to walk a few hundred yards in London to move into a completely different culture. Sensitivity to cultural issues is particularly important, as more psychiatrists will come from Sutton and their patients are more likely to be from the more disturbed boroughs.

The message that has come over from Jeremy Coid and Jeremy Holmes (Chapters 40 and 42) is that it does not make a lot of sense to take personality disorder out of the psychiatric field, to which they will in any case always gravitate with or without associated mental disorders. It is of particular value that Jeremy Holmes has demonstrated what can be done to help them in an ordinary psychiatric district service. Apart from the benefits to knowledge, participation in this sort of development and research generates energy and interest in the therapeutic team.

I agree with Jeremy Coid that we need to get away from single theories and adopt, with Adolf Meyer, a psychobiological approach. You look at your patient from every aspect – biological, psychological and social – and adjust what you can in all areas. It is possible to do this in a general psychiatric inpatient unit, but it is hard. It needs very committed and experienced senior staff across the different disciplines, and persistence to keep the culture going. The pressures of inner city psychiatry make this approach increasingly difficult, and admission becomes even more anti-therapeutic for many people with personality disorders. Although there is everything to be said for keeping these patients out of hospital, it is vital that they are managed by a service which has an interest and an expertise in treating them. It is exciting that new specialist units are developing. I am very pleased that my own recent Trust, Camden & Islington, has developed such a specialist unit. Nonetheless, there will always be substantial numbers of patients with personality disorders admitted into hospital and their management there must be optimised if harm is to be minimised.

I was particularly impressed by the demonstration that the disability and the suffering of these patients is entirely comparable in severity to those with schizophrenia and warrants comparable attention.

Reference

Kennedy HG, Iveson RCY & Hill O (1999) Violence, homicide and suicide; strong correlation and wide variation across districts. *British Journal of Psychiatry* **175**: 462–6.

Panel discussion

Professor John Gunn

I am very familiar with Professor Coid's presentations on these matters and wonder whether I detected a shift in his thinking? Can I provoke you into talking about a particular kind of personality disorder that you did not mention at all today?

Professor Jeremy Coid

I am too frightened to mention it – it is the "P" word, which is not politically correct. I think we used to call it "psychopathic disorder". I am an adherent of Robert Hare's work and the idea that there is something, someone usually in prison, and for brief periods in the community, something called a severe personality disorder, let's call it psychopathic because he does. The Americans are the main workers in the area of personality disorder with a major investment in their own categories, and some of them sit on committees. Most of these categories are actually devised by committees rather than in research exercises. What you are detecting is my moving away, starting off doing research 10 years ago by getting hold of research diagnostic instruments, believing in the avoidant, the borderline, the antisocial, the narcissistic personality disorder, and shifting away from some of those, but I do believe that there is something out there ….

Question: The value of the concept of personality disorder?

Dr Mike Shooter

The important thing is that we are working with a particular person, not a whole race of borderlines or psychopaths or whatever. A classification is justified if it gives you a framework with which to understand and work with a particular patient. I said in the course of my presentation that the worst patient, but the best patient ever given to me, was a rip roaring borderline personality. My consultant had no idea what to do with her, hated her, and threw her glibly to me and said "follow her up in outpatients" which

I did every week for four years. I had no framework to begin with. It was my own article of faith which gradually helped me to understand this particular person, and in the end it worked. Beyond that, I do not see that the concept of personality matters a lot.

Dr Jeremy Holmes

"Is there such a thing as personality disorder" is not a "yes" or "no" question, it is what kind of a thing are we talking about. For instance, let us take social class. Does social class exist? In one sense, it does not, and in another it is an incredibly useful concept to understand all kinds of social phenomena, and I think the same is true for personality disorder. What is difficult about personality disorder, I believe, is you need your Margaret Mahler, you need your developmental perspective, but you also need a sociological perspective. Something is going on in society which has thrown up this concept of personality disorder, as well as something that is going on in the developmental life history of a particular individual, and that is where we struggle, but we have got good models from people like George Brown. His whole research in depression is a sophisticated attempt to bring together these strands.

Dr Tom Parsons

What would you like to say about the training of psychiatrists and the value of more combined psychiatric posts?

Dr Jeremy Holmes

That point links up with what Jeremy Coid said about the virtual absence of training in the diagnosis of personality disorder. But from diagnosing personality disorder we must proceed to its treatment, which is the dominant practical issue. Our personality disorder service in North Devon is multidisciplinary and the training of nurses, psychologists and psychiatrists is deficient for all of them in the area of personality disorder.

Dr Mike Shooter

I would add College support for proper training in the diagnosis and treatment of personality disorder, but I also want to make a plea for proper training in liaising with other disciplines. My own experience of trying to treat anybody with a personality disorder is that the bulk of your time is spent clearing space for therapy, and that involves liaising with the police, schools, social workers, GPs and next of kin, in order to create the space within which you have a context for the treatment.

Question: On the selectivity of specialist services

Professor Coid

I have always wanted to admit patients with personality disorders but increasingly we are overwhelmed with people with schizophrenia who must be given priority. Psychiatry has changed, people are now more selective and defensive against attracting blame. Audit of those who commit homicide and suicide show fewer persons with severe mental disorder than we would expect and far more with substance abuse and personality disorder. These are the dangerous ones. The whole area has been highjacked by the law and order agenda. Is it treatment that we will be giving to these individuals, or surveillance?

43 Descartes has a lot to answer for

Simon Fleminger

Introduction

People with mental disorders suffer more stigmatisation than do those with bodily illnesses. Mental disorders due to organic brain disease are therefore less stigmatised than "functional" mental illness, and this was confirmed in the Royal College of Psychiatrists' survey of public attitudes which identified relatively low levels of stigmatising attitudes towards people with a dementia (see Chapter 3). This view seems partly based on a mind–body dualism; it is OK to suffer a disorder of the body, but not a disorder of the mind.

Of all the mental disorders it is perhaps those with personality disorder who are most likely to be held to blame for their condition. In personality disorder there is therefore the potential for the most marked shift in attitude if an organic brain disease is shown to account for the mental symptoms. In this chapter I will illustrate this shift in attitude with two case examples, both of whom had been turned down by the benefits office for a disability allowance. I will then demonstrate that this polarised view of personality disorder is not justified, because psychological process and brain disorder interact to produce disorders of personality. I will conclude with a recent model of acquired personality disorder, based on the proposed function of the medial orbital frontal lobe.

Case reports

One touchstone of society's attitudes is to be found in the Benefits Office when deciding to whom to allocate Disability Living Allowance. This is illustrated in these two cases:

Case 1

Elliot was being looked after by a sibling by the time he got to see Dr Damasio, a behavioural neurologist in the United States (Damasio 1994). His personality had changed over the previous months and years. First he had lost his job; he would make irresponsible decisions and was no longer a reliable worker. His wife had then left him and it soon became apparent that he could no longer look after himself, and a sibling took him in. On examination he was cool, detached and unperturbed by all that had happened to him. He appeared bright and intelligent with no definite cognitive impairment. It was reckoned by many who had seen him that at best he was lazy and at worst a malingerer. He had been turned down by the disability living allowance board.

Damasio ordered a brain scan, which showed a frontal meningioma which had undoubtedly been responsible for the change in his personality. The decision regarding his disability allowance was reversed, not because of any change in symptoms, though these had deteriorated, but because it was now clear that they were due to organic brain disease.

Case 2

A man was injured in a scuffle; he had fallen back and cracked his head as he fell. It is unlikely that he was unconscious for more than a minute. Following the injury he suffered bad headaches. But more troubling was the personality change. He lost his job, being no longer able to apply himself at work; he would arrive late unless his girlfriend got him out of bed and took him to work. He was argumentative and impulsive, wanting things done for him immediately. He became completely self-absorbed. Perhaps most worrisome of all he became a hostile patient, damning doctors in their presence as useless and becoming threatening. There was no good evidence of any significant cognitive impairment; his professional knowledge was unaffected, as was his memory. A CT brain scan was reported as normal. He was turned down for Disability Living Allowance (DLA), perhaps because it was thought that he was lazy and was more interested in getting compensation than getting back to work.

Review of his history, however, indicated that his personality change had been immediate and for the first few days following the injury he was quite disinhibited and confused. He suffered anosmia. A MRI brain scan, more sensitive than a CT brain scan, was ordered and showed a discrete lesion in the medial orbital frontal region (Figure 1). The Benefits Office reviewed his case and he was now accepted for DLA. There had been no change in symptoms but a brain disorder could now account for his disability.

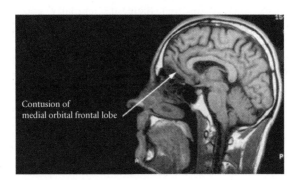

Figure 1. Personality change after brain injury.

Bridging the mind–body gap

There are three strands to the argument that a dualistic approach is not appropriate for mental disorders including personality disorder:

1. Mental symptoms may be indistinguishable regardless of aetiology

Mental symptoms arising from disorders of the mind are often no different from those from disorders of the brain. For example in Parkinson's disease the depression syndrome which may be observed is no different from depression occurring in the absence of organic brain disease. The behaviour and personality traits of people with neurotic illness are very similar to those of people who have suffered a traumatic brain injury (Brooks and McKinlay 1983). Common to both are changeable mood, social withdrawal, and reduced drive.

Traumatic brain injury, particularly if it involves the medial orbital frontal lobe, can produce an acquired anti-social personality disorder essentially indistinguishable from the "idiopathic" disorder (Anderson et al. 1999).

2. Mental symptoms are often the result of an interaction between psychological processes and brain disorder

My interest in interactions between psychological process and brain disorder, between mind and body, arose from the observation that a specific psychological intervention could terminate a delusional misidentification; the patient believed that his house had been replaced by a duplicate. It was the first symptom of a dementia. I formulated a model, based on psychological studies of perceptual and cognitive systems, to illustrate how such an interaction might be effected. The model predicted that there would be an inverse relationship between the degree of organic brain disease and the degree of psychological disorder required to produce a delusional misidentification.

Alastair Burns and I went on to demonstrate that a systematic review of the literature supported this contention (Fleminger and Burns 1993). In some patients without evidence of organic brain disease the delusional misidentification had only occurred within the context of a psychotic illness, for example paranoia. However if there was manifest organic brain disease, for example due to head trauma, then the symptom was often found in patients who otherwise had no evidence of psychosis. In many, however, it seemed to be the combination of both the organic brain disease and the psychological disturbance that was necessary to precipitate the symptom.

In the field of personality disorder there are similarly good accounts of an interaction between brain disease and psychosocial effects in the genesis of the disorder:

(a) If you suffer antisocial personality traits before a severe head injury then you are more likely to develop antisocial personality disorder after the injury (Kozol 1946).

(b) In children it is those with poor parenting plus traumatic brain injury who go on to develop oppositional defiant disorder (Max et al. 1998).

(c) Early neuromotor/obstetric problems, markers of brain disease, plus an unstable family environment predict violence in young men (Raine et al. 1996).

(d) Greater dysfunction of energy metabolism in prefrontal brain regions is found in murderers with no history of psychosocial deprivation (Raine et al. 1998)

In the case of examples (b) and (c) the effect is not simply the additive effect of two independent processes. It is due to a positive interaction: having both risk factors markedly increases your risk.

This firm evidence of a close interaction between brain disease and psychological factors means that it is not possible to entertain the notion of a mind divorced from the body.

3. Cognitive models of mental symptoms demonstrate how the mind and brain interact

We need a good cognitive model of mental symptoms which can explain how brain disorder and psychological process interact. Such an account will help our colleagues and the public appreciate the limitations of mind–body dualism.

Damasio (1994) has proposed a cognitive model which goes some way to explaining the behaviour of people with antisocial personality disorder: the somatic marker hypothesis. It is by no means the only plausible account of what happens in the brain in antisocial personality disorder. It perhaps only explains one aspect of the condition: the person's impoverished ability to take future consequences into account in decisions to act. The somatic marker hypothesis does, however, have the virtue of being testable, and bringing together the biology and psychology of personality disorder.

The model rests on the idea that the higher cognitive functions of the brain are founded on more primitive brain systems involved in emotional processing. Reasoning is therefore not divorced from emotional processing but relies on phylogenetically older systems of the brain which guide behaviour through awareness of pleasant or unpleasant bodily states. These systems enable the animal to know, on the basis of past experience, what action is most likely to be successful.

Damasio gives the example of a bee looking for nectar in a meadow full of flowers. Which colour flower is most likely to be rewarding? By integrating the results of sampling of numerous flowers the bee develops a continuously updated probability profile. On the basis of this the flowers which are most likely to be rewarding are selected.

A person negotiating his way through society needs a similar guidance system. For example should he borrow money from his best friend's worst enemy? The best outcome of this quandary is not available from conscious interrogation of all the various possible outcomes; there are too many permutations and combinations stretching too far into the future. We need a system which has learnt from past experience of decisions taken in similar circumstances. Some of the outcomes will not have transpired till months or years after these earlier deeds. The good, bad and indifferent outcomes of each past deed are integrated to give the best bet on future consequences of similar options now being considered. On the basis of this a signal is sent, a *somatic marker*, to guide decision making.

Damasio suggests that it is the unconscious experience of our somatic state, a somatic marker, which guides our decision making and actions. Thus a decision to act in a way which in the past has been followed by a poor outcome will be met with an antagonistic somatic marker; a "red" signal. It will be suppressed.

This somatic marker system relies on information flowing between conscious processing of higher cognitive functions in the cerebral cortex, and the limbic system. The former comprehends the question and its social context, considers the options, and acts on the decision; the latter provides the somatic marker. He suggests that the medial orbital frontal cortex is the interface between these two systems, and when it is damaged somatic control of actions is lost. We may "know" what to do, but won't do it if the somatic marker is set at red; and just as troubling we may "know" what not to do but will nevertheless do it if the somatic marker is set at green. This then explains his observation that such patients have preserved social knowledge, but fail to act appropriately on the basis of this knowledge. The result is irresponsible behaviour and antisocial acts.

Two predictions follow from the model, both of which have been confirmed (Damasio 1996):

1. In patients with medial orbital frontal cortex lesions information from conscious processing fails to get through to the limbic system. They therefore have impaired autonomic responses to stressful events.

2. They fail to learn on a gambling task and continue to select high-risk cards which result in losses over the longer term.

How does this model help to bridge the mind–body gap?

1. The highest cognitive and personality attributes are founded on primitive brain systems which rely on bodily experiences.
2. The model suggests that the development of a healthy somatic marker system relies on good parenting. To develop, the system must be exposed to a family environment in which actions usually predict outcomes. In this way the connections will develop and learning be enabled. But in a chaotic household a child's reasonably consistent responses may be met with affection on one occasion and anger the next, depending on the unpredictable state of mind of a parent. Or conversely, quite contrary responses may be followed by the same response. This will stunt the development of the system and any outputs will probably be ignored as unreliable.

More recently Damasio and colleagues (Anderson et al. 1999) have looked at brain injuries to this region occurring early in life and suggested that when the lesion is early, the impact is wider. The two cases showed insensitivity to future consequences of actions, similar to people damaged in adult life, but in addition showed defective social and moral reasoning. The result was a picture more typical of idiopathic antisocial personality disorder.

The broader range of problems with early damage indicates the overlap between processes involved in decision making and those for empathy and morals. Better understanding of the biological and psychosocial contributions to these important social functions will perhaps suggest treatment strategies for these conditions. They are at present difficult to treat and accordingly suffer greater stigmatisation.

References

Anderson SW, Bechara A, Damasio H et al. (1999) Impairment of social and moral behaviour related to early damage in human prefrontal cortex. *Nature Neuroscience* **2**: 1032–7.

Brooks DN & McKinlay W (1983) Personality and behavioural change after severe blunt head injury – a relative's view. *Journal of Neurology, Neurosurgery and Psychiatry* **46**: 336–44.

Damasio AR (1994) *Descartes' Error*. New York: Grosset/Putnam.

Damasio AR (1996) The somatic marker hypothesis and the possible functions of the prefrontal cortex. *Philosophical Transactions of the Royal Society B* **351**: 1413–20.

Fleminger S & Burns A (1993) The delusional misidentification syndromes in patients with and without evidence of organic cerebral disorder: a structured review of case reports. *Biological Psychiatry* **33**: 22–32.

Kozol HL (1946) Pretraumatic personalty and psychiatric sequelae of head injury. II Correlation of multiple specific factors in the pretraumatic personality and psychiatric reaction to head injury, based on analysis of 101 cases. *Archives of Neurology and Psychiatry* **56**: 245–75.

Max JE, Castillo CS, Bokura H et al. (1998) Oppositional defiant disorder symptomatology after traumatic brain injury: a prospective study. *Journal of Nervous and Mental Disorder* **186**: 325–32.

Raine A, Brennan P, Mednick B & Mednick SA (1996) High rates of violence, crime, academic problems and behavioral problems in males with both early neuromotor deficits and unstable family environments. *Archives of General Psychiatry* **53**: 544–9.

Raine A, Stoddard J, Birhle S & Buchsbaum M. (1998) Prefrontal glucose deficits in murderers lacking psychosocial deprivation. *Neuropsychiatry, Neuropsychology and Behavioural Neurology* **11**: 1–7.

44 Antibodies to personality disorder

Anthony Bateman

Introduction

Memory, specificity, and recognition of "non-self" lie at the heart of immunology. Early in life contact with an external infectious agent imprints information within a developing, physiological system and imparts a memory. Triggering of that memory by the invasion of the same or similar agent results in the rapid awakening and mobilisation of a dormant army of defenders. The defenders are antibodies which recognise the infectious agent as "non-self". The antibodies sacrifice themselves by combining with the invader, known as an antigen, and the pair die together in service of the whole organism. This principle forms the basis of vaccination in which a relatively harmless form of an antigen is used to imprint "memory". The body's defences are placed on alert so that any subsequent contact with similar invaders leads to an explosive production of defenders to prevent the infection taking hold.

In a similar vein we can understand the development of personality and protection from disorder. Memory, specificity, and recognition of the self and non-self are at the core of personality development. Just as antigens stimulate antibodies so psychological processes of the mother or care-giver stimulate responses in the developing infant which are remembered and repeated. The responses are adaptive and gradually become the best way the child has for dealing with situations that recur. This forms the basis of transference as posited by psychoanalytic theory.

Overall the immunological system is developmental, protective from infection, and reliant on a dynamic interchange between the internal and external worlds which in itself is dependent on differentiation between self and non-self. Personality is also developmental, protects the individual from psychological trauma, and has a relationship between internal and external or self and non-self at its core. The personality is as varied and individual as the immunological response, begins in infancy, depends on both environmental influences and internal factors, and may be acquired both passively and actively.

Before we can understand factors protecting against personality disorder we must clarify what is meant by the term personality disorder.

Personality disorder (PD)

All are agreed that personality and its development are complex, poorly understood, and that no one factor accounts for their variance. Attempts to categorise personalities, for example in ICD-10 and DSM-IV, are united only by their inadequacy. For greater precision people talk of traits or dimensions. It seems that traits may well predispose or even determine what type of personality disorder an individual can develop. Children with anxious traits develop PD with anxiety problems such as avoidant or obsessive–compulsive personality whilst those with traits of impulsivity develop antisocial or borderline PD. But whatever the categorisation of PD, there is little doubt that it is basically a disorder of relationships. All definitions contain statements about interpersonal and social situations. I intend to take borderline personality disorder (BPD) as my prototype. In this condition the patient shows "stable instability", comprising intense but unstable personal relationships; self-destructiveness; constant efforts to avoid real or imagined abandonment; chronic dysphoria such as anger or boredom; transient psychotic episodes or cognitive distortions; impulsivity; poor social adaptation; and identity disturbance.

Personality development

Personality develops via a multitude of influences. Whilst these are large in number, each one is small in effect. They may be grouped either as genetic or as psychosocial factors. Twin studies allow us to partial out the relative contribution of environmental and genetic factors. There is no doubt that dispositional traits show heritability. Many of the traits of BPD have been shown to have some inheritability. But the problem is not only that personality is clearly partially inherited, like some antibodies, in a passive manner and that it is partially environmentally determined, but that multiple genetic and environmental factors contribute to each trait and that whether a vulnerability to a trait is switched on may also depend on environment. Conversely traits may be switched off by environmental influence. Let us take the example of naturally shy monkeys. When baby monkeys who are naturally shy are fostered by confident monkey mothers they quickly outgrow their shyness.

In summary, we have a situation in which genetic and environmental influences intermingle in a complex way with neither having primacy. Personality is both within and without the genes, and it is the environment that can provide the antibodies to disorder. So, what are these antibodies?

Antibodies to personality disorder

In effect antibodies to personality disorder are certain traits that develop during infancy and childhood as a result of family environment, experience of trauma and deprivation, and social and cultural influence. We are now beginning to realise that the mother–infant interaction is one of the most potent relationships governing the personality and that not only is resistance to infection transferred from mother to baby but psychological resilience can be transferred too. So what factors are important? In essence these are what I am going to call basic "prototraits" which eventually give rise to behavioural phenotypes which we can observe. There are many of these "prototraits" and I am only going to discuss three of them in relation to borderline personality disorder. These are attachment styles, intersubjectivity, and tolerance of arousal.

Attachment

Attachment theory, developed by John Bowlby (1969), a psychoanalyst, postulates a universal human need to form close affectional bonds. At its core is a reciprocity of early relationships, most often the mother–infant relationship. Attachment behaviours of the infant such as proximity seeking, smiling, and clinging are reciprocated by adult behaviours such as touching, soothing, vocalisation, holding, and so on. There is a "musical dance" between mother and infant. The deftly learned steps are so subtle that we are only just beginning to appreciate their complexity. The goal of the attachment system is the experience of security, which is the primary regulator of emotional experience. We are not born to regulate our own emotional reactions. A regulatory system evolves in which an infant's signals of moment to moment change are understood and responded to by the caregiver, thereby achieving regulation. Experience of this mother/caregiver–infant interaction are aggregated into representational systems or internal working models. Later we rely on these models to predict reactions and to respond to emotions, particularly within relationships. Again this forms the basis of transference. In fact we can reliably measure these internal working models in action using the strange situation test (Ainsworth et al. 1978). Infants briefly separated from their caregiver in a situation which is strange to them react in different ways. Secure infants explore their surroundings readily in the presence of their caregiver, are anxious in the presence of a stranger, are distressed by their caregiver's absence, rapidly seek re-contact with the caregiver on her return and shortly afterwards continue their exploration. Some infants are made less anxious by separation, do not seek proximity following separation and seem not to differentiate between caregiver and stranger. These infants are anxious-avoidant. A third group appear to show limited exploration, are highly distressed by separation and cannot settle afterwards. The caregiver's attempts to reassure fail and the infant's anger and anxiety appear to prevent him from deriving comfort from proximity. These infants are known as anxious-resistant. Finally a group exhibit undirected behaviour, for example becoming disorganised, resorting to hand clapping, head banging, or even freezing. A history of repeated separation, intense marital conflict, and severe neglect or physical or sexual abuse have all been associated with this pattern.

These infant patterns of attachment have been shown to be stable across the lifespan to the extent that individuals have been followed over the years. Prospective longitudinal research has shown that children with a history of secure attachment are independently rated as more resilient, self-reliant, socially orientated, empathic to distress, and to have deeper relationships (Sroufe et al. 1990). In fact the attachment style at 1 year is the single best predictor of psychopathology at 5–6 years. Other longitudinal studies have shown a 68–75% correspondence between attachment classifications in infancy and classifications in adulthood (Becker-Stoll et al. 1999). It is possible to classify attachment patterns in adults through the Adult Attachment Interview (AAI) (Main and Goldwyn 1994). Further, attachment relationships play a key role in the transgenerational transmission of deprivation or personality resilience. Secure adults are 3–4 times more likely to have children who are securely attached to them. Even more startling is the fact that the pattern that the mother remembers as having with her own mother is the best predictor of the attachment pattern she will have with her own baby. This is true even when parental attachment is measured before the birth of the child. Children may have different attachment patterns with each parent or different caregivers.

Attempts to link attachment styles of infancy to BPD have met with some success. There is evidence of a link between childhood sexual abuse and BPD (Paris et al. 1994), although not all individuals who experience abuse develop BPD so there are clearly other factors. Most studies show rates of reported abuse of between 25% and 60%. AAI narratives of BPD show a predominance of preoccupied attachment styles, and within this the confused, fearful, and overwhelmed sub-classification appears to be most common. Other work has emphasised both the preoccupied and ambivalently attached features of BPD (Gunderson 1996). For example the need of borderline patients to seek proximity is well known, with patients telephoning frequently, demanding help, and even clinging to their helper and refusing to leave out-patient clinics and in-patient wards.

But, directly applied, normative observations of attachment are probably insufficient to provide an account of the development of BPD even though patients are clearly insecure in their attachment. Firstly, anxious attachment patterns in infancy may correspond to relatively stable adult strategies. Secondly, angry protests of an obstinate but clinging infant may fit neatly as an analogy of the aggressive stance of the borderline, but the borderline frequently attacks her own body rather than the mind of someone else. It seems there must be more to it, and in order to increase our understanding of the different developmental processes I shall now turn to intersubjectivity, a further prototrait.

Intersubjectivity

Whilst attachment patterns are observable, internal psychological processes accompany their development. Of major importance for the personality is the development of intersubjectivity. Intersubjectivity is the ability of an individual to understand another person's mind. The capacity to say accurately "I feel that you feel that I feel etc." is more complex than it sounds. Inability to understand others and their reactions is at the heart of personality disorder as well as some other problems. In some personalities there is a failure of empathy. This is prominent in anti-social, narcissistic, and borderline personalities. In others there is a more specific failure to understand another's thoughts, for example schizotypal personality. It is probable that the development of a full capacity to understand another is a complex interaction of different developmental systems involving the self, the other, and inanimate objects.

At 9 months a child will point at something and continue pointing until the mother looks in the right direction. The child will then stop pointing. In order to do this he needs to be able to understand that his mother's gaze links with recognition of the direction of the object.

Around 15 months empathy develops. For example a child's way of comforting himself was by sucking his thumb and pulling his ear. On seeing his father was upset he put his own thumb in his mouth and went over to his father and started stroking his father's ear. Again, to do this requires recognition of the feeling of the father, a linking of that feeling to an experience of ones' own, and the implementation of a response that has been found to be helpful for oneself. In this particular example it may be that the self and other remain partially undifferentiated since the child sucks his own thumb and pulls his father's ear!

A 3-year-old watches his friend hide a chocolate in a box saying that he will come back later to eat it. After he leaves the room the experimenter moves the chocolate and places it in a fruit bowl amongst the apples. The observing child is asked "where will your friend look for the chocolate when he returns to the room?" The 3-year-old predicts that his friend will look in the fruit bowl as he himself knows that is where it is. He makes the mistake of believing that his knowledge is shared with his friend. He cannot differentiate between his knowledge and that of his friend. Four- to five-year-olds will accurately predict that their friend will look in the place in which they left the chocolate. The three-year-old has not yet developed a theory of mind but the four- to five-year-olds have.

As I have mentioned, an impairment in intersubjectivity is present in personality disorders to a greater or lesser degree (Fonagy and Target 1996). The unstable sense of the self found in borderline patients results from an absence of reflective capacity. Inner representations of one's own internal states and those of others are a prerequisite of a stable sense of identity. Maltreatment, frequent misinterpretations of the child's state by the caregiver, and frank abuse impair this development. The consequence is an adult who does know who or what he is, what he does or does not feel. This results in an attempt to establish an identity through the use of others. Borderline patients see whole aspects of themselves in others and try to control them as if they were part of their own internal representation, losing the potential for a "real" relationship between two people. If aspects of oneself are experienced as being in others, separation becomes frightening, and Gunderson (1996) has highlighted the intolerance of aloneness and terror of abandonment of borderline patients.

Tolerance of arousal

Emotional instability is another common symptom of BPD and has even formed the core of some theoretical views. Linehan (1993) argues that the central problem of the borderline individual is affect regulation. Parental responsiveness to a child's feelings is important if a child is to learn to control emotion. There are two aspects to this that I would like to mention. Firstly, parents continually try and expand a child's tolerance of anxiety, for example by gradually increasing separation. The child replaces the parent with a substitute or transitional object which at one moment represents the mother or caretaker thereby allaying anxiety and yet at another is unnecessary and merely a blanket or teddy bear. Overprotection or neglect of the child distorts this process and prevents autonomy. Secondly, persistent invalidation of a child's feeling and internal state leads to confusion of feelings and inability to distinguish one feeling from another. If the child feels angry at something and that feeling is invalidated how can the recognition of appropriate and inappropriate anger develop?

Consistent with this view is the fact that borderline patients are known to often present in states of high anxiety or to show sudden outbursts of rage. Ability to tolerate such feelings requires mentalisation which acts as a buffer when actions of others are unexpected (Fonagy 1991). A capacity to think about feelings allows a space between feeling and action and forestalls automatic conclusions about intentions. Clearly the traumatised individual is going to be disadvantaged as his or her internal working models are based on early experience in which malevolence is not just possible but probable. It may be impossible for a therapist, for example, to persuade a patient that his interpretation of motive is wrong. Indeed to try and do so may be experienced as an attempt to destroy his mind. The borderline patient cannot imagine easily that someone else could have a construction of reality different from his own, which is experienced as compelling and accurate.

Conclusion and antibody development

Returning now to protection against personality disorder, no single factor alone can account for the variance of personality and its disorders. The interaction of the environment and our genes determines our final character. I hope that I have made the case that it is the dynamic interplay between infant and mother that is formative and protective. Failure to develop robust and resilient prototraits leads to disorder. It is the study of attachment and other "prototraits" that will be productive for our future understanding of personality, not only to help us to protect against disorder but also to inform our treatments, which at present are relatively inadequate.

Taking a developmental and relational view of personality, as I have done, leads firmly to a psychotherapeutic approach as the core of treatment (Bateman and Fonagy 2000). All psychotherapies rely on the development of a constructive relationship as a vehicle for effective change. Failure actively or passively to acquire psychological antibodies during childhood may be ameliorated through a psychotherapeutic vaccination. Psychotherapy stimulates relational problems in a sort of test tube and is able to look at other ways of reacting in the future. It also insists that an individual

243

develops an understanding of the mind of another and thereby develops intersubjectivity. In this way an individual who is faced with a relational or social situation which in the past has led to distress and personal damage may find a new way to negotiate the problem – a pathway that has been stimulated, remembered, and understood through the treatment itself. This may allow borderline patients not to harm themselves, not to destroy relationships but, above all, to gain pleasure in relationships with others.

References

Ainsworth MDS, Blehar MC, Waters E & Wall S (1978) *A Psychological Study of the Strange Situation*. Hillsdale, NJ: Erlbaum.

Bateman AW & Fonagy P (2000) Effectiveness of psychotherapeutic treatment of personality disorder. *British Journal of Psychiatry* **177**: 138–43.

Becker-Stoll F, Zimmerman P & Fremmer-Bombik E (1999) Discontinuity and continuity in adult attachment representation: a 12-year longitudinal study. Presented at Society for Research in Child Development Biennial Meeting, Albuquerque, New Mexico, April.

Bowlby J (1969) *Attachment and Loss*, Vol 1: *Attachment*. London, Hogarth Press and Institute of Psychoanalysis.

Fonagy P (1991) Thinking about thinking: some clinical and theoretical considerations in the treatment of a borderline patient. *International Journal of Psychoanalysis* **72**: 639–56.

Fonagy P & Target M (1996) Playing with reality: I. Theory of mind and the normal development of psychic reality. *International Journal of Psychoanalysis* **77**: 217–33.

Gunderson JG (1996) The borderline patient's intolerance of aloneness: insecure attachments and therapist availability. *American Journal of Psychiatry* **153**: 752–8.

Linehan MM (1993) *Cognitive–Behavioural Treatment of Borderline Personality Disorder*. New York: Guilford Press.

Main M & Goldwyn R (1994) Adult attachment rating and classification system. Unpublished manuscript, University of California at Berkeley.

Paris J, Zweig-Frank H & Guzder J (1994) Psychogical risk factors for borderline personality disorder in male outpatients. *Journal of Nervous and Mental Disease* **182**: 375–413.

Sroufe LA, Egeland B & Kreutzer T (1990) The fate of early experience following developmental change: longitudinal approaches to individual adaptation in childhood. *Child Development* **61**: 1363–73.

Commentary on Section 5B

Christopher Cordess

In Chapter 43 Simon Fleminger traces our (empirically established) greater prejudice and stigmatisation of mental disorders, as opposed to physical disorders, to the entrenched mind–body dualism of our cultural and professional ways of thought. He cites personality disorder as a particularly striking case of dualistic thinking, and argues, cogently, that such dualism is incompatible with contemporary knowledge regarding the complex interactions of brain and mind (i.e. psychological processes) in the aetiology of personality disorder. He proposes, possibly optimistically, that with greater understanding should come a reduction of stigmatisation of the personality disordered patient. This effect may be tempered, however, by the fact, as emphasised by Bateman in Chapter 44, that personality disorder is essentially a relationship problem which impinges upon others and frequently offends society – which, naturally, tends to respond in kind.

Fleminger gives examples – one from Damasio (1994) and one from his own practice – in which a tumour and a traumatic injury to the medial orbital frontal region of the brain, respectively, produced disorders of personality which, aside from the history (of late onset) and test results, produced a clinical picture and mental symptoms indistinguishable from the more common type of personality disorder which is traditionally considered to be a "disorder of the mind". As if to underline our dualistic thinking, personality disorders where no organic or neuropsychological cause has been detected have been referred to as "idiopathic" in the neuropsychiatric literature.

Fleminger cites his own investigations of the interaction of psychological processes and the effects of brain disease, and consequent interactive treatment interventions. He briefly reviews the "cognitive model" of (unconscious) "somatic markers" described by Damasio (1994), which is a general theory but which specifically informs us about the behaviour of people with antisocial personality disorder. This theory relies on the view that emotional processing is represented by phylogenetically older, somatic, systems in the brain which, however, underpin and are essential to the function of the higher cognitive functions. Reasoning and rationality are intertwined with, and dependent upon, emotional processes, as – in psychological and neurophysical terms – information flows back and forth between emotional representations in the limbic system and consciously processed higher cognitions in the cerebral cortex. I think it true to say that the perceived view now is that cognitive and emotional functions are distributed over a large number of mutually complementary and interdependent critical and subcritical systems and processes (Damasio 1994). In brief, emotion and reason are interdependent in health and are separable only in pathological states. This is a remarkably similar non-dualistic, integrated model to the one described by Bateman from a more psychological starting point. In fact, it has an uncanny resemblance to the early psychoanalytic model of the topographical division between conscious ("secondary process") and unconscious ("primary process") mental function, but with the (considerable) increased biological specificity of locating function (and error) in this system in the medial orbital frontal cortex. Fleminger concludes that the development of a healthy somatic marker system relies on good parenting. To develop, the system must be exposed to a parental and social system in which "actions reasonably reliably predict outcomes". This coincides with the emotional "validation", "intersubjectivity" and "tolerance of arousal" – and possible confusion of emotions – discussed by Bateman, which I refer to below.

Anthony Bateman has a way of describing and summarising the most complex bodies of observational and experimental research, and clinical experience and clinical theory, in easy to follow, everyday language. He represents a growing body of practitioners who integrate psychodynamic and psychiatric knowledge in a powerful combination. He uses the active and passive acquisition of physical antibodies by the infant from the mother, or by vaccination, as a metaphor for the psychological development of human personality, ideally in relationship with the parent, but, where that goes wrong, in a later therapeutic one. He traces the roles of what he calls "proto-traits", selecting three – "attachment style", "intersubjectivity" and "tolerance of arousal" – in the development of "normal personality" and "borderline personality disorder" (BPD), respectively. He regards personality disorder essentially as a disorder of interpersonal and, therefore, social relationships which is better accounted for by traits or dimensions than by attempted specific categorisation.

In aetiological terms he is clear that personality development is dependent upon both genetic, heritable dispositions and traits on the one hand, and environmental influence on the other, in an interactive and complex intermingling – with neither having primacy, but in which one can help "trump" the other: for example strong genetic resilience factors may "make up" for a poor environment, or, particularly "containing" parenting may compensate for genetic vulnerability. So far, it is the environment which is most mutable and can be adjusted to provide the necessary antibodies by internalisation of "infant – mother – infant" experience, although genome research long in the future may have relevance for making adjustments to flawed personality development.

Bateman describes Bowlby's attachment theory as based upon a universal human need to form close affectionate bonds. We are not born to regulate our emotional reactions within such relationships, and need to learn such regulation by experiencing emotional security within the reciprocity of interaction – the "musical dance" – between mother and infant. We thereby acquire "internal working models" with which we can predict reactions and respond within future interpersonal relationships. He gives an account of the variation in these "internal working models" and consequent attachment styles which can be demonstrated empirically; there may be, for example, (stable) secure or (unstable) anxious–avoidant or anxious–resistant attachments formed; or, worst, the infant may develop a "disorganised" form of attachment, which has been linked to a history of repeated separations, or severe physical or sexual abuse. These attachment patterns in infants have been shown to be remarkably consistent over the lifespan, on follow-up in longitudinal studies, and clearly therefore have major import in the understanding of personality development and personality disorder. Specifically, so-called "preoccupied" and "ambivalently attached" sub-categories of attachment, as well as the "disorganised" form are predictive of some BPD. However, Bateman concludes that "directly applied, normative observations of attachment" are probably insufficient for a total account of the development of BPD.

Bateman describes the internal psychological processes which accompany "attachment" in terms of "inter-subjectivity", and its developmental importance in regard to understanding the feelings and thoughts of others – and the significance of the failure of such developments in the various sub-types of personality disorder.

Specifically, the unstable sense of self found in BPD patients may be considered to result from an absence of reflective capacity, or "reflective self function" which, in turn, is traceable to failures of representations of self and others. Maltreatment, failures of "atunement" and misinterpretation of the child's subjective state by the carer, or frank abuse, may all impair normal development. The consequence may be a borderline personality in which a person does not know who or what she is, or what she feels. As a consequence others may be "recruited", by whom she can live – as it were – vicariously, by massive projection and introjection: such a "solution" is hopeless for the development of a relationship between two distinct people and explains the instability of relationships of those with BPD, as well as their alternation between terror of aloneness and abandonment, on the one hand, and chaotic "fused" relationship states on the other. Borderline personality disorder, that is, can be conceptualised partly as a failure to develop inter-subjectivity.

A related "proto-trait" is that of "tolerance of arousal" (indeed "enjoyment" of emotional intensity), and its opposite, the failure to regulate arousal and related emotional states. Such failure also is a core failure in those suffering from BPD. The "normal" development of "affect regulation" (Linehan 1993) relies upon gradual experiences of separation and loss which can be mourned – frequently for the child via the use of transitional objects – and which are thereby tolerated, albeit relatively or imperfectly. For Donald Winnicott this was the gradual impinging of an adult state of "disillusion" upon an infantile state of "illusion". Similarly, a degree of attainment of inter-subjectivity of feeling will "validate" and give empowerment to a capacity for regulation of affects and emotions. By contrast, persistent failure to recognise feelings, or their invalidation, will lead to later confusions of emotions when high states of arousal occur. Mentalisation and self-reflection will not have developed sufficiently to act as a "buffer" under degrees of psychological stress.

Bateman thereby stakes out the ground for a predominantly psychotherapeutic approach as the core treatment for personality disorders, in which, according to this view, there has been a failure by the primary carer to impart a "psychological survival kit". All the psychotherapies and sociotherapies have their place, and emphatically not any single mode. He picks up the metaphor of vaccination for stimulation of childhood antibodies to physical disease where maternal transmission has not occurred, and likens it again to the psychological situation described, and the possibility of "vaccination" by psychotherapy.

Implicit in the whole approach is the need for education and services based upon the significance of these developmental processes and the instigation and resourcing of preventative measures – a tall order for a society which, overall, with its fragmentation and breaking down of community structures, appears rapidly to be heading in the opposite direction.

The conclusion of both these excellent papers could be summarised by Fleminger's final two sentences. "Better understanding of the biological and psychosocial contributions of these important social functions will perhaps suggest treatment strategies [and, one might add, preventative measures] for these conditions. They are at present difficult to treat and accordingly suffer greater stigmatisation". Both contributors have contributed to our better understanding from, perhaps, as non-dualist a point of view as 21st century man is presently able to achieve.

References

Damasio AR (1994) *Descartes' Error*. New York: Grosset/Putnam.
Linehan MM (1993) *Cognitive–Behavioural Treatment of Borderline Personality Disorder*. New York: Guilford Press.

45 Where to treat? Its relevance to treatability

Robert Bluglass

My current interest in this subject is, of course, inspired by the two years that I recently spent as a member of the team appointed to investigate the serious irregularities in the Personality Disorder Unit at Ashworth Special Hospital. At the beginning of 1997 a patient on the Personality Disorder Unit at Ashworth absconded, and a document which found its way to the Secretary of State for Health listed allegations which maintained that several patients on the wards, including a number with horrific histories of violence and antisocial behaviour, were out of the control of the staff and engaged in a variety of illicit activities.

In particular it was alleged that staff misappropriated prescription drugs and sold them to patients; one ward was a distribution centre for drugs to the rest of the PDU; random drug tests were advertised in advance and easy to evade; large amounts of cash circulated on the ward; an ex-patient of the unit visited the ward in the company of his young daughter and this child was allowed to play unsupervised with two patients, one of whom had a record of serious sexual offences against young girls. The father of the girl regularly brought in pornography, which was copied by patients, and traded. Patients were able to smuggle in alcohol, sometimes with the complicity of staff. In addition room searches were farcical, some rooms had allegedly not been searched for over a year and patients were often warned of impending searches, giving time to move offending material; patients were able to select compliant nurses to escort them on outside trips. These allegations were so serious that the Secretary of State initiated a judicial inquiry under the chairmanship of His Honour Peter Fallon QC, the recently retired Senior Circuit Judge and Recorder of Bristol (Fallon et al. 1999a,b).

We were asked to investigate these allegations and in the light of our findings to review the management of the PDU, its security arrangements and aspects of the management of the hospital. Our remit was then widened, when the Inquiry was announced in Parliament, and then again when our remit was reviewed by the succeeding Secretary of State for Health, Mr Frank Dobson and his Junior Minister Mr Paul Boateng. This allowed us to consider the nature and treatability of psychopathic disorder and to make recommendations for future care and management with knowledge of the views of a range of specialists and other colleagues on these contentious topics.

We were thus able to carry out a very detailed, thorough and objective investigation of Ashworth which confirmed that most of the allegations that had been made were largely accurate and there were also a considerable number of other deficiencies in management and in professional responsibilities.

When we reviewed the history of the development of the concept of psychopathic disorder it became crystal-clear that this is a topic that has been characterised by scepticism, uncertainty and lack of agreement since it was first given a legal status by the Percy Commission in 1954 (HMSO 1957). The realisation that the inclusion of psychopathic disorder in the Mental Health Act of 1959 would mean that unknown numbers of such patients may be admitted to Broadmoor and other hospitals resulted in a political knee-jerk reaction on the part of the then Minister, Enoch Powell, which reflected the stigma, ambivalence and nervousness towards them. This resulted in the 1961 Inquiry into the Special Hospitals which recommended that special units should be set up, ostensibly for research and assessment, but primarily to hive this group off to others to contain. In the event only one such unit was created, in North London, which was not in the end used for this purpose.

This concern can be understood. The enthusiasm of the time to incorporate psychopathic disorder in the 1959 Act owed much to the late Sir David Henderson's classic definition which concluded that the inadequacy or failure of psychopaths to adjust to ordinary social life is "not a mere wilfulness or badness which can be threatened or thrashed out of an individual so involved, but constitutes a true illness for which we have no specific explanation" (Henderson 1939). He pointed out to his opponents that the failure of their punitive methods supported his arguments but he also acknowledged that psychopathy is frequently not amenable to medical treatment. Consequently, these patients were seen, at least by some, to have been imposed upon the hospitals even though a strategy for treatment had not yet been devised.

At the time of our Inquiry into Ashworth it was evident that there was a wide diversity of opinion about the treatability of those categorised a suffering from psychopathic disorder. In 1992 Dr Rosemarie Cope surveyed all British consultant forensic psychiatrists for their views on diagnosis and treatability. Ninety percent responded. As far as treatability was concerned she found that there were firmly held and widely differing views. Only a minority of respondents, about 10%, were totally dismissive of psychopaths and their treatability. There was a similar proportion of enthusiasts who stated equally vehemently that psychiatrists had a duty to treat this group of patients who caused suffering to themselves and society. Most respondents were somewhere in between, with a range of views, according to the type of case, about where treatment should take place, under what legislation and by whom.

In the Ashworth Inquiry we decided that if we were to make recommendations about the future management and/or treatment of those with severe personality disorder (as we came to call them) we should take evidence from those with expertise or experience in this field who were known to have opinions on this subject. We decided to devote two weeks of our public hearings to the examination of experts who had previously agreed to submit a paper to us. They had been asked to give their views on the following issues:

1. The validity of the diagnosis of severe personality disorder.
2. The value of treatment of severe personality disorder.
3. The services needed to meet the needs of individuals suffering from severe personality disorder.
4. The relevance of the legal category of psychopathic disorder; and any changes deemed desirable in the current legal, clinical and administrative arrangements for managing these individuals.

Fifteen senior academic and clinical forensic psychiatrists and psychologists kindly agreed to cooperate with us, and we were particularly grateful to them for agreeing to submit to cross-examination from leading counsel and the panel – possibly not an easy experience, but the majority clearly enjoyed it. It was a method that allowed elucidation of opinions and a record to be taken and subsequently published as part of the evidence received by the Inquiry (Fallon et al. 1999a,b).

The evidence confirmed Dr Cope's findings that there continues to be a wide diversity of opinion among experts about the treatment and management of those with severe personality disorder.

But there was considerable agreement on a number of issues. Much of this evidence reflected agreement with conclusions recorded by Dolan and Coid (1993) in their excellent book. We found much agreement that some people in the severe category that concerned us are more treatable than others and that they are those who are less seriously disordered and with a lower propensity to violence. Some are sometimes treatable and their treatability depends upon the behaviour that has brought them to attention, the history and nature of the recent presenting episode and the presence or absence of co-existing conditions. Some patients are more treatment-resistant than others but need 'management', and to achieve some success in developing a therapeutic strategy, compliance is important.

We also concluded from the evidence of our experts that in developing a new strategy, the sensitive balance between therapy on the one hand and security on the other, which had failed on two occasions, must crucially be achieved in the future. We found that many psychiatrists, including some working in secure settings, believed that psychological methods of treatment are the most effective and that pharmacological methods are generally ineffective although necessary in some patients, particularly those with co-morbidity. We also considered that the principles developed in the therapeutic community model have much to offer for some patients.

We gave much time to arriving at our conclusions for the management of those with severe personality disorder in the future, bearing in mind the views expressed by our experts and our conclusion that new units are necessary in the future for those few in the severe category who are likely to be treatable. Firstly we concluded that:

1. Hospital management and treatment is appropriate for "compliant" patients and those who do not suffer from treatment-resistant anti-social severe personality disorder.
2. We do not accept from the evidence that all persons classified by whatever means as suffering from a personality disorder are necessarily suffering from a disease, equivalent to a physical disease, or that they are always appropriately to be dealt with in the health services (with the risk that this legitimises their detention). Some will of course benefit; it is a matter for individual assessment.
3. Management in prison units is more appropriate for some, particularly those who are non-compliant and treatment-resistant.
4. The diagnosis, classification and treatment needs of individual cases must be based upon standardised protocols and be administered by specially trained and approved personnel.

We considered it important to recognise that not all of those with a severe personality disorder are necessarily dangerous. Between 2% and 3% of the general population are said to be classifiable as anti-social personality disorder. They may suffer personally as a result and may be a source of difficulty from time to time to others but they may not commit an offence punishable by imprisonment or demonstrate a risk to others. Those who are dangerous, who present a real and continued physical or psychological risk to others, do not necessarily have a severe personality disorder and no such assumption should be made unless it has been demonstrated by testing. We therefore came to the conclusion that dangerousness and severe personality disorder should be the subject of separate evaluation and assessment in those who have committed an offence punishable by imprisonment.

In order to avoid the "lottery", the gamble as to whether or not an offender is sent to prison or is made the subject of a hospital order, we recommended that the courts should no longer have the option of making a hospital order on a person who has offended and has a severe personality disorder. The prison service would, in the future, take responsibility for those assessed as unwilling or unable to benefit from hospital care. Others after conviction who are appropriately assessed for treatment (agreed standards and protocols etc.) would be transferred on a transfer direction and sent back when the time was right. Both the NHS and the prison service should develop special treatment units for those with severe personality disorder and work closely together.

In order to protect society from those who are dangerous, as we have defined it, who may or may not have a severe personality disorder and have not attracted an indefinite sentence, we have recommended the introduction of a reviewable sentence. This would be available for dangerous offenders for offences where the punishment for the offence is not fixed by law or where an indefinite sentence is not available to the trial judge. This would allow a reviewable sentence to be passed, based upon tariff principles, renewable for periods up to two years at a time.

Where is the most appropriate setting for the management of offenders with severe personality disorder? It was our conclusion that a hospital setting is appropriate for those who justify a medical model of management on the basis of assessment for treatability and that small special units within the NHS, linked to other facilities providing high security, are the best model. Such units would have a significant level of input from psychologists.

We already know from recent surveys that the prevalence of personality disorder is high in prisons in England and Wales (Singleton et al. 1998). There are already special units for those who present a high risk or threat, and we are suggesting that special units for those who are difficult to manage but who are untreatable or treatment-resistant should be provided in prisons. We were not persuaded that there is a justification for creating a new facility that is neither prison nor hospital as has been suggested by planners in the Home Office. Nor do we think that there is any justification for creating a new offence or grounds for detention for those who have not committed an offence but who are perceived by a public official to be a cause for concern, or a potential risk. We are not persuaded even if the person has a past record of dangerous offences. Our proposals can only be applicable and are only meant to be applicable to those who are appearing before a court. My colleagues and I are therefore concerned with the proposals which have recently been put forward in a discussion document by the Home Secretary and the Secretary of State for Health. Their proposals appear to perpetuate the misconception that the only way to detain dangerous people is by linking their behaviour to a mental disorder in order not to contravene the European Convention on Human Rights. If some personality disorders are treatable conditions they are stigmatised by this inevitable link to dangerousness. It is of course also unacceptable to require psychiatrists to make crucial decisions that will ultimately determine whether or not an individual loses his liberty.

Finally I would leave the last word to a much revered predecessor, one of the fathers of modern forensic psychiatry, Dr Peter Scott CBE, whose cautionary comments of 1975 ended our Report on the Personality Disorder Unit at Ashworth Special Hospital. Dr Scott was sceptical about the decision to develop Regional (Medium) Secure Units. In his Denis Carroll Lecture of 1975 he maintained that psychiatry had failed (a) the dangerous offender and (b) the unrewarding, degenerate, "not nice" offender (Scott 1975). He defined the two groups as follows: a dangerous offender is one who risks or brings about destruction which is severe, irreversible, unpredictable and untreatable. No matter how destructive a person has been in the past, he is not dangerous if he is treatable. The unrewarding patient is essentially one who does not "pay" for his treatment, either (i) by dependence or (ii) by getting better, or (iii) in either process by showing gratitude to his carers, cheerfully if possible. The "not nice" patients are the ones who habitually appear to be well able to look after themselves but do not, who break the institutional rules, get drunk, upset other patients, or even quietly go to the devil in their own way quite heedless of nurse or doctor.

Dr Scott went on to observe that detaining custodial institutions have two aims: one therapeutic, the other custodial. These can and should be complementary, but there is a tendency for these functions to polarise out and eventually split like a living cell into two separate institutions. He warned that the solution to the Special Hospital problem in the 1970s was not to build new institutions (meaning then the proposed medium secure units) but to put the funds into improving care in prisons. The medium secure units would, he predicted, be selective, excluding the most difficult patients such as psychopaths and those requiring high-security or long-term care. In due course new problems would arise and the tendency to divide would return.

References

Cope R (1992) A survey of forensic psychiatrists' views on psychopathic disorder. *Journal of Forensic Psychiatry* **4**: 215–35.

Dolan B & Coid J (1993) *Psychopathic and Antisocial Personality Disorders.* London: Gaskell.

Fallon P, Bluglass R, Edwards B & Daniels G (1999a) *Report of the Committee of Inquiry into the Personality Disorder Unit, Ashworth Special Hospital Cm 4194-1.* London: The Stationery Office.

Fallon P, Bluglass R, Edwards B & Daniels G (1999b) *Report of the Committee of Inquiry into the Personality Disorder Unit, Ashworth Special Hospital Cm 4195,* (Vol. II) London: The Stationery Office.

Henderson DK (1939) *Psychopathic States.* New York: Chapman and Hall.

HMSO (1957) Royal Commission on the Law Relating to Mental Illness and Mental Deficiency, (Chairman, Lord Percy of Newcastle). Report Cmnd 169. London: HMSO.

Scott PD (1975) *Has Psychiatry Failed in the Treatment of Offenders?* The Fifth Denis Carroll Lecture. Institute for the Study and Treatment of Delinquency, London.

Singleton N, Meltzer H, Gatward R, Coid J & Deasy D. (1998) *Psychiatric Morbidity Among Prisoners.* London: The Stationery Office.

46 The "therapeutic community": Outcome evaluation

Kingsley Norton and Fiona Warren

Personality disorder

Personality disorder (PD) is defined by the International Classification of Diseases (World Health Organization) as: "deeply ingrained and enduring behaviour patterns, manifesting themselves as inflexible responses to a broad range of personal and social situations. They represent either extreme or significant deviations from the way the average individual in a given culture perceives, thinks, feels and particularly relates to others. Such behaviour patterns tend to be stable and to encompass multiple domains of behaviour and psychological functioning. They are frequently, but not always, associated with various degrees of subjective distress and problems in social functioning and performance".

Diagnosing PD is a complex task, since all aspects of personal functioning need to be considered and many sources of information regarding the patient may need to be utilised. Evidence accumulated needs to demonstrate: (1) markedly disharmonious attitudes and behaviour; (2) an enduring pattern of abnormal behaviour not limited to episodes of illness; (3) a behaviour pattern that is clearly maladaptive to a broad range of personal and social situations; (4) attitudes and behaviour that may lead to considerable personal distress; (5) an association with significant problems in occupational and social performance. Inevitably there is a degree of subjective bias which is always present in making judgements about what is, for example, a "markedly disharmonious attitude" or a behaviour pattern which is "clearly maladaptive". As a result of all the above, the diagnosis may be unreliable.

There are many categories and sub-categories of PD (see Table 1). However, these heterogeneous categories are polythetic and not mutually exclusive. It is common for there to be PD sub-category co-morbidity (Dolan et al. 1995). Sadly, research has also shown that patients with PD are unpopular (Lewis and Appleby 1988). Some psychiatrists appear willing to stigmatise such individuals, through an unwillingness to make a diagnosis of personality disorder or to view them as potentially untreatable. It is difficult to imagine that such an unsatisfactory, if not unprofessional, state of affairs could exist with respect to many other diagnoses, which form part of the International Classification of Diseases (ICD).

Table 1. Classification of personality disorders in ICD-10 and DSM-IV: comparison of current classification of personality disorder subtypes (after Tyrer 1991)

ICD-10		DSM-IV	
Code	**Description**	**Code**	**Description**
F60.0	*Paranoid* – excessive sensitivity suspiciousness, preoccupation with conspiratorial explanation	301.00	*Paranoid* – interpretation of people's actions as deliberately demeaning or threatening
F60.1	*Schizoid* – emotional coldness detachment, lack of interest in other people, eccentricity and introspective fantasy	301.20	*Schizoid* – indifference to relationships and restricted range of emotional experience and expression
	No equivalent	301.22	*Schizotypal* – deficit in interpersonal relatedness with peculiarities of ideation, appearance and behaviour
F60.5	*Anankastic* – indecisiveness, doubt, excessive caution, pedentry, rigidity and need to plan in immaculate detail	301.40	*Obsessive-compulsive* – Pervasive perfectionism and inflexibility
F60.4	*Histrionic* – self-dramatisation shallow mood, egocentricity and craving for excitement with persistent manipulative behaviour	301.50	*Histrionic* – excessive emotionally and attention seeking
F60.7	*Dependent* – failure to take responsibility for actions, with subordination of personal needs to those of others, excessive dependence with need for constant reassurance and feelings of helplessness when a close relationship ends	301.60	*Dependent* – persistent dependent and submissive behaviour
F60.2	*Dysocial* – callous unconcern for others, with irresponsibility, irritablity and aggression, and incapacity to maintain enduring relationships	301.70	*Antisocial* – evidence of repeated conduct disorder before the age of 15 years
	No equivalent	301.81	*Narcissistic* – pervasive grandiosity, lack of empathy and hypersensitivity to the evaluation of others
F60.6	*Anxious* – persistent tension, self-consciousness, exaggeration of risks and dangers, hypersensitivity to rejection, and restricted lifestyle because of insecurity	301.82	*Avoidant* – pervasive social discomfort, fear of negative discomfort, fear of negative evaluation and timidity
F60.30	*Impulsive* – inability to control anger, to plan ahead, or to think before acts, with unpredictable mood and quarrelsome behaviour	301.83	*Borderline* – pervasive of mood and self-image
F30.31	*Borderline* – unclear self-image, involvement in intense and unstable relationships	301.84	*Passive aggressive* – pervasive passive resistence to demands for inadequate social and occupational performance

Problems with sub-categories

The frequently encountered co-morbidity of PD categories, in psychiatric and forensic patient samples, together with the lack of mutually exclusive sub-categories of PD, suggest that a unitary concept of PD may be more clinically useful (Coid 1990). The fact that sub-category co-morbidity rates show a gradient (from primary to secondary to tertiary healthcare levels and also with increasing levels of security), however, raises the possibility that the co-morbidity is a marker of overall PD severity (Dolan et al. 1995).

Defining severity is in itself problematic, since there is no single adequate severity measure or consensus about which battery of measures to apply (Norton and Dolan 1995). Many workers describe severity in terms of associated (rather than core) PD features, such as criminal behaviour or deliberate self-harming. Optimally, a small number of self- and observer-related instruments could measure the range of relevant domains of personal functioning, including both core and selected associated features. Without a satisfactory pre-treatment measure of severity, which is also sensitive to change, evaluating treatment outcome of personality disorder is highly problematic.

A pragmatic solution to the problem of measuring severity in PD has been suggested by defining a threshold for "severe" PD (SPD). Membership of more than one of the three "clusters" of DSM PD sub-categories and their defining characteristics thus qualifies a patient for SPD (Tyrer and Johnson 1996). Any patient fulfilling membership of two or more PD sub-categories *from more than one cluster* fulfils the definition of "severe". This issue of severity is topical, with the Government having published its document "Managing Dangerous People with Severe Personality Disorder [DSPD]: Proposals for Policy Development" (Home Office and Department of Health 1999). DSPD, with little agreement on the "S", and problems with judging accurately the "D" (let alone the "PD"), could exercise both clinical and research minds for years to come.

Problems with PD outcome literature

Most sub-categories of PD receive scant attention in terms of treatment and prognosis. Only two have been studied in depth: "borderline" and "anti-social". With the former, there are formidable terminological problems, since the adjective "borderline" is used both to refer to a psychoanalytic concept (Kernberg 1984) and as part of a DSM classification of Axis II Developmental Disorders (American Psychiatric Association). Anti-social personality disorder, however, is not without its own share of terminological vicissitudes, viz. "dissocial", "psychopathic", "sociopathic" disorder, which overlap but are not synonymous terms.

Embarking on fresh outcome research in the field of personality disorder is not helped by the poor quality of earlier methodologies and the unreliability of their associated findings. Currently there are inadequacies in the definition of personality disorder, overlapping criteria for its sub-categories, unreliable measures of baseline status, and inadequate measures of change (on one item of the antisocial personality sub-category criteria of DSM, for example, it is not possible to change because it concerns historical facts about the patient). Most previous studies have had small numbers (including high attrition rates), retrospective design, no control or comparison groups, and often inappropriate conclusions based on the presented data and its analysis.

Some of the above inadequacies in the PD literature are a reflection of the relative youth of the field of study and may be little different from those of other "young" sub-specialties. Certain of them, however, are PD-, SPD- and DSPD-specific methodological problems which future research must negotiate. First, there is the PD patient's relative incapacity to articulate his/her problems verbally (rather than nonverbally, for example, via interpersonal conflict with clinician or researcher) in ways that a clinician or researcher can recognise and measure. Second, based in part on the above difficulties, PD patients often challenge authority figures (including healthcare professionals and researchers) and may not comply with consent or other research procedures, such as form-filling, and may even "drop out" altogether. Third, PD patients' adequate treatment is usually lengthy and labour-intensive, leading to problems with recruiting adequate numbers to study in a feasible space of time. Fourth, there is a need for long-term follow-up to ascertain that core personality change has resulted and/or to demonstrate that change is sustainable. Fifth, the most severely disturbed PD patients require complex, as well as long-term, treatment interventions which do not lend themselves to an easy randomised controlled trial (RCT) methodology because of difficulties (ethical and otherwise), for example, not being able to maintain a pure, "no treatment" control group over an extended study period.

There is an ethical obstacle to randomisation in the absence of a demonstrated alternative treatment for SPD patients, many of whom are at considerable risk of destructive "acting out" (towards themselves and/or others) and who would be unable to receive therapeutic community (TC) treatment. In addition, experimental RCTs ideally have at least some blindness. This is not feasible for a treatment, such as at Henderson Hospital, which is both intensive and lengthy (average 7 months and a maximum of one year). As already mentioned, it would be unlikely that sufficient influence could be ethically exerted to ensure that the "no-treatment" group was just that. A "treatment as usual" comparison is a more feasible approach. Alternatively, if waiting lists for patients to be admitted are sufficiently long (itself an undesirable state of clinical affairs), the "waiting list condition" could be used as a control group, since ethical obstacles would be less serious.

In terms of a democratic TC treatment, such as that provided by Henderson Hospital, there are additional problems. Randomisation could introduce change to the treatment being studied, especially if it were to be carried out "post-selection". The selection process involves other patients and is part of a therapeutic alliance-building endeavour; hence it forms part of the treatment proper. Randomisation occurring after this point (i.e. after treatment had in effect started) would thus raise ethical issues concerning the potential harm to patients through disappointing reasonable expectations and breaking any alliance that had been formed.

A very thorough review of the TC and other literature in respect of "psychopathic and antisocial personality disorders" concluded that "the randomised double-blind control trial of treatment outcome is not yet appropriate for studying psychopathic disorder" (Dolan and Coid 1993). However, there have been RCTs as revealed by a recently commissioned, as yet unpublished, systematic literature review, evaluating evidence for the efficacy of TCs in psychiatric and other settings (Lees et al. 1999). Only 10 RCTs were identified but there were also 10 cross-institutional or comparative studies and a further 32 studies utilising some form of control group. Of these 52 studies, 41 related to democratic TCs, of which Henderson Hospital is an example.

A meta-analysis of the 29 studies which were of sufficient quality showed strong support for the effectiveness of TC treatment (Lees et al. 1999). Of the 29 studies, 19 indicated a positive effect, within the 95% level of confidence. The summary odds-ratio (0.57 and an upper confidence interval of 0.61) calculated across all 29 studies, as is the convention with meta-analyses, underlines the strength of this finding. It is worth noting also that the RCTs were spread across different types of TCs, suggesting that no one subset of studies strongly affected the overall summary result.

Henderson Hospital and treatment outcome

Treatment approach

Henderson Hospital's outcome studies suffer from almost all of the methodological flaws referred to above, at least to some degree. In spite of this, there has been a discernible trend over time for an improvement in the sophistication of the methodology employed. First and foremost there has been a more detailed description of the treatment method, which is embraced by the term "democratic therapeutic community" (DTC), than was available hitherto (Norton 1992).

Patient population

The population of patients treated at Henderson has also been defined more rigorously by an outcome study of 588 referrals to the service funded by South Thames (West) Regional Health Authority R & D Programme. In terms of sociodemographic characteristics, the population can be seen to be mainly single adults (average age 28; range from 17 to 45 years) who have had substantial prior psychiatric history and/or contact with the Criminal Justice System (see Table 2).

Table 2. Demographic characteristics of admissions to Henderson Hospital

Feature	Admissions 1991–1994 (n=238)	
	n	%
Gender (Female)	127	53.4
Ethnicity (White)	225	96.2
Marital Status (Single)	186	81.6
Employed	25	10.7
Inpatient treatment	148	65.5
Outpatient treatment	169	74.1
Previous convictions	100	42.7
Suicide attempts	133	60.2
Overdoses	147	68.1
Self-mutilation	124	56.9
Alcohol abuse	124	55.1
Drug abuse	98	43.9

The preferred diagnostic criteria in PD classification systems have each changed over the years, leading to some difficulties with comparing successive outcome studies. Currently patients are described in terms of their DSM sub-category diagnoses as measured by the "Personality Disorder Questionnaire" a self rating instrument (see Table 3).

Table 3. Personality disorder sub-category diagnoses in admissions to Henderson Hospital

Diagnosis	Admitted (n=186)	
	n	%
Paranoid	142	76.3
Schizoid	96	51.6
Schizotypal	131	70.4
Antisocial	115	61.8
Borderline	159	85.5
Histrionic	105	56.5
Narcissistic	87	46.8
Avoidant	126	67.7
Obsessive	87	46.8
Dependent	109	58.6
Passive-aggressive	75	40.3
Self-defeating	19	10.2
Sadistic	37	19.9

The most prevalent sub-category diagnosis is borderline personality disorder (87%), followed by paranoid personality disorder (76%), histrionic personality disorder (76%) and antisocial personality disorder (61%). On average, patients received seven of the 11 sub-category PD diagnoses each, with only 5.9% of patients attracting sub-category PD diagnoses from within a single cluster (74% of referrals would qualify for a severe personality disorder diagnosis as defined by Tyrer and Johnson – see earlier). The population can also be described in terms of its antisocial behaviour, with up to 59% of admissions having received convictions as adults and 20% being on probation at the point of referral (Dolan et al. 1994).

Outcome studies

The early outcome studies for Henderson Hospital treatment focused on indirect measures, such as hospital readmission, criminal conviction and re-employment. They are summarised in Table 4.

Table 4. A summary of outcome studies from Henderson Hospital

Study	n	Follow-up period	Criteria of success	Success rate (%)	Description of same
Rapoport (1960)	64	1 year	Improved clinically since admission	41	All discharged men
Tuxford (1961)	86	2 years	In employment	55	All male probation
			No recidivism	61	& borstal discharges
Taylor (1963)	?	9 months	In employment	60	Discharged men
Whiteley (1970)	112	2 years	No recidivism	43.6	Discharged men
			No re-admission	57.5	
			Neither of the above	40	
Copas & Whiteley	104	2 years	No recidivism	42	Discharged men
(1976)	87		or re-admission	47	
	104		"	33.6	Same 104 as above
Copas et al. (1986)	194	3 years	"	41	Male and female
		5 years	"	36	discharges
Controls	*51*	*3 years*	"	*23*	*Non-admitted controls*
		5 years		*19*	
Dolan et al. (1991)	62	8 months	Improved psychological functioning on SCL-90	55	Male and female discharges
Dolan, Warren & Norton (1997)	70	1 year	Clinically significant change in borderline	42.9	Male and female discharges
Controls	*67*		personality disorder symptomatology than in untreated controls	*17.9*	*Male and female non-admitted controls*

The outcome of Henderson Hospital treatment has also been evaluated prospectively and in terms of "core" PD phenomena. One year after referral or discharge from treatment, 137 patients were followed up using Borderline Syndrome Index (BSI) questionnaires to assess borderline personality disorder symptomatology (Dolan et al. 1997). The 70 patients admitted showed a statistically significant reduction in borderline symptomatology compared to their pre-admission scores. Changes were positively correlated with length of stay ($p < 0.001$). The magnitude of change was clinically significant in 43% of cases. The non-admitted sample of 67 referrals showed some decrease in score, as might be expected from "treatment as usual" in their local services during the year following referral. However, the changes in the group admitted were significantly greater than those found in a comparison group of non-admitted referrals ($p < 0.001$) (Figure 1). The non-funded referrals showed the worst outcome; of these only 18.2% showed any clinical improvement after one year (see Table 6).

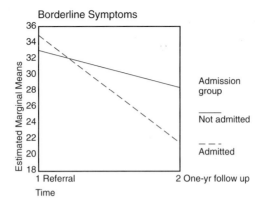

Figure 1. Change in borderline symptoms between baseline and one year follow-up; admitted versus not admitted comparisons.

Table 5. Mean (SD) Borderline Syndrome Index scores at referral and one-year follow-up

Sample	Referral	Follow-up	Mean change	95% CI difference from treated sample	Mann–Whitney U-test of difference (*p*-value)
Admitted (*n*=70)	34.6 (9.4)	20.3 (14.8)	14.3 (13.7)	–	–
Non-admitted (*n*=67)	33.3 (10.6)	26.9 (13.4)	6.4 (12.2)	3.5 to 12.3	0.0013
Non-admitted subgroups					
Non-funded (*n*=22)	33.5 (11.6)	28.4 (14.9)	5.1 (10.6)	2.9 to 15.5	0.004
Did not attend/ cancelled (*n*=27)	30.5 (11.2)	24.3 (13.6)	6.14 (13.1)	2.1 to 14.2	0.016
Not selected (*n*=18)	37.6 (6.6)	29.3 (10.9)	8.3 (12.7)	−1.1 to 13.1	NS

Table 6. Charge in individuals' BSI scores

Sample	Reliable improve-ment (%)	Clinically significant change (%)	Both reliable and clinical change (%)	95% CI difference in proportions from admitted sample	Chi-squared (*p*-value)
Admitted (*n*=70)	61.4	42.9	42.9	–	–
Non-admitted (*n*=67)	37.3	22.4	17.9	0.1 to 0.4	0.0015
Non-admitted subgroups					
Non-funded (*n*=22)	22.7	18.2	18.2	0.05 to 0.45	0.036
Did not attend/					
cancelled (*n*=27)	40.7	29.6	18.5	0.06 to 0.43	0.025
Not selected (*n*=18)	50.0	16.7	16.7	0.05 to 0.47	0.041

Impulsivity is a defining characteristic of some personality disorder sub-categories and can contribute substantially to the difficulty of the clinical management. Its presence and potential change in response to treatment was therefore studied. It was hypothesised that since Henderson Hospital treatment incorporates a treatment structure for setting limits on a range of impulsive and destructive behaviours, patients might demonstrate lower rates of such behaviours post-treatment and lower rates than those in the comparison group who did not receive specialist treatment. One hundred and thirty-five referred PD patients completed an assessment of a range of impulsive feelings and behaviours at referral and one year follow-up. Comparisons were made within and between groups of patients admitted (*n* = 75) and not admitted (*n* = 60). The following are results of work in progress.

The Henderson treated group showed significant reductions in both total impulses between pre- and post-test. The second hypothesis, however, was fully supported by the results, which showed highly significant differences between change scores for the admitted and non-admitted groups for both impulses and behaviours (see Figures 2 and 3).

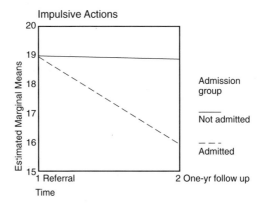

Figure 2. One-year outcome of impulsivity: comparison of patients admitted to Henderson Hospital and those not admitted.

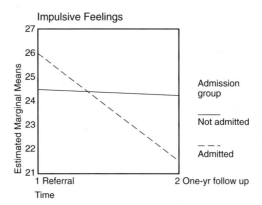

Figure 3. One-year outcome of impulsivity: comparison of patients admitted to Henderson Hospital and those not admitted.

Change during treatment

Studying the pattern and timing of change during treatment might shed light upon whether observed changes at follow-up are a result of the treatment. If the latter, then it would be predicted that change would be incremental and that different aspects might change at different rates. Therefore some of the measures used at referral and follow-up were repeated at 3 monthly intervals during treatment. Repeated measures analysis of the during-treatment to follow-up scores show highly significant main effects of time for borderline symptoms, self-esteem, anxiety and depression. Figures 5–7 display the group scores at each time point from baseline through treatment to one year post-discharge for the admitted sample of the PD patients previously referred to. This gives some idea of the profile of change during the treatment. Again, these analyses represent work in progress on this study.

It had been demonstrated previously that self-esteem was improved during admission to Henderson. This finding was replicated in the current study (see Figure 4). There is also statistically significant improvement in the Borderline Syndrome Index scores (see Figure 5). Depression and anxiety also reduce over time in treatment (see Figures 6 and 7).

Overall, it seems that there is a genuine improvement in the core borderline PD symptomatology, depression, anxiety and self-esteem over time, through treatment to outcome. These results lend support to the finding that there was a greater improvement in borderline symptomatology between referral and one-year follow-up in those who received Henderson treatment compared with those who did not (Dolan

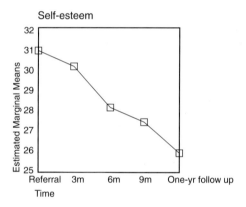

Figure 4. During-treatment change in self-esteem.

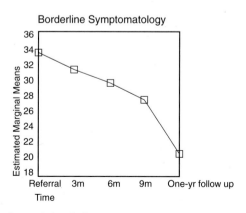

Figure 5. During-treatment change in borderline symptoms.

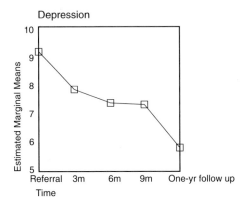

Figure 6. During-treatment change in depression.

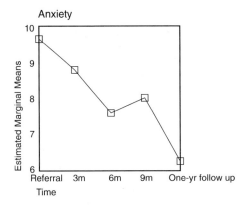

Figure 7. During-treatment change in borderline anxiety.

et al. 1997). The outcome results that compare those admitted with those who did not receive treatment in terms of depression, anxiety and self-esteem at one-year follow-up are not yet available. The during-treatment changes are interesting since the pattern and rate of improvement seem similar across measures. It is also noteworthy that there is an increase in anxiety immediately prior to leaving the community but that this then improves between leaving and one-year follow-up.

Further work will be conducted to make statistical comparisons between the changes evident from this work and the one-year period of "no treatment" received by the comparison group. This latter period may be seen as an opportunity for "spontaneous remission" in those who do not receive the specialist treatment. Should there be a treatment effect, we would expect the during-treatment reductions in the admitted group to be greater than the no-treatment change in the comparison group. Further work is required to elucidate the inter-relationship between self-esteem and borderline psychopathology, both during treatment and beyond the end of treatment.

Cost offset

The cost offset of specialist treatment of personality disorder at Henderson Hospital has been evaluated (Dolan et al. 1996). Information on the psychiatric and penal service usage in the one year prior to admission and the one year subsequent to discharge from treatment was obtained from the patients, their referrers and/or their general practitioners. In the one year before admission to Henderson, a cohort of 24 patients had used a total of £335,196 worth of psychiatric and prison services (average £13,966 per patient – 1992/3 "costs"). In the one year after discharge, no patient spent time in prison or in a secure psychiatric unit, although more outpatient treatment was consumed, perhaps a marker of more appropriate use (rather than misuse) of such services, and indirectly of change. The total cost of service used was £31,390 (average £1,308 per patient). This represents an annual saving post-discharge of £303,806. The 24 residents were in treatment for an average of 231 days, thus the actual cost of their treatment was £25,641. Assuming that services continued to be used at the same rate, the cost of admission to Henderson would be recouped in under two years and represent savings thereafter, assuming that improvements were sustained (see Tables 7–9).

Table 7. Service usage in the year before admission to Henderson Hospital (24 patients at 1992/3 tariffs)

Service	Units	No. of patients	No. of units	Unit mean (£)	Total cost (£)
In-patient beds	Day	17	1568	153.2	240,218
Secure psychiatric beds	Day	2	140	173	24,220
Out-patient assessments	Each	6	6	179	1,074
Out-patient therapy	Episode	12	12	586	7,032
Day hospital	Day	3	404	71	28,684
Prison	Week	4	88	386	33,968
Total costs (£)					**335,196**
Cost per patient (£)					**13,966**

Table 8. Service usage in the year following admission to Henderson Hospital (24 patients at 1993/4 tariffs)

Service	Units	No. of patients	No. of units	Unit mean (£)	Total cost (£)
In-patient beds	Day	3	73	179	13,932
Henderson Hospital	Day	1	50	110	5,500
Out-patient assessments	Each	2	2	166	332
Out-patient therapy	Episode	12	12	790	9,480
Day hospital	Day	1	28	70	1,960
Total costs (£)					**31,390**
Cost per patient (£)					**1,308**

Table 9. Average length and cost of stay at Henderson Hospital (23 patients)

	Minimum	Average	Maximum
Length of stay	1 day	361 days	225 days (7.5 months)
Admission cost	£111	£40,071	£25,000

Conclusions

Taken together, the meta-analysis of TC treatment and the particular outcome studies from Henderson Hospital demonstrate evidence for "treatability" of at least some patients who fulfil the diagnostic criteria for PD or SPD. The quality of much of the research in the field of PD can be criticized on a number of grounds, including the paucity of RCT methodology. Those RCTs that exist, however, support the view that the TC method can indeed be an effective treatment. It is important therefore that the myth of "untreatability", which a minority of psychiatrists would seem to apply to all patients with PD, is finally dispelled. Likewise, the small number of clinicians who refuse to consider PD as a medical diagnosis and therefore do not diagnose it should themselves now be offered remedial help or else risk professional ostracization.

We conclude with two views on stigma from ex-members of Henderson Hospital's democratic therapeutic community:

"Anyway, having heard I was being treated as a borderline personality, I think my attitude to myself and the attitude of those around me changed significantly. Actually that's not quite true. The only people who I noticed both at the time and with hindsight, who treated or spoke to me differently, were ironically the ones that should have had some awareness of personality. The professionals began gradually, yet dramatically, to become increasingly dismissive of me." (MB)

"Being labelled as having a 'personality disorder' was for me unhelpful and an inaccurate description of what I experienced. I have faced stigma and discrimination from having 'mental health problems'. However, if this happens and is perpetuated within the medical profession itself, how can views within 'wider society' be expected to change? Labels are for clothes – not for people." (Name withheld)

References

Coid JN (1990) Psychopathic disorders. *Current Opinions in Psychiatry* **2**: 750–6.

Dolan B & Coid J (1993) *Psychopathic and Antisocial Personality Disorders: Treatment and Research Issues.* London: Gaskell.

Dolan BM, Evans C et al. (1994) Funding treatment of offender patients with severe personality disorder: Do financial considerations trump clinical need? *Journal of Forensic Psychiatry* **5**: 263–74.

Dolan B, Evans C et al. (1995) Multiple Axis-II diagnoses of personality disorder. *British Journal of Psychiatry* **166**: 107–12.

Dolan B, Warren, F et al. (1996) Cost-offset following specialist treatment of severe personality disorders. *Psychiatric Bulletin* **20**: 641.

Dolan B, Warren F et al. (1997) Change in borderline symptoms one year after therapeutic community treatment for severe personality disorder. *British Journal of Psychiatry* **171**: 274–9.

Home Office and Department of Health (1999) Managing Dangerous People with Severe Personality Disorder: Proposals for Policy Development. July 1999.

Kernberg O (1984) *Severe Personality Disorders: Psychotherapeutic Strategies.* New Haven, CT: Yale University Press: 179–96.

Lees J, Manning N & Rawling B (1999) *Therapeutic Community Effectiveness.* CRD Report 17. York: NHS Centre for Review and Dissemination.

Lewis G & Appleby L (1988) Personality disorder: the patients psychiatrists dislike. *British Journal of Psychiatry* **153**: 44–9.

Norton K (1992) A culture of enquiry – Its preservation or loss. *International Journal of Therapeutic Communities* **13**: 3–25.

Norton K & Dolan B (1995) Assessing change in personality disorder. *Current Opinion in Psychiatry* **8**: 371–5.

Tyrer P, Casey P & Ferguson B (1991) Personality disorder in perspective. *British Journal of Psychiatry* **159**: 463–71.

Tyrer PJT & Johnson T (1996) Establishing the severity of personality disorder. *American Journal of Psychiatry* **153**: 1593–7.

Commentary on Section 5C

Anton Obholzer

Chapters 45 and 46, perhaps because they come from such different perspectives, complement each other very well. Chapter 46, though giving credit to the view that random control treatment studies are important in helping to evaluate outcomes, is essentially about creativity and the art of helping the personality disordered to help themselves. It thus comes from that quadrant of psychiatry that is concerned with group and social processes and the unspoken, often unconscious, factors that are at work in therapeutic communities.

In Chapter 45, Bluglass by contrast represents the "hard" end of investigative fact-finding – perhaps not surprising as he was reporting on the findings of the Fallon enquiry into Ashworth. Yet, as mentioned, the two chapters fit together very well, for, in my view, in order to have a well-functioning institution, you need clarity about concrete conscious issues – the structure, the setting, the roles, the expectations and outcome hoped for – and then within the above-named emotional container you need an ideal, a vision, concepts of constructive partnership in the service of the common goal and, perhaps most importantly, awareness of what the factors are that sabotage such a venture.

The two authors in Chapters 43 and 44 also represented different ends of the spectrum, namely neuropsychology and psychoanalysis, and again they agreed that both elements were required to work together if understanding was to be achieved and therapeutic progress was to be made.

The realisation that an integrative approach is more fruitful than the polarization we have witnessed over the past decade or two is of course not new. Both Maxwell Jones at Dingleton and Tom Main at the Cassel Hospital were very aware of the need to integrate structure and a creative therapeutic culture. It is interesting to speculate why that understanding was lost and instead replaced with a polarised factionalism of those who believed that personality disorders were treatable and those convinced that they were not.

My hypothesis is that the very nature and relative intractability of the condition, needing long-term and intensive therapy, made for a process of staff being disheartened. This "disheartening" then led to either a turning against those that "resisted one's best efforts", a situation most beautifully described in Tom Main's paper "The Ailment" (Main 1989), or else led to a state of mind of being "devoted" to the concept of treatability, though there was precious little evidence to back one's views.

It is also easily forgotten that what might be called a "personality disorder state of mind" is an innately dangerous condition to be exposed to – not only for the patient who is personality-disordered, but also for all who come into contact with him or her. This particularly affects staff working in institutions housing such individuals, and accounts, in my view, for the dangerous and perverse situations, such as described by Bluglass in Chapter 45, that occur in institutions where both patients and staff are cut off from external moderating influences, and are instead constantly exposed to what can only be described as noxious processes. Just as there is a warning on every cigarette packet from HM Chief Medical Officer of Health "Smoking can seriously damage your health" so there should be a warning on every staff contract, particularly in "total" institutions working with the personality-disordered, saying "unless strict training and staff support measures are adhered to, working in this field can seriously damage your state of mind, your health and your career."

So what are the risks of working in this field? From a psychoanalytic perspective it is particularly the risk that personality "enclaves" in the worker, that in ordinary everyday circumstances are dormant or manageable, are charged with the excitement, dangerousness and perversion that is an everyday occurrence in the workplace dealing with personality disorders, and that they grow, become unmanageable and lead to a change and corruption of the overall personality that in the long term is irreversible.

Some may regard this view as far-fetched; I see it as a public health matter, no different from the need to be aware of the risks inherent in certain industrial processes – be it working with asbestos or with personality disorder. For, as Norton and Warren write in Chapter 46, what is on offer in a therapeutic community or, I believe, equally in a therapeutic situation is the fact that the toxins of the behaviour are noted, named and not gone along with, and an attempt is made to substitute the toxin with a capacity to metabolise the behaviour onto something less severe and damaging. Would it be wrong to describe a therapeutic community as the equivalent of a therapeutic renal dialysis device? – I believe not. The question of course is what happens to the artificial kidney or its socio-technical counterpart – the workers in the system?

Coming from a different perspective, namely that of industrial psychology and of organisational consultancy, it is interesting to observe that here too some have now reached the conclusion that intelligence as measured by the IQ test is not enough, and in fact a poor indication of success in life, both personally and in business. What is required is intelligence paired in tandem with what Daniel Goleman (1997) calls "emotional intelligence". I quote "The new measure takes for granted having enough intellectual ability and technical know-how to do our jobs; it focuses instead on personal qualities, such as initiative and empathy, adaptability and persuasiveness".

Could it be that what is required to run an effective business is also what is needed to run an effective personality disorder treatment unit? If so, what is required is intelligence and structure on the one hand, and emotional intelligence and creativity, adaptability and persuasiveness on the other.

References

Goleman D (1997) *Emotional Intelligence: Why It Can Matter More Than IQ*. London: Bloomsburg.
Main T (1989) *The Ailment and Other Psychoanalytic Essays*. London: Free Association Books.

Part 6

The Law and mental illness

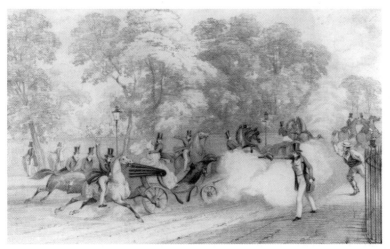

Edward Oxford 1840

47 The need for risk assessment: Myth versus reality

David Tidmarsh

This chapter is a personal account by a retired forensic psychiatrist of his impressions over a professional lifetime of the literature about the risk of violence by the mentally ill. The early literature, almost all from the USA, describes a low risk of violence by patients discharged from hospital before and soon after the second world war. There the surprisingly low risk of violence by patients released from maximum security hospitals as a result of the Baxstrom and Dixon decisions encouraged the policy of deinstitutionalisation. However, in the UK the high profile case of Graham Young led to a more cautious approach. Since then evidence from discharge studies has shown a higher than expected risk of violent offending amplified dramatically by the abuse of substances. The evidence for an increased risk has been reinforced by studies of birth cohorts, population surveys and studies of offender populations. Though in absolute terms this risk is very small, this evidence comes at a time when risks in other branches of medicine have declined and society has become reluctant to accept even the lowest of risks. It is in this climate that politicians are now seeking to regulate psychiatric practice.

When I was initially approached about this chapter I had only the vaguest idea about what I was letting myself in for, let alone who else would be contributing to this book. I now suspect that I was selected as one of the few psychiatrists who would still be prepared to put forward some antediluvian notions which could then be triumphantly exposed by the subsequent contributors. What I intend to do is to go over some recent history which explains why the question of risk has become such a prominent issue in psychiatry. It might be useful to let you have a few biographical notes so that you can see where my ideas have come from and thus provide myself with the usual excuses. The first is that my father was born in 1872, so that Victorian concepts were very much alive in the family and, possibly because we lived near Downe in Kent, Darwin rather than Freud was an early influence. It was economics that led me into psychiatry. Returning from National Service abroad in the early 1960s I found that jobs were hard to come by and that most of my contemporaries had emigrated. At a course at the National Heart Hospital I met by chance a psychiatric registrar studying for his medical membership. He told me that even registrar jobs in psychiatry were easy to obtain and that if I could spell schizophrenia I would probably be taken on. I could and I was. This may not indicate the stigmatisation of psychiatric patients but it certainly showed that psychiatry was not highly regarded at that time.

There followed several happy years at Horton Hospital in Epsom much influenced by Henry Rollin. Here, with a catchment area which contained such disparate elements as Hampstead, Paddington and Wimbledon, one certainly learnt about the ecology of mental illness and perhaps equally about the attitudes of the psychiatrists in these areas. Suffice it to say, although we held our outpatient clinics at Paddington General

Hospital, so near to St Mary's, we had no academic connection with that teaching hospital nor with the observation wards that sent us their more unpromising patients. With its inner city catchment area, Horton at that time took a disproportionate share of Section 136 and Section 60 patients, and my proficiency at spelling schizophrenia increased by leaps and bounds, as did my awareness of the causes of criminality in these revolving door patients. In those days, before registrar rotations were the fashion, we tended to stay longer in one hospital. This allowed us to follow patients much further along the course of their illness than trainees can nowadays, so that, for instance, one could follow cases of Huntington's chorea from the first hesitant misdiagnosis all the way through to inpatient incapacity and death. Likewise those with schizophrenia who had been given another diagnosis and a rosy prognosis elsewhere and had then deteriorated into chronicity. The sheer number of patients, the diversity of their backgrounds and their stereotypical symptoms left one in no doubt that one was dealing with an illness. It was also obvious from the low mortality in the long stay wards that only a small proportion of these patients could become long stay and therefore that they must have spent most of their lives in the community. It is only recently that Paul Mullen has provided quantitative support for this, albeit in Australia (Mullen et al. 2000). These patients had GPs, there were social workers and we did see them in the out-patient clinic. Community care is not new: it is just that the balance has shifted somewhat.

Outside the hospital, and perhaps particularly at the Hampstead end of our catchment area, Szasz, Laing and Cooper reigned supreme. For them schizophrenia did not exist, or, if it did, it was not an illness. One suspects that people with schizophrenia were not so much stigmatised as sanctified. I have to confess that I have not read everything that they wrote, but I think it is inconceivable that any of them would have attributed dangerousness to any form of mental illness. And in parentheses, if one is looking for really malicious stigmatisation, as opposed to the casual unthinking variety, the way that Laing blamed parents for the illnesses of their children must be a prime example and I suspect his views still linger on.

After Horton I spent two years studying homeless people at the Camberwell Reception Centre with Dr Sue Wood, a sociologist, loosely attached to Professor Wing's Social Psychiatry Unit at the Institute of Psychiatry. We demonstrated that the reception centre had as large a turnover of mentally ill people and far more mentally disordered people than any of the large psychiatric hospitals in London, a fact which was of course well known to the GPs working there. The Maudsley, a mile or two away, was less keen to become involved. Incidentally it was there that I first heard the expression "bin doctor", and I realise now that there are other sources of stigma than the public at large.

It is perhaps just as well that I was only vaguely aware of Szasz's definitions of psychiatrists as "agents specially trained to silence all those who transgress against the prevailing power interests in contemporary society" or perhaps as "professional degraders of stigmatised individuals" (see Roth 1976). Had I known and believed this, I might well have hesitated about taking up a consultant post at Broadmoor, which I did in November 1973. This in retrospect was an interesting time for Broadmoor.

After the 1959 Mental Health Act the demand for beds in Special Hospitals had increased dramatically and admissions to Broadmoor had risen from their long-term average of 67 a year to a peak of over 170 in 1971. Despite the increased turnover, the inpatient population had fallen, thus relieving the gross overcrowding. With the combination of conventional psychiatry and the cooperation of consultants in what we still called county hospitals, who were happy to take our patients, everything seemed to be going well and the dangerousness of Broadmoor patients appeared to have been overestimated. Then came Graham Young. He was convicted in 1972 of murdering two workmates by poison and administering poison to four others. After his conviction it was revealed that he had been in Broadmoor since the age of fourteen after administering poison to three of his close relatives and that he had started administering poisons again only weeks after his conditional discharge (Holden 1974). The media had a field day. This case, albeit one with an obscure and atypical diagnosis, shattered complacency and led to a severe loss of confidence in psychiatrists and the immediate setting up of the Aarvold Committee, which in due course strengthened the safeguards surrounding the discharge of restricted patients. It also put risk back on the agenda. My own experience was salutary. One of the patients on my ward was already in the transfer pipeline when I arrived, and left a few weeks later. Very quickly he formed a relationship with a female and killed her. His was a case of delusional jealousy.

Elsewhere, however, there were fewer anxieties. In 1973 John Gunn, now Professor Gunn, published a book *Violence in Human Society* and allocated only one page to schizophrenia, and the psychiatric textbooks written at that time said virtually nothing about risk. The next year Steadman and Cocozza (1974) published their follow-up study of the 967 patients released from maximum security hospitals in New York State as a result of the 1966 Baxstrom decision. They proved to be remarkably non-violent, and the same was true of the 586 patients released as a result of the 1971 Dixon case in Pennsylvania (Thornberry and Jacoby 1979). Studies of this kind gave academic respectability to the policy of deinstitutionalisation. However, differences in the perception of the dangerousness of the mentally ill remained, and in 1979 the whole question of dangerousness was reviewed at a symposium organised by Broadmoor. My job was to review the literature (Tidmarsh 1982). This was extremely sparse but what emerged was that pre-war, and therefore of course pre-chlorpromazine, studies of discharged psychiatric patients showed an arrest rate well below that for the normal population and violence was hardly mentioned. As time went on rates of violent offending increased until they were above those for the normal population but not alarmingly so. It was, I think, Nigel Walker who pointed out that the safety of the Baxstrom patients could be explained by their age, their institutionalisation and their supervision in the community. These factors would also explain the low rates for patients discharged from more conventional hospitals and more recently for the patients discharged from the Friern Hospital (Trieman et al. 1999). At this conference I was able to quote Patrick McGrath, who had said in 1968 that of 293 murderers released from Broadmoor none had killed again. However, later figures were rather more disturbing. Thus 20 of 1,946 patients who left Broadmoor between 1960 and 1978 went on to commit homicide. However, more of these 20 were personality disordered than mentally ill.

How has the picture changed in the last 20 years? There are I believe three themes. First are the changes which could plausibly have led to an increase in offending. These would include the changes in the law in the USA which made dangerousness a necessary criterion for admission to hospital. If one only admits patients with a dangerousness label it is hardly surprising that a greater proportion of discharges will be dangerous or that in the USA there has been a steady rise in the offending of discharged patients. Although this has never been the case here, many social workers interpreted the Mental Health Act as if it were. Then there is the decrease in the number of beds for psychiatric patients which in the last 10 years has led to bed occupancies of well over 100%, a quite ridiculous situation, which, I believe, must lead to too high a threshold for admission and the discharge of many patients whose psychosis and behaviour have not been stabilised. Perhaps more important is the availability of drugs of abuse. When I started psychiatry the admission of a heroin addict created a furore around the whole hospital. We now hear that 30% or more of admissions for schizophrenia have a dual diagnosis, and if there is one thing certain about the offending of the mentally ill it is that drugs amplify it. We hear rather little about what is being done to prevent this malignant complication.

The second theme is the increasing sophistication of research strategies, the methodological issues of which are now much clearer thanks, for instance, to Link and Stueve (1994) and have moved beyond just following up discharged patients, though even this has become more sophisticated. Of recent follow-up studies I will only quote Lindqvist and Allebeck (1990), who showed that the rate for violent offences for patients with schizophrenia discharged from hospital was four times higher than the general population of Stockholm, Link et al. (1992), who identified the association between psychotic symptoms and violence, and Mullen et al. (2000), who more recently found that psychiatric patients have a higher rate of offending than normal controls in Australia. There, offending rates had increased, but no more than in the control population, and they made the important point that those first admitted in 1985 spent hardly longer in the community than those admitted for the first time 10 years previously, so that care in the community could not be blamed. Other studies, however, have not shown increased rates.

Modern research strategies include the enumeration of the mentally ill in various populations of offenders, the following up of birth cohorts and population surveys. The prevalence of schizophrenia in the community is about 0.4%. If a greater proportion is found an explanation is required, though this need not be an entirely psychiatric one. It may only be because of selection pressures: thus homeless psychotic people are likely to be remanded in custody, so a survey in a remand prison, as opposed to a survey of all those remanded for a particular offence, will increase the figures. Examples of an increased prevalence free from this kind of bias are the 10% of people with schizophrenia found in released life sentenced prisoners being supervised by probation officers (Taylor 1986) and the 4% of all homicides in England and Wales (Shaw et al. 1999). The converse of this is the finding by Humphries et al. (1992) that a fifth of 253 patients in their first schizophrenic episode had behaved in ways threatening to the lives of others before their admission to hospital. It is interesting that delusions of poisoning, known as a risk factor to Mowat as long ago as 1966, were again identified. The authors were surprised how often life-threatening behaviour had not led to admission or indeed prosecution and were alarmed at the late presentation to the psychiatric services of these very ill people.

The major study of an unselected birth cohort comes from Denmark (Hodgins et al. 1996) and showed convincingly that patients of all diagnostic groups who had had psychiatric hospital admissions had a higher rate of offending than the population at large. Interestingly it was women in the major mental illness group whose risk was increased the most – a finding now emerging from other studies.

However, perhaps the most convincing evidence of a link between psychosis and violence comes from the Epidemiologic Catchment Area surveys of communities in the USA, which, for example, showed that some 18% of those who met the DSM criteria for schizophrenia and who were both hallucinated and deluded had been violent in the previous year – four times as many as those without these symptoms. Here of course one must not forget that the rates were very much higher for those with substance abuse (Swanson et al. 1996).

The impact of all this research was such that as early as 1981 Steadman went back on his Baxstrom views and could say that research supported public fears to "an extent rarely acknowledged by mental health professionals" and that "it no longer seems defensible for mental health professionals or social scientists to attend a neighbourhood meeting to assuage prospective neighbours of a hostel by assuring them that mental patients are less dangerous statistically than their present neighbours". By coincidence it was on 30 March that year that John Hinckley shot and wounded President Reagan (Low et al. 1986). However, since then Steadman seems to have changed his mind yet again on the basis of the similarity of the rates of violence of discharged patients and a community sample in his MacArthur study (Steadman et al. 1998).

This research has perhaps been focused on relative rather than absolute risk, which is of course small. Hodgins et al. (1996) found that, though this was four times the rate for those without mental disorder, only 6.7% of men with a major mental illness in the Danish birth cohort had been convicted of a violent offence in a 12-year period. In England and Wales there are between 20 and 40 people killed each year by psychotic individuals. Taylor and Gunn (1999) have pointed out that this is a very small number compared with the number of those killed on the roads. This is true and no doubt comforting to those unlikely to be in contact with severely disturbed patients, but it is not the whole story. Thus there is the fact that homicide is not the only crime of violence committed by the mentally disordered. It accounts for perhaps a fifth of special hospital patients and even fewer of those detained in other hospitals. Then there is the lack of evidence that psychotic homicide is getting any less. This is in stark contrast to death rates in other medical areas, for instance anaesthetics, and suggests that the psychiatric services as a whole have not given priority to safety. I have argued elsewhere (Tidmarsh 1997) that today's psychiatric services are willing to accept risks to the public that are high in comparison with risks not acceptable to, for instance, those siting a new factory. I note, in passing, that though the Paddington rail crash killed 31 people, in the two years before nobody was killed on the railways. Nor is today's psychiatric treatment for violent offenders particularly effective. Thus for instance a study of patients with schizophrenia treated in one highly respected Regional Secure Unit showed that 49% were convicted of a violent offence during a mean follow-up of 3.9 years (Baxter et al. 1999).

My third theme is the gradual acceptance of the importance of how the public perceives risk, which is emphatically not in purely statistical terms. It has become fashionable to list factors that make a risk less acceptable to the public. I will quote one given by Calman et al. (1999): involuntary, inequitably distributed so that some benefit while others suffer the consequences, inescapable, unfamiliar, man-made rather than natural, causing irreversible damage, posing danger to children, causing dread, damaging identifiable rather than anonymous victims, poorly understood by science and, lastly, subject to contradictory statements from responsible sources. I would add risks that were once seen as controlled but are now seen as uncontrolled. This list was not compiled with psychiatric patients in mind but I think you will agree that psychotic violence would score high on a scale of these items. Whether the public is prepared to accept what is, after all, a very low risk is a political decision not a scientific or medical one.

The political decisions have now been taken for us. Governmental insistence on the Care Programme Approach with risk assessment built in, the National Confidential Inquiry into Suicide and Homicide by People with Mental Illness and the much maligned statutory homicide inquiries are all part of this response. Facing an audience of doctors, it would be easy to say that these political responses were driven entirely by the media. I am sure that this was part of it but I would like to think that it is also possible that the findings of research were also important, likewise an understanding that risk is not just a matter of numbers. There are I believe two myths: the first is that the mentally ill are extremely dangerous and should all be locked up and the second is that they are completely harmless and their reputation is all due to labelling, the media and Sir Alfred Hitchcock. The truth is that some mentally ill people in some circumstances can be dangerous. Institutional denial of this fact helps nobody. I would like to end with a notion plucked from the Maastricht Treaty. This is known as the Precautionary Principle and it requires society to take prudent action when there is significant scientific evidence (but not necessarily absolute proof) and when inaction could possibly lead to harm. This prudent action includes risk assessment and, more important, risk management, but does not mean locking up all our patients.

References

Baxter R, Rabe-Hesketh S & Parrott J (1999) Characteristics, needs and reoffending in a group of patients with schizophrenia formerly treated in medium security. *Journal of Forensic Psychiatry* **10**: 69–83.

Calman KC, Bennett PG & Coles DG (1999) Risks to health: some key issues in management, regulation and communication. *Health, Risk and Society* **1**: 107–16.

Gunn J (1973) *Violence in Human Society*. Newton Abbot: David and Charles.

Hodgins S, Mednick SA, Brennan PA, Schulsinger F & Engberg M (1996) Mental disorder and crime. *Archives of General Psychiatry* **53**: 489–96.

Holden A (1974) *The St Albans Poisoner*. London: Hodder and Stoughton.

Humphries MS, Johnstone EC, MacMillan JF & Taylor PJ (1992) Dangerous behaviour preceding first admissions for schizophrenia. *British Journal of Psychiatry* **161**: 501–5.

Lindquist P & Allebeck P (1990) Schizophrenia and crime. A longitudinal follow-up of 644 schizophrenics in Stockholm. *British Journal of Psychiatry* **157**: 345–50.

Link BG & Stueve A (1994) Psychotic symptoms and the violent/illegal behaviour of mental patients compared to community controls. In: Monahan J & Steadman HJ (eds). *Violence in Mental Disorder: Developments in Risk Assessment*. Chicago: University of Chicago Press.

Link BG, Andrews H & Cullen FT (1992) The violent and illegal behaviour of mental patients reconsidered. *American Sociological Review* **57**: 275–92.

Low PW, Jeffries JC & Bonnie RJ (1986) *The Trial of John W Hinckley*. New York: Mineola.

Mowat RR (1966) *Morbid Jealousy and Murder*. London: Tavistock.

Mullen PE, Burgess P, Wallace C, Palmer S & Ruschena D (2000) Community care and criminal offending in schizophrenia. *Lancet* **355**: 614–17.

Roth M (1976) Schizophrenia and the theories of Thomas Szasz. *British Journal of Psychiatry* **129**: 317–26.

Shaw J, Appleby L, Amos T, McDonnell R, Harris C, McCann K, Kiernan K, Davies S, Bickley H & Parsons R (1999) Mental disorder and clinical care in people convicted of homicide: national clinical survey. *British Medical Journal* **318**: 1240–4.

Steadman HJ (1981) Critically assessing the accuracy of public perceptions of the dangerousness of the mentally ill. *Journal of Health and Social Behaviour* **22**: 310–16.

Steadman HJ & Cocozza JJ (1974) *Careers of the Criminally Insane. Excessive Social Control of Deviance*. Lexington: Lexington Books.

Steadman HJ, Mulvey EP, Monahan J, Robbins PC, Appelbaum PS, Grisso T, Roth LH & Silver E (1998) Violence by people discharged from acute psychiatric inpatient facilities and others in the same neighbourhoods. *Archives of General Psychiatry* **55**: 393–401.

Swanson JW, Borum R, Swartz MS & Monahan J (1996) Psychotic symptoms and disorders and the risk of violent behaviour in the community. *Criminal Behaviour and Mental Health* **6**: 309–29.

Taylor PJ (1986) Psychiatric disorder in London's life-sentenced offenders. *British Journal of Criminology* **26**: 63–78.

Taylor PJ & Gunn J (1999) Homicides by people with mental illness: myth and reality. *British Journal of Psychiatry* **174**: 9–14.

Thornberry TP & Jacoby JE (1979) *The Criminally Insane. A Community Follow-up of Mentally Ill Offenders*. Chicago: Chicago University Press.

Tidmarsh D (1982) Implications from research studies. In: *Dangerousness: psychiatric assessment and management*. London: Gaskell.

Tidmarsh D (1997) Psychiatric risk, safety cultures and homicide inquiries. *Journal of Forensic Psychiatry* **8**: 138–51.

Trieman N, Leff J & Glover G. (1999) Outcome of long stay psychiatric patients resettled in the community: prospective cohort study. *British Medical Journal* **319**: 13–16.

48 Stigmatising "Care in the Community": Community care and risk management

Philip Fennell

I plan to address the role that Law in the UK can play in both reducing and increasing stigma. My general argument will be that psychiatric medicine is gradually being colonised by criminal justice models of risk management. This will have implications for the nature of the doctor/patient relationship. I will also make some general statements about proposals that are currently being made by the Government about dangerous people with severe personality disorder.

Goffman said that stigma is not simply an attribute that somebody has, it is a process that sends out messages about what society regards as normal. By identifying people as abnormal and having "spoiled identity", we are reinforcing the normality of everyone else. Stigma theory, according to Goffman, is an ideology which explains a person's inferiority and the danger that they represent to society. The paradox with present Government policy is that it is committed to guarding against total exclusion, yet it is also employing the same mechanisms of engendering social solidarity as governments which are not worried about social exclusion, e.g. deciding that certain people need to be cleared off the streets, deciding that risk needs to be managed more effectively, etc. The important effect it has on the service user, the patient, is that we see that person through the lens of the label that we have given them, and that has consequences for their behaviour; they may start to react in ways which we might not desire them to.

Stigma performs an important function in shaming. Criminal justice process uses shaming. Penal values are based around the idea that if you identify wrongdoers and subject them to some kind of stigma this may *encourager les autres* and will provide important social messages. How does this all relate to mental disorder? I have gone back to 1890 in my historical analysis, looking at legal textbooks on lunacy and how lawyers saw mental disorder. There is an apt quote from Pope's treatise on *The Law and Practice of Lunacy*:

"In so far as they are irrational, the insane though in the State are not of the State. On the other hand, although not of the State the insane are yet in the State. Hence the State has relations with them though not those which it has with its citizens proper."

So you get this distinction being drawn between citizens proper and the insane. And then what we are really worried about:

"(They are) possessed of a physical force without a regulating mind; subject to the natural instincts untutored by discipline; uncontrolled by the fear of punishment; some classes of the insane threaten continual danger to those with whom they are brought in contact."

Morris (1994), in her book *The Dangerous Classes*, writes about the social control of risky populations in early Victorian times: the underclasses, people who wouldn't get married and things like that. There we see a precursor of the idea of risk management and the management of so-called dangerous populations.

Now, we are told, Government policy on psychiatric practice is to be based on the three Ss: *safe*, *sound* and *supported*. But there is another key ingredient, not mentioned in this alliteration, and that is *therapy*. The whole trend of the reform proposals that we have seen in the Government's Green Paper is to downgrade the so-called treatability test, which has been used not just in connection with people with personality disorder. People often forget that the treatability test is an essential requirement for a renewal of detention of people with mental illness. But it is downgraded in the Green Paper.

Community care

Tidmarsh, in Chapter 47, reports convincingly concerning the way in which research on risk has influenced public policy, but it has also been greatly media-driven and driven by the effects of the homicide enquiries. I am the first to acknowledge the need for the relatives of victims and for people who have suffered as a result of criminality by mentally disordered people to have a proper examination of what went wrong so that lessons may be learned. However, it is undeniable that the constant procession of these enquiries reinforces an association between criminality and mental disorder, which I believe to be exaggerated. What we then see is a development of risk control policy. How do we control risk? The best way is to have the possibility of detaining the person who is risky. Detention is the bedrock of all policies of risk management of dangerous populations. You have to have the possibility of detaining the person. If you release them into the community you have to have the possibility of redetaining them or of getting them to accept the therapy that you are offering to them in the community. No longer do you have the safeguard that anything that goes on within the institution is in a regulated zone where people can be treated without consent. You have problems of how you control people once you put them into the community. I would suggest that the only real way we have thought of doing this is by recalling people to detention; the model which is used for conditionally discharging restricted patients.

In my contention, we are seeing a convergence between the penal system and the psychiatric system, and I'll skim over the features of this convergence very quickly. The first of them is that the criminal justice system increasingly contains the possibility for indeterminate detention, discretionary life sentences, mandatory life sentences under the "two strikes and you are out" and, enhanced sentencing under the Criminal Justice Act as dangerous offenders. Advantages that used to be peculiar to the mental health system, such as indefinite detention of someone who poses a risk, are being transplanted into the penal system. But we are also seeing penal values coming into the psychiatric system. The so-called hybrid order, if it is ever used under the Crime (Sentences) Act 1997, is designed to ensure that a person will serve a minimum period in detention before they are released if they are no longer mentally disordered.

This invites us to question the extent to which penal policy values are infected, if you like, by medical ideas and health care values are infected by penal policy values. Think of some of our key concepts in health care values: the principle of therapeutic intervention, including the philosophy "above all do no harm"; the principle of confidentiality; and the idea that the doctor/patient relationship is a therapeutic alliance. Penal policy values include ideas like stigma and shame: you shame offenders who have transgressed; a tradition that there should be some proportionality between the sentence and the gravity of the offence. Ideas of selective incapacitation and preventive detention are increasingly fashionable. And finally, and very importantly in the modern time, ideas of victim protection and ideas that victims should have rights in the process are coming to the fore.

Risk management

How do we manage risk effectively? The bedrock of risk management is what we have under the Mental Health Act: renewable detention. Potentially indefinite detention, through restriction orders without limit of time, is an obvious example of that. But risk management and therapy are not the same thing. There is a definition of treatment in the Mental Health Act 1983 which says that "medical treatment for mental disorder includes nursing care, habilitation and rehabilitation", so it is very wide. Nevertheless, I would argue that risk management can be achieved by indefinite detention without any commitment to therapy – for what the expert committee on the Mental Health Act calls "positive clinical measures".

Risk management is based on graduated relaxation of security. You place an individual in a special hospital and move them to a secure unit; then to a local hospital and finally to a community. That approach is fostered by our legal system of transfers and granting leave, etc. But of all these options, community care carries the highest risk unless you can provide for recall at the discretion of the Home Office as a restricted patient, or at the discretion of the clinician. One of Dr John Hamilton's projects, after the infamous Halston judgement, was to produce a short clause to amend the Mental Health Act which would simply have allowed for a conditional discharge-type arrangement for non-offender patients. If we had that we could probably have saved an awful lot of paper between then and the present day because in effect that is what is happening now. So if we want effective risk management we need extended detention, we need continuing controls over patients who are discharged into the community (and the Patients in the Community Act 1995 was an effort to achieve that), but we also want easy recall to detention in hospital of those whose conduct in the community gives rise to concern. If one was sitting in the Home Office or the Department of Health looking at a pure risk management model, these are the things one would want: medicalisation of the penal system, indeterminate detention, continuing supervision, and sex offender training programmes.

Since this chapter is about the Law and mental illness, I wondered whether I would be allowed to mention personality disorder. But I think it is important to recognise that there is a moral hierarchy of mental disorder in this whole stigma business. If you are mentally ill you are so (*pace* Ronald Laing) "by visitation of God". But if you are personality-disordered somehow the presumption seems to have come in that these are the bad mad, the people whose madness is their own fault. That perhaps they could have done something about it. What we see then is the convergence between the penal and the therapeutic regime: convergence between the type of rights patients get and the type of rights prisoners get, and a convergence in review procedures.

If we look at the process of law reform, the homicide enquiries have given a new primacy to risk management, which you can see in the new care programme approach document available on the web. We have the Human Rights Act 1998, which is requiring public authorities to act compatibly with rights under the Human Rights Convention; and we have the essential project of law reform, which is the uncoupling of detention and compulsory treatment. Always there has been some kind of link, except with guardianship under the Mental Health Acts 1959 and 1983, between compulsory community treatment and detention in hospital. Extended leave under Section 17 and the new arrangements under the Patients in the Community Act all presuppose that the person has been detained under one of the long-term sections in the Mental Health Act. When the Minister of Health appointed the expert committee in 1997 he read them the political equivalent of the riot act. He told them three times, lest they might not register it, that they would be expected to ensure that non-compliance with agreed treatment plans in the community was not an option, i.e. whatever you do, make sure you deal with the question of compulsion in the community effectively. The expert committee decided that whilst they were singularly lacking in detail, one might say, on compulsory community treatment, they should take seriously the exhortation to do a root and branch review of the Mental Health Act. And their principles were based on the idea of non-discrimination – that wherever possible the principles governing mental health and physical health were to be the same. They also put patient autonomy at the top of their list. The recognition of enhancement of patient autonomy was a fundamental principle which should go in a new law, and it should only be disregarded in very well-defined circumstances.

How were they to achieve this non-discriminatory approach? They decided to try and make the possibilities for treatment of psychiatric patients without consent pretty much the same as for treatment of people with physical illnesses, i.e. based on the incapacity of the person concerned. But they couldn't simply say "We will only detain the incapacitated", because lots of people may have mental capacity according to the legal tests on mental capacity but they may pose quite a high risk. How did the committee square this circle? What they did was to propose a two-tier approach. If you are incapable you can be admitted in the interests of your health or safety or for the protection of others. If you are capable you have to present a substantial risk of serious harm. The risk threshold is higher if you are capable. They also mention the legal principle of reciprocity and entitlement to services. This is the so-called *quid pro quo* of community compulsion: that in order to justify compelling people to accept treatment and services in the community you have to give them some sort of an entitlement to those services. That is to be done through the national service frameworks and through guidance and documents of that nature. A final protection envisaged is speedy independent review.

No longer will we have the four-part classification of mental disorder that exists at the moment in the Mental Health Act. It will be mental disorder of a nature or degree requiring clinically supervised care and treatment. Mental disorder means anything in the DSM-IV, which covers everything from mild anxiety to homicide. This is rather alarming to those of us who have perused it, and one would worry about a definition of mental disorder which was so potentially broad and all-inclusive were it not accompanied by other safeguards. And the essential safeguard would be the requirement for properly supervised care either in hospital or the community. The care and treatment has got to be in the patient's best interests. It must be the least restrictive alternative. As I mentioned earlier, the differential test of whether you get sectioned depends on whether you have capacity or not. If you haven't got capacity you can be detained if necessary for your health, safety or the protection of others, or you can be subject to compulsory community treatment. If you have got capacity you need to show a substantial risk of serious harm to your own health or safety, or to the safety of other people, or of being seriously exploited; and there must be positive clinical measures: i.e. the condition must be treatable. One of my arguments against this is that I don't see a great deal of difference between admitting somebody because it is necessary for their health, safety or the protection of others, and a substantial risk of serious harm, and I don't think you would be admitting an incapable person unless there was such a substantial risk of serious harm to other people.

The Green Paper was in favour of a broad definition of mental disorder, but what is needed is a statement that it is the presence of mental disorder requiring specialist mental health treatment. It agrees with the principle of the least restrictive alternative. But that is not a new concept – it appeared in the previous two Mental Health Acts. It cannot be implemented without compulsory powers. Its principles are very watered down: preference for informal care; patients to be involved as far as possible; safety is of key importance; treatment is to be in the least restrictive setting. But there is no "treatability" in all that. The treatability test is conspicuous by its absence, although the Government White Paper of December 2000 requires that there be a care and treatment plan to address either the disorder itself or behaviours arising from the disorder. Hence, what is being treated is not just mental disorder but the risky behaviour that may arise from it. When we get to the Dangerous Severe Personality Disorder (DSPD) proposals, these removed the notion of treatability where possible. We have detention on grounds of risk; we see the paper applying mental health approaches in conjunction with criminal justice terminology by talking about diagnosis of risk. We have proposals for third-way institutions, neither health nor criminal justice but something in between, and the first of these have been established at Whitemoor Prison and Rampton Hospital. So what these DSPD proposals represent, in my view, is the apotheosis of risk management without any fear of commitment to the treatability test or any of the things which make psychiatrists' contribution to risk management the valuable thing that it is. Thus we are again seeing a convergence between the values of the criminal justice system and those of the mental health system. And we have seen a battle fought out in this Green Paper as to what should be its central concept. Should it be incapacity? Should it be risk? Generally, the White Paper has come down in favour of risk.

What are the consequences of this convergence? I am a medical lawyer, and if you look at what medical law embraces it is the care of patients suffering from physical illness, with the concept of treatment without consent where there is incapacity. It deals with the psychiatric system where detained psychiatric patients may be treated without consent subject to the second opinion procedure. It also embraces the prison system where prisoners receive attention to their health care needs. We are beginning to see attempts to put the health care grid on the penal system, most recently evidenced by Ian Brady's attempt to use medical law-based rights effectively to starve himself to death. The consequence of this convergence between the psychiatric system and the penal system will be the risk management movement pulling the psychiatric system more towards the criminal justice end of the spectrum rather than towards the health care end. The model of legal rights and duty is much more recognisable to penologists and criminologists than it is necessarily to health care lawyers.

Are human rights a countervailing force? Human Rights papers under the Convention have been very important in shaping our mental health law. The rights to review of detention in the United Kingdom were influenced by the case of K v UK, which said that you can't recall a restricted patient, unless it is an emergency, without objective medical evidence that they are mentally disordered. An important safeguard for conditional discharge of restricted patients is the case of Stanley Johnson in the UK, where the Court of Human Rights held that deferred discharge of a restricted patient must not be unreasonably delayed, although the authorities did have the right to defer the discharge to enable suitable arrangements to be made. The Human Rights Act will potentially uphold ideas of patients' rights to question decision making which affects their future.

Deprivation of liberty

Article 5 of the European Convention deals with deprivation of liberty – nobody can be deprived of their liberty unless certain grounds are present. And the ones that are relevant for us are these:

- Detention on grounds of unsoundness of mind; where you need objective evidence of mental disorder which is sufficiently serious to justify detention in hospital.
- Detention following conviction of a criminal offence under Article 5 (1A), with the safeguard of a criminal trial.
- Detention for the prevention of crime; but this is only allowed for the purpose of bringing someone before a court which will try them for an offence.

The situation, then, is that the Human Rights Act is the last possibility of restraining the DSPD proposals, because if you are detained as being of unsound mind you have to be detained somewhere in a clinical setting which will not be antitherapeutic. If you are detained on grounds of having committed a criminal offence you can be detained, and can continue to be detained, on grounds of dangerousness without infringing the Convention. But the DSPD proposals are being put forward as a way of detaining people without necessarily having to offer them a therapeutic intervention which will address their core disorder; without subjecting them to a treatability test. And my argument is that a treatability test is what justifies psychiatric involvement in these cases. If you can't offer some prospect of positive clinical measures then what you are offering is growing old in custody, not some positive therapeutic intervention.

Reference

Morris L (1994) *Dangerous Classes: The Underclass and Social Citizenship.* London: Routledge.

49 Fashions in forensic care: Implications for sense of self

Annie Bartlett

Introduction

The origins of this chapter lie in a project undertaken a few years ago in a secure hospital. I and two colleagues undertook a period of observation in three separate wards in the hospital. We each spent six months doing what might charitably be termed "hanging about" and more seriously entitled "participant observation". Fieldwork required us not only to observe what went on but also to think about ourselves in relation to the staff and the patients that we encountered. We all reflected on our identities. I noticed that parts my core identity fell away. During fieldwork I ceased to be a doctor, both in the sense of thinking and behaving like a ward-based psychiatrist. But I still was a doctor. I ceased also, for the purposes of fieldwork, to have a life outside the hospital, as I chose not to divulge real aspects of my social identity. But that life outside the project continued. I became a blank canvass onto which staff and patients projected fantasies, with varying degrees of approximation to my real existence. This seemed similar in some respects to the experience of the patients I met, on whom a forensic identity had been foisted. When they entered a secure hospital they had had a similar but different journey to mine. I wondered how they thought about themselves, which parts of themselves they took with them, which parts, like me, they left behind or sealed off behind a cloak of privacy.

These research observations seem to me to be of clinical relevance as well. Specifically this chapter considers the parallel processes which create the "self" of forensic patients and the "selves" of the staff involved in custodial care. To do that it is necessary to use clinical material to look at ourselves and our patients under the microscope.

Being a forensic patient

Recently I sat in interview with a patient of mine who did not like me. He wanted to change his "consultant", his term, the only part of my identity that seemed either conspicuous or to matter to him. As far as I could tell, the reason he wanted another consultant was because I was saying things to him, about himself, that he found intolerable. He wanted to be discharged immediately. I explained that our risk assessment of him suggested that that would not be wise, indeed not in keeping with current practice. To discharge him would have been cavalier. He denied the relevance of his past violence, saying it was all a long time ago. Speaking of the recent past, he said he had not been violent or if he had, it was not in the way I described. He argued that his current leave arrangements meant he could not see his mother, who was ill, or his children. His lack of contact with them caused him anguish. In his view a discussion of dangerousness was irrelevant to the things that were most important to him. As the conversation progressed he became more anxious. He sweated. He overrode my comments as if to stem the tide of unacceptable remarks about himself. I was stressing his patient "self". He was impatient, stressing the normality of his real life and relationships. This is a run-of-the-mill interview. It is a variation on the idea of breaking bad news, telling people, not in this case that they have terminal illnesses, but that they cannot easily stop being forensic patients. Both the adjective "forensic" and the noun "patient" are important. He and I were both deaf in that interview. He would not hear about the unacceptable dangerous parts of himself. I could not hear (and perhaps should not have heard) that I was being unfair, unreasonable, and unnecessarily coercive in keeping him in hospital. Here were parallel processes. This excerpt of interview highlights identities commonly invoked in clinical work, the "consultant" and the "dangerous forensic patient". In neither case do the identities invoked sit easily with who either of us think we are.

Becoming a forensic patient would rank pretty low on the list of ambitions parents have for their children. Being a mental health patient is bad enough but being a forensic patient is stigma "squared", even if the club's membership is growing. There are two elements to this. The first is what may happen to you when this attribution "forensic" is made. You may be locked up in very secure places for a long time far away from your roots. This is real and indisputable. Second, people may construe you differently by virtue of the term "forensic patient"; you embody negative attributes where the relationship of such attributes to your real history may be both inexact and arbitrary. This is evident in the process of forensic referral. The threshold for referral is very varied. In one place you might need to commit rape and in another just damage property. The referred patient, even if not accepted by a forensic service, has moved part way along the line towards a forensic identity.

From clinical experience it is apparent that it will be difficult to get accommodation once a forensic label is ascribed. Bed and breakfasts will not want someone "dangerous" near children. Hostels are more wary; the person becomes, as a patient of mine did recently, someone who needs an extra form when applying for work. The anxiety of helping agencies in this new climate of risk management is intense. Staff fear the media spotlight rather than the dangerous individual.

But the transformation of identity from "patient" to "forensic patient" is not independent of actual characteristics although there may be little agreement between therapist and patient about which characteristics matter, and how. The reductionist medical approach will emphasise issues of diagnosis – someone may become a "schizophrenic" rather than a person with schizophrenia. The current vogue for risk assessment will create "high-risk" or "low-risk" cases – never "no risk". Such terms, as in my own service, may never have been operationalised. The recording of inaccurate and perhaps misleading risk data can satisfy a managerial need, not a clinical one. The person reading the court or tribunal report about themselves may disagree with much that is written. In practice they may see little advantage in pointing out this disagreement. The staff have peered through an "institutional filter" that emphasises issues of risk in a way that would have been unthinkable 15 years ago.

So the experience of being a forensic patient may leave a person not recognising themselves on all those all important bits of paper. Other desirable parts of the self may be difficult to maintain. The issue of parenting illustrates this well. Since the Fallon report (Fallon et al. 1999) there have been changes in the rules about child visitors to secure hospital units. It has become more difficult for family links to be maintained. One patient reported to me that a previous consultant had said to him that he was not a father, he was his, the consultant's patient. The remark is cruel. But its implication is in keeping with patient reality. At times it may be appropriate to restrict contact between patients and potential victims, e.g. children and partners; often it is a product of institutional, blanket rules. Very few women in the Special Hospitals, if any, have sexual designs on children, but the post-Fallon recommendations have been applied wholesale.

Forensic patients can respond to their new identity in several ways. They can refuse to play ball. They can refuse patienthood. They can blame the system, say it is unfair, and if they had gone to prison they would be out now. The punishment – hospital, does not fit the crime. They can deny the appropriateness of a mental health label. They would prefer to be a "prisoner" or an "inmate". They can avoid therapeutic engagement. This may follow from their chosen identity or it may be a way of shielding parts of themselves from the intrusive, unblinking gaze of the multidisciplinary team who have a tendency to chat amongst themselves about people's innermost feelings. They may deny the seriousness or relevance of past violence to the present or the future. The conceptual framework of risk, where the past predicts the future, may seem genuinely unreal.

This is a rather bleak view of the therapeutic challenge many forensic patients present. But an essential prerequisite of forensic work is to avoid self-delusion. It may be convenient to see custodial care as a benign process acting in the patient's best interests. From the patient's point of view that is unlikely to be obvious. Two book titles came to mind as I was writing this paper. One was *Born a Number* (Harding 1985), written by a man some years ago with experience of the secure hospital system. The other was published recently by a woman detained many times in hospital, entitled *Am I Not a Person?* (Hart 1998). The titles, thought up a decade apart, speak for themselves. They emphasise the difficulty of maintaining an acceptable sense of self as a mental health patient.

Being a coercive practitioner

Perucci (1974) wrote about contamination. Just as patients were liable to stigma, he suggested, so too were staff. This is an important dimension of staff experience of the care of the mad. Staff who work with the dangerously mad may themselves come to be seen by the outside world as a necessary evil. Nowhere is the truth of this more evident than in the special hospitals. Staff in the special hospitals know how easy it is to become associated with negative patient characteristics. To a certain extent they do daily battle with a one-dimensional image of themselves. In recent years they have been portrayed in the media as physically brutal (Brindle 1992a), sexually abusive of women (Brindle 1992b) and conniving at the sexual abuse of children (Harding 1997). Each of these terms is interestingly indicative of a particular kind of offence, often linked with special hospital admission. This view of forensic practitioners may be shared by people working in other parts of the mental health system. Being seen from outside is one aspect of the forensic self, another is the forensic practitioner's self-image.

Some years ago a woman was referred to me with a history of significant violence to health care professionals. She showed intense feelings even within a first interview preoccupied with establishing basic history. When next seen I deliberately had a colleague with me. I thought that the interview might get out of hand. It went badly, neither I nor my colleague were able to meet her needs. Having left the building feeling rejected and unhelped, she returned with broken glass. We had waited behind seeing that she had loitered by the building, seeming uncertain about going home. She came back into the building, visibly aroused. She shouted to see me on my own, and brandished the broken glass. I ran away. She than cut herself, not me. Later she was very distressed about the incident. I saw her again and she went home. She had convinced us of the extent of her distress. We did not call the police nor did we "section" her. Later contact with her confirmed that she had intended to kill me. Our risk management may seem rather relaxed. Would it have been prudent to admit for assessment to tide her over the crisis? Looking back at this defining moment in Joanna Bloggs' psychiatric career, we were right to let her go home. Her subsequent history confirms that. But I worry now that I would not have the courage to do the same again. You can see the tabloid headlines "Woman stabs innocent passers-by with glass from psychiatric outpatient department. Staff took no action after an earlier incident that day." The radical changes in risk management means that were the same incident to occur again, I would probably behave differently. I would be more coercive. I would be backed up by the Mental Health Act, by good practice guidelines and no doubt by my colleagues. I would like myself less but I would still do it. It would be "effective clinical risk management", just what we are supposed to be doing. But this seemingly neutral term, this technical procedure is designed both to disguise the moral and ethical decision making that it embodies, and the fact that real people, like the "I" of the story, make decisions.

My argument is not against all coercion in psychiatry. It is sensible at times to use the powers of the Mental Health Act. But more of our patients, more of the time will be involved in clinical situations where their views may be respected by us as individuals, but will be over-ridden by us as professionals operating in line with current practice guidelines. It is our professional selves that have changed.

Increasingly custodial care?

Thus far, the argument has been based on anecdote. But there are several potential sources of information which would enable us to decide whether mental health care has become more custodial. These include the Department of Health's statistics about bed occupancy, the size of forensic services, the direction of government policy initiatives and the experiences of patients and staff who work within forensic services. Some of this information is inconsistent, ambiguous and difficult to interpret.

The Department of Health (1999) figures suggest there has been an increase over a 10-year period (1987/88–1997/8) in both Part II and Part III sections. There is recent fluctuation and a flattening out of the overall rate of increase. Sections 2 and 3 show large increases, 8,700–12,000 and 2,500–8,750 respectively. Section 3 shows a threefold increase. The numbers admitted informally and then sectioned have risen. Court and prison disposals have increased, but mainly through the use of Section 48. Judges do not seem minded to increase the rate at which restriction orders are imposed.

But scarcely a week of the *British Medical Journal* goes by without the appearance of a new forensic post. Looking back on the service to South West Thames in 1988 there were two consultants and a handful of inpatient beds. In 1999 there were 43 medium secure beds, 15 minimum secure beds and a large number of community forensic patients served by five consultant-led teams. Many would applaud such apparently appropriate expansion, including Trust management. There appears to be a general trend leading to a national increase in medium secure beds and a small decrease in special hospital beds. This implies an increase in the number of individuals dealing with patients detained for long periods of time.

Policy initiatives in the last decade have not been all one way. The now historic Reed Report (Department of Health and Home Office 1992) was heartening; its liberal principles make interesting reading now. It would seem that whatever the appropriate level of security was thought to be in 1992 it is likely that it is greater nowadays. The recent moves to increase the surveillance and coercion of patients stem from the debate over care in the community. Central government reinforces the idea of dangerous mental illness (Department of Health 1998); it is keen on the introduction of community treatment orders. Practice guidelines ensure not only better delivery of care but also better "keeping tabs on people". Supervision registers, though widely mocked, still exist. The Supervised Discharge order is in much the same vein. Most recently, and indeed infamously, the policy initiative to change patterns of care for those with severe personality disorders has caused outcry from psychiatry and civil liberties organisations alike. The fictitious category "dangerous and severe personality disorder" (DSPD) has been introduced as if it were a diagnostic entity (Home Office 1999). The government wishes to incarcerate the unconvicted in conditions that will almost inevitably lead to a demoralised work force and a client population with very little to lose.

In sum, the evidence above points towards a shift, piecemeal, towards more coercive care both in forensic and other branches of psychiatry.

Implications for staff

Like other people forensic practitioners try to avoid the stresses and strains of the job. The intelligent empathy needed to work with the difficult to engage is potentially exhausting. Deflection of intolerable affect from detained patients can be done in several ways. Forensic clinicians are keen to assess and less able or less keen to treat. Contact with patients can be minimal. At least one clinical director in London in a Forensic Service has no inpatient beds at all. Medico-legal work is less demanding than treatment. Courts make decisions. The Home Office can be blamed for a patient's slow progress on a Restriction Order, the climate of risk for a more cautious approach to dangerous patients. In this way one's awareness of responsibility for the system in which one participates can be decreased.

Psychiatrists as a group have objected to many of the changes that have come about. Representations to the Home Office about DSPD have been particularly energetic. Yet we will not be witnesses to further change but probably active participants.

Herbert Reed (1991) wrote a poem called "The Naming of Parts", in which the elements of a gun are named so that you know what you are using. In naming parts you recognise something for what it is, and your relationship to it. So, in acting clinically there is a need to spell out not just the practice issues, but also the moral and ethical ones intrinsic to shifting concepts of "dangerousness". Only then can individual clinicians know what they are doing, and whether the changes in practice indicated above are compatible with their sense of self as doctors.

References

Brindle D (1992a) Staff who tell of cruel patient treatment risk death threat. *Guardian*, March 10.

Brindle D (1992b) Women patients were left naked. *Guardian*, March 3.

Department of Health and Home Office (1992) *Review of Health and Social Services for Mentally Disordered Offenders and Others Requiring Similar Services (Reed Report)*. London: HMSO.

Department of Health (1998) *Modernising Mental Health Services: Safe, Sound and Supportive*.

Department of Health (1999) In-patients formally detained in hospitals under the Mental Health Act 1983 and other legislation, England: 1988–89 to 1998–99. *Department of Health Statistical Bulletin*.

Fallon P, Bluglass R, Edward B and Daniels G (1999) *Report of the Committee of Inquiry into the Personality Disorder Unit, Ashworth Special Hospital*. Vol. 1. London: HMSO.

Harding L (1985) *Born a Number*. London: Mind.

Harding L (1997) Prison or hospital. *Guardian*, February 17.

Hart S (1998) *Am I Not A Person?* Nottingham: Word Factory.

Home Office (1999) *Managing People with Severe Personality Disorder: Proposals for Policy Development.* London: Home Office.

Perucci R (1974) *Circle of Madness: On Being Insane and Institutionalised in America.* Englewood Cliffs, NJ: Prentice Hall.

Reed H (1991) Naming of Parts. In: J Stallworthy (ed.). *Collected Poems.* Oxford: Oxford University Press.

50 Mental health legislation is discriminating and stigmatising

George Szmukler

The non-consensual treatment of patients suffering from "mental disorder" is regulated by specific mental health legislation. Legislation for a minority group of persons by definition "discriminates" between them and the majority. Does it in the process act to discriminate against that minority or does it protect them? I argue that mental health legislation does the former, although ostensibly promoting the latter. (Detailed expositions of the arguments can be found in Campbell & Heginbotham (1991), Campbell, Rosenman (1994) and Szmukler and Holloway (1998, 2000).)

Paternalism, "capacity" and "best interests"

A patient with a 'physical disorder' such as cancer may refuse treatment even if the disease is life-threatening. Because we respect personal autonomy we accept the decision unless there is reason to believe that the patient's decision-making capacity is impaired. Paternalistic interventions in medicine (with, as we shall see, the notable exception of psychiatry) are only allowed when a patient lacks the mental capacity to make treatment decisions for himself or herself, and treatment is in the patient's best interests.

There is no statutory law on capacity, and the common law is at present widely regarded as unsatisfactory. However, following a report on mental incapacity by the Law Commission (1995) and a period of consultation (Lord Chancellor 1997), the Government is proposing legislation which will clarify the meaning of *capacity* and *best interests* and define the powers of others to act on behalf of incapacitated patients (Lord Chancellor 1999). *Capacity* involves the patient's ability to understand and retain information about the nature of the treatment and the consequences of accepting it or not, and to reason with that information. "*Best interests*" attempts to determine what the patient might have chosen in this situation if he or she had capacity, based on past statements (as in an advance statement) or according to those who know the patient well. When a future period of incapacity is predictable, a patient may also appoint a person to take healthcare decisions on his or her behalf according to stated preferences or principles. The patient's values are thus given weight, important in a multicultural society. However, the new legislation regarding decision-making for those with mental incapacity will not cover those with "mental disorder". Evidently there is something different between mental capacity in "physical" and "mental" disorders, but there is no attempt to define what this might be.

In contrast to impairment in decision-making by patients with "physical disorder" as above, under the Mental Health Act 1983 (and that of 1959), as well as mental health acts in most countries, non-consensual treatment of those with "mental disorder" is governed by an entirely different set of tests. *Capacity* plays *no role* in decisions to initiate treatment against a patient's wishes. Instead the MHA 1983 allows involuntary treatment if the person: is suffering from a mental disorder; the disorder is of "a nature or degree which makes it appropriate ... to receive medical treatment ..."; and it is "necessary for the health or safety of the patient or for the protection of other persons ..."

For the moment let us stay with the health or safety of the patient only. Two significant observations can be made. Firstly, different rules apply to those suffering from a "mental disorder" compared to those with a "physical disorder" when their decision-making capacity is in doubt (that is, usually, when they don't agree with the proposed treatment). Secondly, compared with the rules for those with "physical disorders", the rules for those with "mental disorders" fail to respect the autonomy of the patient in the same way. The patient's reasons for rejecting the treatment are not explored (as they must be in determining *capacity*), nor is the question of whether treatment is in the best interests of the patient. The sole consideration is the patient's "health or safety", presumably from the perspective of the clinician (or other representatives of society). But we accept that patients with physical disorders, provided they have capacity, can make decisions that may be seriously detrimental to their health or safety. Health and safety are not the ultimate values. For persons with capacity, their personal values are given dominion. Those with mental disorder are not given this privilege; they may be treated against their will. There seems to be an underlying assumption that *"mental disorder" necessarily entails mental incapacity*, so the question does not need to be asked. And also, that the values espoused by a person with a disordered mind are not to be taken seriously in determining where their best interests lie. These assumptions are patently untrue.

By failing to respect the mentally disordered patient's autonomy, by not presuming capacity unless there is reason for doubt, by assuming that mental disorder entails incapacity, and by enshrining these prejudices in separate legislation which applies uniquely to those with "mental disorder" (which remains undefined), mental health legislation *discriminates against* those with mental disorders and *stigmatises* them. The discrepancy in the degree of respect for the autonomy of patients in two current draft bills – the Draft Mental Incapacity Bill (2003) and the Draft Mental Health Bill (2002) – is painfully obvious. The latter explicitly elevates risk reduction above autonomy.

"Incapacity legislation", such as the government is proposing for those with physical disorders, but which covers non-consensual treatment for *all patients with mental incapacity*, from whatever cause (head injury, post-ictal confusion, learning disabilities, schizophrenia, Alzheimer's disease, psychotic depression, and febrile toxic states) is the only fair legislation. Only then may an important source of discrimination against a stigmatised subset of incapacitated patients cease.

Protection of other persons

Equally if not more discriminatory are those aspects of mental health legislation referring to the *"protection of other persons"*. Those with mental disorders are virtually unique in being liable to detention (in hospital) because they present a risk of harm to others, but before they have actually committed a violent act. This constitutes a *form of preventive detention* to which our society, in other contexts, has an understandable aversion on civil liberty grounds. Under existing legislation, the detention of dangerous persons is *not* based on the *level of risk* they pose, but on whether they are called mentally disordered or not.

Although some groups of persons with mental illness are more likely to be violent than the normal population, especially in association with substance misuse (Steadman et al. 1998), persons with mental disorder perpetrate only a small fraction of serious violence in our society (Swanson et al. 1990). There is no evidence that violence is more predictable in those with mental disorder compared to the rest of the population. Indeed the most predictably dangerous persons are those with a track record of dangerous behaviour, most of whom are not mentally ill – habitual spouse abusers, dangerous drivers (especially in association with alcohol), regular substance misusers, and those with a short temper who regularly place themselves in situations where they are likely to be provoked. Even if it were more predictable, this would still not justify a lower threshold for detention for those with mental disorder compared to the rest of us. Nor does "treatability". Groups of non-mentally disordered dangerous persons might respond just as well, if not better, to psychosocial "treatment" programmes aimed at reducing dangerous driving or domestic violence. The fact that treatment-resistant mentally ill patients who are deemed dangerous are detained the longest shows also that "treatability" is a lame justification.

Mental health legislation confuses *paternalism* and the *protection of others*. They are quite separate ends. The former is concerned with the health interests of the patient and empowers others to act when the patient lacks the capacity to act in his or her best health interests. The *protection of others* turns on the *risk of harm*. This risk may not have much to do with illness or with a patient's capacity to make treatment decisions. If a patient lacks capacity and treatment is in his or her best interests, non-consensual treatment is justified. Whether there is a danger to others or not may not be especially relevant, although it would of course be taken into account in best interests considerations and might prompt particularly urgent action to ensure the safety of patient and others.

For all other persons, those with mental disorders *who retain capacity* as well as everyone else in the population, the liability to preventive detention should be equal. There are two questions to ask about a potentially dangerous person, whose order is crucial. *First*, what is the risk? Risk should be ascertained without reference to whether the person suffers from a mental disorder or not, and in an appropriate judicial setting. If the risk is deemed unacceptable, a *second* question arises – what can be done, if anything, to reduce it. At this point treatment might be offered to the dangerous mentally disordered person if this carries a likelihood of reduction of risk. If no "treatment" or similar intervention exists, or if it is rejected, then a custodial disposal will be necessary. This of course amounts to a *generic dangerousness or preventive detention* provision against which many will recoil. I am not arguing for or against generic dangerousness legislation; only that the same laws should apply to the mentally disordered as to the rest of us. Either we have generic legislation applicable to all of us or we have no preventive detention for anyone, including those with mental disorder. The present situation is clearly discriminatory against those with mental disorder – at an equal level of risk, the mentally disordered person is much more likely to be detained.

Why has this prejudicial situation arisen and why is it so rarely challenged? I believe it reflects deeply ingrained fears of the mentally ill and stereotypes of dangerousness which are so inherent in 'folk' notions of mental illness that their uncoupling is not even thought about. By failing to note the distinction between health interests and the protection of others, and by getting the order of the two key questions wrong, we allow the continuing possibility of abuses of civil liberties. The Government proposed such an abuse where the application of a state-defined "diagnosis" ('dangerous severe personality disorder') and an ascription of dangerousness would be enough to indeterminately detain someone even in the absence of a previous violent offence or the possibility of effective treatment (Home Office and Department of Health 1999). Persons with mental disorder do not receive the protections from preventive detention that the rest of us do. Mental health legislation supports this, thus reinforcing an underlying stereotype that the mentally ill are inherently dangerous, and is thus stigmatising.

Mental health legislation is unnecessary. An "*Incapacity Act*", such as that proposed for non-mentally disordered persons (Lord Chancellor 1999), should be suitable for all patients with incapacity. In so far as "protection of others" is concerned, the same legislation should apply to those with mental disorders as to the rest of us, together with the protections the rest of us insist upon. It is for these reasons that Holloway and I have argued that "dismantling mental health legislation may be the single most important action we can take to finally give equal rights to persons with mental illness and to eliminate stigma" (Szmukler and Holloway 1998).

References

Campbell T (1994) Mental Health Law: institutionalised discrimination. *Australian and New Zealand Journal of Psychiatry* **28**: 554–9.

Campbell T & Heginbotham C (1991) *Mental illness: Prejudice, Discrimination and the Law*. Dartmouth: Vermont.

Home Office and Department of Health (1999) *Managing Dangerous People with Severe Personality Disorder: Proposals for Policy Development*. London: The Stationery Office.

Law Commission (1995) *Mental Incapacity*. Law Commission Report No. 231. London: HMSO.

Lord Chancellor (1997) *Who Decides? Making Decisions on Behalf of Mentally Incapacitated Adults*. (Cm 3803). London: The Stationery Office.

Lord Chancellor (1999) *Making Decisions: The Government's Proposals for Making Decisions on Behalf of Mentally Incapacitated Adults* (Cm 4465). London: The Stationery Office.

Rosenman S (1994) Mental health law: an idea whose time has passed. *Australian and New Zealand Journal of Psychiatry* **28**: 560–5.

Secretary of State for Health (1999) *Reform of the Mental Health Act 1983: Proposals for Consultation*. London: The Stationery Office.

Steadman H, Mulvey E, Monahan J et al. (1998) Violence by people discharged from acute psychiatric inpatient facilities and by others in the same neighborhoods. *Archives of General Psychiatry* **55**: 393–401.

Swanson JW, Holzer CE Ganju VK & Jono RT (1990) Violence and psychiatric disorder in the community: evidence from the Epidemiologic Catchment Area surveys. *Hospital and Community Psychiatry* **41**: 761–70.

Szmukler G & Holloway F (1998) Mental health legislation is now a harmful anachronism. *Psychiatric Bulletin* **22**: 662–5.

Commentary on Part 6

Christopher Cordess

In Chapter 47, David Tidmarsh provides a personal view of psychiatric attitudes to risk over his own professional lifetime of some 40 years. He believes that there are two myths – each equally dangerous in themselves – the one "that the mentally ill are extremely dangerous and should all be locked up" and the second "that they are completely harmless and that their reputation is due to labelling, the media and Sir Alfred Hitchcock". Whereas nowadays, driven by increasing political coercion, we increasingly err towards the "locking them all up" end of the spectrum, Tidmarsh believes that during his earlier career psychiatry lived within a professional mix of ignorance and denial of any enhanced dangerousness of the mentally disordered – for which we are now, as a profession, paying a high price.

He charts the course of received psychiatric "wisdom" from the historically significant studies of the non-violence at follow up of large cohorts of patients released from penitentiaries as a consequence of the Baxstrom (in 1966) and Dixon (in 1971) decisions in the USA – which underwrote the de-institutionalisation movement from psychiatric hospitals – to the quite different viewpoints of the present. He considers broadly four factors in what is a major volte face: the reduction in beds and the shift towards dangerousness as a criterion for admission; the increase in the use of drugs of abuse especially in combination with an "Axis I" (i.e. mental illness) disorder; improved methodologies of research which now "capture" the increased prevalence of violence amongst the mentally disordered; and the perceptions of the public (fuelled by the media), which in my view represents the greatest change of all. I think of the amount of energy which the police force now expends, for example, upon combating and "correcting" public fears of stranger violence as opposed to crime prevention.

The main research studies (quoted by Tidmarsh in his chapter) which have established the increased prevalence of violence in the mentally disordered are well known, for example those by Hodgins et al. (1996), Swanson et al. (1996), Shaw et al. (1999), and Mullen et al. (2000).

Tidmarsh quotes Calman et al. (1999) on the general features of risk of any sort which make it less acceptable to the general public: "involuntary, inequitably distributed so that some benefit while others suffer the consequences, inescapable, unfamiliar, man-made rather than natural, causing irreversible damage, posing danger to children, causing dread, damaging identifiable rather than anonymous victims, poorly understood by science, and lastly, subject to contradictory statements from responsible sources". They apply, as Tidmarsh describes, to psychotic violence – but even more, I would say, to the violence associated with personality disorder, and we need to take notice of them in our attempts to better understand the sources of stigmatisation of our patients as well as ourselves. The fact that in absolute terms the mentally disordered are responsible for a tiny percentage of public violence, compared, say, with motor vehicle accidents, does not seem to mitigate public opinion.

What is intriguing about Tidmarsh's choice of quotations is that two of them, which he employs as intended "weapons" of his own against the anti-psychiatry movement of Szasz, Laing and Cooper, return – in the present political climate of "invitations" to psychiatry to play the role of agent of social control – to haunt even mainstream psychiatry: Szasz defined psychiatrists as "agents specially trained to silence all those who transgress against the prevailing power interests in contemporary society" – not a bad description of the original D and SPD proposals which, hopefully, psychiatrists will refuse to be part of – and, as "professional degraders of stigmatised individuals" (see Szmukler's critique of specific Mental Health Legislation in Chapter 50).

In Chapter 49, Annie Bartlett writes from an anthropological point of view of the roles and identities we adopt as forensic psychiatrist and forensic patient, and the misunderstandings and stigmatisations that are thereby enforced, and which we and our patients enact. It could have been couched in terms of "projections" and "transferences" – of patients projecting their transferences on to us and us on to patients – but is perhaps the more incisive for eschewing these familiar and – it has to be said – sometimes jaded terms.

Forensic psychiatry, by its nature and increasingly, deals with the highly stigmatised – a double jeopardy of both "mental health patient" and "forensic" to boot: and patients categorised under both or either term, as Bartlett describes, have been partially construed through an "institutional filter that emphasises issues of risk in a way that would have been unthinkable 15 years ago".

Correctly she notes that central government serially reinforces the idea of dangerous mental illness: it seeks now to introduce community treatment orders, and increasingly practice guidelines aim better to "keep tabs on people"; similarly Supervision Registers and Supervised Discharge give greater powers of surveillance and coercion and are part of the Law and Order rhetoric of political vote catching. The latest proposals for detention of those within the fictitious category of D and SPD have brought especially energetic protestations by psychiatrists to Home Office Ministers and officials – but, Bartlett notes, I hope incorrectly, "We will not (just) be witnesses to further change but probably active participants". This will be ultimately depressing if it becomes true, and we are so supine as a profession as to collude with what we have actively protested as ethically unacceptable. The Nuremberg issue of the *BMJ* in 1996, quoted by Heath (2001), warned of "the dangers whenever political forces directly enlist the medical profession in an agenda of social and economic transformation". It should be noted that "D and SPD" has been removed as an entity from the Draft Mental Health Bill (2002), but the (lack of) definition of mental disorder within the Bill and the removal of the "treatability" clause leave open the possibility of a "catch-all". Meanwhile, the D and SPD units continue to be built and the protocols worked on.

Bartlett seeks to reinstate the subjective experience of the forensic patient – the preservation of a sense of self – in the highly objectifying, dehumanising, contemporary world of risk preoccupation. Similarly, she demonstrates, too, the dangers for professionals of forgetting their essentially humane calling in the world dominated by "effective clinical risk management" – and, I would add, inappropriately applied management speak, bureaucracy and impoverished discourses of "evaluation", whose final achievement may be to kill off the finer and valuable points of the whole substance and subject they seek to regulate. Rather as the era of prevention of risk of infection of foods by pesticides, in agriculture, gave way to the rebound and iterative fear of the toxicity of the preventative agent, and the consequent idealisation of "organic" foods – i.e. a law of diminishing returns – so does present coercive health legislation risk "backlash" by public and staff alike.

Bartlett invites us to follow "The Naming of Parts", the title of a poem by Henry Reed: "Each of the elements of a gun are named so that you know what you are using . . . So, in acting clinically [especially in the contemporary political climate] there is a need to spell out not just the practice issues, but also the moral and ethical ones intrinsic to shifting concepts of 'dangerousness' [and the primacy of third party protection, rather than the primacy of one's duty to one's patient]. Only then can individual clinicians know what they are doing, and whether the changes in practice . . . are compatible with their sense of self as doctors".

Both George Szmukler and Philip Fennell (in Chapters 50 and 48), from their very different perspectives, address the stigmatising effects of mental health legislation. For Szmukler specific mental health legislation for persons with "mental disorders" differentiates them unfairly from persons with "physical disorders" for whom there is no equivalent "physical health legislation". It is unacceptable because it discriminates against them, and therefore stigmatises them uniquely: it does so by ignoring "mental capacity" and thereby devaluing autonomy; by permitting non-consensual treatment (even of those who would be judged competent); and by allowing for preventative detention.

Fennell, by contrast, accepts the need for mental health legislation, but presently sees a "convergence between the psychiatric system and the penal system ... with the 'risk management movement' pulling the psychiatric system more towards the criminal justice end of the spectrum rather than towards the health care end." The future is indeed bleak if, to quote Fennell, some of our "key concepts in health care values: the principle of therapeutic intervention, including the philosophy of 'above all do no harm'; the principle of confidentiality; and the idea that the doctor/patient relationship is a therapeutic alliance" (rather than one of detection and disclosure) are to go by the board. He sees the criminal justice and penal systems as consciously stigmatising, seeking to convey social messages of deterrence by a process of "shaming". How then can we de-stigmatise our mentally disordered patients, including those within the criminal justice system, in the light of this politically driven convergence upon increasing numbers of people who are essentially the marginalised and unwanted?

Fennell writes "if one was sitting in the Home Office or the Department of Health looking at a pure risk management model, these are the things one would want: medicalisation [he means psychiatrisation] of the penal system, indeterminate detention, continuing supervision, and sex offender training programmes". All these are either in place, or will be, if the proposed new Mental Health Act is enacted. In the original "Reforming the Mental Health Act: Part II: High Risk Patients" (2000), which has evolved into the Draft Mental Health Bill (2002), we are informed that "Arrangements for the assessment of those already serving prison sentences will also be improved by the creation of a new power for the Home Secretary to direct such individuals for assessment". Such "directions" join the already compulsory Sex Offenders Treatment Programme (SOTP), which has become mandatory but which has not been evaluated, or, at best, outcome studies have not been published. Apparently imprisonment now includes not only the restriction of freedom, but a "brave new world" compulsion to enter into bureaucratically and State-devised, coercive "treatment" programmes, driven and predominantly manned, not by well-trained clinicians (with their own professional and ethical codes) but by prison system employees.

Fennell is generally critical of the Government White Paper, "Reforming the Mental Health Act: Part I The New Legal Framework" (2000); the Draft Mental Health Bill (2002) will not allay his fears. Firstly, he criticises the proposed very broad definition of mental disorder as "any disability or disorder of mind or brain, whether permanent or temporary, which results in an impairment or disturbance of mental functioning" (i.e. scrapping the current four-part subclassification); and, secondly, the "downgrading" – more accurately the expulsion – of the "treatability" test which is currently a required criterion within the current Mental Health Act (1983).

With the broadest possible definition of mental disorder and no treatability requirement, indefinite detention for all manner of indiscretions, including the political, becomes a terrifying possibility. Fennell comments on how government policy on psychiatric practice is sloganised (as if selling a soap powder) as based on the three Ss: "Safe, sound and supported" – essentially, and admittedly, a policy of public protection and social control of perceived risk, with little commitment to clinical care or, it seems, understanding of an ethic of treatment. At the pragmatic level it is unlikely to assist in the recruitment and retention of staff to already depleted psychiatric services.

The expert Committee for the new Mental Health Act (later called the Richardson Committee) which the Government set up in 1997, according to Fennell, "took seriously the exhortation to do a root and branch review of the Mental Health Act", basing their principles on ideas of non-discrimination and autonomy, and focusing heavily on capacity. Depressingly the White Paper and the Draft Mental Health Bill embrace few of these principles, but focus instead on risk above all other concerns.

Both Szmukler and Fennell are united in their condemnation of the proposals originally contained in the Government White Paper "Reforming the Mental Health Act: Part II" (and now the Draft Mental Health Bill) for what Szmukler calls "the state-defined 'diagnosis' of dangerous and severe personality disorder (D and SPD)", which for Fennell is "the apotheosis of risk management without any fear of commitment to any of the things which make psychiatrists' contributions to risk management the valuable thing that it is". For Fennell "the D and SPD proposals are being put forward as a way of detaining people without necessarily having to offer them a therapeutic intervention; without subjecting them to a treatability test". "But", he continues, "a treatability test is what justifies psychiatric involvement in these cases: If you can't offer some prospect of positive clinical measures then what you are offering is growing old in custody, not some positive therapeutic intervention." As stated previously, although the specific label "D and SPD" does not appear in the Draft Mental Health Bill (2002), the units for housing such people are in place, and the "catch-all" nature of the lack of definition allows for detention of personality disordered people on the basis of risk. He sees Article 5 of the Human Rights Act as "the last possibility of putting a stall on the D and SPD proposals".

Szmukler, on the other hand, regards neither "*treatability*" of those mentally disordered who may be regarded as potentially violent nor "predictability" of violence in the mentally disordered as necessarily relevant in relation to their detention, since he maintains that this detention is essentially discriminatory anyway. Why not, he asks, detain *anyone* on the basis of risk – habitual spouse abusers, dangerous drivers or substance abusers, the great majority of whom are not mentally ill – rather than the mentally disordered who make up such a small absolute number of those who are seriously violent or represent high risk? Logically, and I believe correctly, as Szmukler recognises, this argument could be used to promote the introduction of provisions for generic dangerousness or preventative detention regulations – against which he says, many will recoil. I suppose I fear that, after the DSPD debacle, present government thinking might well pick up the rhetorical question concretely, miss its irony and attempt to introduce just such legislation! At least psychiatrists wouldn't be directly implicated.

The government, indeed, proposes new legislation (following the report on mental incapacity by the Law Commission, and a period of consultation (Lord Chancellor 1997 – cited in Chapter 50)) which will "clarify the meaning of *capacity* and *best interests* and define the powers of others to act on behalf of incapacitated patients (Lord Chancellor 1999 – cited in Chapter 50). However, Szmukler is critical of the fact that "this new legislation regarding decision making for those with mental incapacity will not cover those with mental disorder". Szmukler regards "incapacity legislation" such as the government is proposing for those with physical disorders as the only fair legislation for all patients with mental incapacity from whatever cause. He lists head injury, post-ictal confusion, learning disabilities, schizophrenia, Alzheimer's disease, psychotic depression, or febrile toxic states. The alternative – as we have now, and look set to continue – is necessarily stigmatising of mental disorder. He concludes that for the reasons he has given in his chapter, he and Holloway in their 1998 paper have argued that "dismantling mental health legislation may be the single most important action we can take to finally give equal rights to persons with mental illness and to eliminate stigma".

Although logically compelling, I find Szmukler's argument breaks down essentially for pragmatic reasons – that, at least at the present time, the assessment of capacity is undeveloped and likely to be unreliable, and in all the conditions and mental states cited would be likely to be variously assessed by different practitioners (and courts). For example, current models of capacity are biased towards cognition and ignore modern emotion theory (Appelbaum and Grisso 1995; Charland 1998).

Tidmarsh has given us the historical context; Szmukler and Fennell have provided sophisticated and stimulating commentaries upon the follies that our government, on "our" behalf, are about to enact, and Bartlett has depicted the "risks" of engaging in this essentially socially controlling and dehumanising change of policy and culture. Mental health patients and staff alike – beware!

References

Appelbaum P & Grisso T (1995) The Macarthur treatment competence study. I: Mental illness and competence to consent to treatment. *Law and Human Behaviour* **19**: 105–25.
Charland L (1998) Is Mr Spock mentally competent? Competence to consent and emotion. *Philosophy, Psychiatry and Psychology* **5**: 67–81.
Heath I (2001) A Warning to the GMC. *British Medical Journal* **322**: 439.

Part 7

Creativity and mental disorder

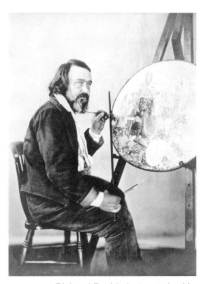

Richard Dadd photographed in
Bethlem Hospital, *c.* 1856, at work
on his painting

51 Genius and the mind

Andrew Steptoe

Genius is a word that is much used and abused. While few would object to calling Shakespeare or Michelangelo geniuses, the term is also applied to celebrity chefs ("a genius in the kitchen") and to footballers with great ball control skills. The mantle of genius appears to be bestowed on any individual whose creativity or skill is admired, and acknowledged to be above the level of most contemporary practitioners of the same activity. Posterity often makes different judgements. For example, painters like Alexandre Cabanel and Bouguereau were highly esteemed in mid-nineteenth century Paris, but are now recognised as much lesser talents than Manet, Monet or Renoir. There seems much to be said for Francis Galton's notion of genius as "the opinion of contemporaries, revised by posterity".

The theme of this session is creativity and mental disorder, and the relationship between mental illness and the creative process is discussed by Anthony Storr in Chapter 52. This presentation will outline more generally our understanding of the origins and development of exceptional creativity. I will then illustrate a way in which we may try to understand some of the psychological characteristics of the great creators of the past, by applying the concepts of present-day psychology and psychiatry.

The origins of creativity

A bewildering range of views about the origins of creativity have been proposed over the years (Steptoe 1998a). The ancient Greeks held that natural talents might be endowed at birth, and that inspiration was one of the gifts given to an infant by the gods. This interesting idea meant that an exceptional ability might be present from the earliest stages of life, yet not be inherited. The notion that genius is genetic has an equally long history, but has gained strength over recent years through the development of behaviour genetics, and the recognition of genetic influences on a range of psychological processes. Scientific work on hereditary genius was initiated by Francis Galton, who used a family history approach to argue that exceptional creativity in a particular domain ran in families: the Bach family of musicians is a good example. Of course, it can be argued that such families create the ideal environmental conditions for the stimulation of interest, skill and understanding in a particular domain, and some authorities have argued that exceptional creativity arises almost entirely from these nurturant processes (Howe 1999).

A second argument for genetic factors is that they help to explain how some rare creative forces apparently emerge at a very early age out of nowhere. How else can one account for the extraordinary Srinivasa Ramanujan, who was born into humble circumstances in rural southern India, where even paper to write on was a luxury, and who became one of the greatest mathematicians of the twentieth century? The behavioural geneticist David Lykken has used the term "emergenesis" to describe the unique combination of genes that might lead to qualitative shifts in talent or capability in a particular individual (Lykken et al. 1992). These genes might be present in other family members, though not in the combination necessary to generate the high levels of invention, persistence or concentrated interest in the field, necessary for great work.

Psychological theories about exceptional creativity have also taken a number of forms. The psychodynamic tradition has construed creativity as a manifestation of psychosexual or developmental disturbance. A famous example is Freud's "analysis" of Leonardo da Vinci, when he argued that Leonardo's creativity stemmed from neuroses related to homosexuality. There are many other analyses or psychobiographies of writers, politicians and artists; indeed, 40 years ago the analytic approach was so dominant that Hitschmann (1956) asserted that "only an analyst is competent and qualified to write the biographies of great men". Such approaches rely on the acceptance of psychodynamic models, and have also been criticised on two other grounds. One is "eventism", or placing undue weight on the significance of particular incidents in a person's life, rather than their day to day experience. The second is that analysis represents a form of reductionism, in accounting for creativity in terms of internal psychological processes, without taking the crucial social and cultural milieu into account (Anderson 1978; Amabile et al. 1996).

Psychoanalytic theories can be seen to some extent as refinements of the romantic view of creativity as a product of emotional turmoil and distress. The image of the artist as hero, struggling in a garret to forge his or her work out of the debris of a tempestuous love life or traumatic childhood, emerged in the early nineteenth century, and appeared to be exemplified by individuals such as Byron and Beethoven.

Recent years have seen renewed emphasis on an almost opposite perspective, which is that creativity and inventiveness emerges from a craft background, and from the refinement of skills in specific genres developed over years of practice (Ericsson 1996). Historians of art, for example, have learnt a great deal about the apprenticeship system in Renaissance studios, where techniques were acquired painstakingly over many years. For example, extensive drapery studies were carried out by Leonardo da Vinci and other apprentices in the studio of the sculptor and painter Andrea del Verrochio. Cloth was dipped in plaster or clay, then placed in a fixed set of folds, so that it could be copied by apprentices under different lighting conditions (Rubin and Wright 1999). Work such as this led to very exact techniques and beautiful images that are not in some senses original at all. Even mature Renaissance artists did not paint as their inspiration took them, but operated within strict guidelines set by patrons (Baxandall 1972). Several contracts for the painting of altarpieces and other works have survived from fifteenth century Florence, and show how artists were was given exact instructions about the size of the panel, its subject, the types of paint and colour to be used, and so on. Painters like Domenico Ghirlandaio were often supervised in their work by a member of the commissioning body, to make sure that they did not deviate from the agreed design and worked according to the agreed time schedule.

Another example of creativity emerging from practical skill and a craft tradition comes from music. Johann Sebastian Bach was born in 1685, and by the age of 15 had begun a professional musical career. This meant that he became deeply versed in the musical genres of the time, both sacred and secular, with musical fashions, and with the practical constraints of producing new music to be played at most once or twice, usually without much rehearsal time. Throughout his life he was obliged to compose specific kinds of music speedily, as demanded by his patron or by the church calendar. As well as composing, he was required to perform regularly, train choirs, and teach non-musical subjects such as the Catechism. During his early years in Leipzig, he had to combine his duties in St Thomas's Church and the choir school with composing a cantata every week. On Monday morning, he sat down with a sheaf of blank paper, and within a couple of days had to select the text for next Sunday's cantata, prepare the paper physically by ruling musical staves, and then compose fifteen or twenty minutes of choruses, solos and chorales. The next couple of days were taken up with copying the individual parts for the choir, soloists, orchestra and continuo, and with teaching the choir their music. On Friday and Saturday there were rehearsals, and the new cantata was performed at eight o'clock on the Sunday morning. The cycle then began again the day after for next week's work. Bach is thought to have composed over fifty cantatas a year for at least three years. These cantatas are not trivial pieces, but works of profound insight and musical genius. Bach could only have undertaken such a rigorous workload by taking a practical task-orientated approach, and by using his years of training to work out his musical ideas without waiting for inspiration to strike.

Psychological processes of creativity

However, the fact that someone practices a craft successfully does not make them inventive in their profession. Some special talents are required to turn routine output into masterpieces. Psychological research has endeavoured to understand the cognitive processes underlying what we would generally call inspiration. Unfortunately, there is a major difficulty in investigating the exceptional creators of the arts, literature and sciences – namely, that many of the most interesting practitioners are no longer alive, and direct evidence of cognitive processes is scanty. Academic psychologists have sought to circumvent this problem by studying more mundane forms of creativity: investigating the most successful graduates from art schools, people on creative writing courses, and so on (Sternberg 1999). Much of this research is focussed on divergent thinking, and on associative thinking and the capacity of creative individuals to make connections between apparently unrelated topics. The role of imagery in innovative thinking and creativity has also been recognised, and is mentioned by a number of great thinkers such as the mathematician Poincaré (Miller 1996). The capacity to concentrate hard, and to think about problems at a subconscious level while going about other activities, are characteristics of almost all highly creative people.

One can see how such processes might operate in practice in fields such as musical composition. Every composer works within a genre with defined conventions and musical structures, whether it be the classical idiom, atonalism or an esoteric form of jazz. Most composers also have an individual style, which can be seen as a repertoire of particular musical gestures, rhythms or harmonies that characterise that person's work. A new composition typically involves innovative gestures or themes within the harmonic world of that individual, coupled with new combinations of existing phrases or passages. For some composers, this process evidently involves extensive trial and error, working out different possibilities on paper; this is why the sketches of people like Beethoven are so interesting. Other composers appear to have worked out the problems in their heads before committing themselves to paper. For example, contemporaries describe Mozart as being preoccupied with music most of the time, walking around in a distracted fashion, or sitting quietly looking at nothing. This was the time during which he was actually composing. Then he would go to his desk, pick up his pen, and ask his wife to chat to him while he wrote the music down. Many of his autograph manuscripts were written without any corrections or mistakes. He clearly had many of his scores well worked out in his head before he set pen to paper (Steptoe 1996a).

Research on creative people of the past: Mozart as an example

In the second part of this chapter, I want to ask whether we can use any of the concepts and methods of present-day psychology to throw light on the emotional states of creative individuals in the past. To what extent can we use the historical record to understand the states of mind of the greatest creators? It is difficult to talk in generalities about these issues, since there are so many differences between the lives and experiences of exceptional creators. I will therefore concentrate on a single individual – Wolfgang Amadeus Mozart – in order to illustrate an approach that might prove fruitful for other individuals in the historical record (Steptoe 1996b, 1998b).

One feature that emerges very strikingly from any reading of Mozart's life is that he had an extraordinarily stressful life, yet continued to perform and compose at an astonishing rate. Over the last 10 years of his life, he wrote six operas (including *The Marriage of Figaro, Don Giovanni* and *The Magic Flute*), 17 piano concertos, six symphonies, 15 string quartets and quintets, together with a wide range of other instrumental, chamber and vocal work. At the same time, he earned most of his money by playing rather than composing, so had regular concert and teaching demands.

Yet these years were also full of emotional distress stemming from many sources. Mozart and his wife Constanze had six children over these years, four of whom died in infancy. The family always lived in small lodgings of four or five rooms where the composer worked and taught as well as lived, so was constantly surrounded by domestic activities and small children. There were bouts of serious illness, both for Mozart himself and Constanze, who also had very difficult pregnancies. In 1787, Mozart's father Leopold, with whom he had an intense emotional relationship, died, as did two of his close friends. To this can be added serious periodic financial difficulties, changes in popularity, and shifts in the macroeconomic environment that made his existence as an independent musician increasingly precarious.

However, one cardinal tenet of contemporary research on emotional stress is that bad events and experiences in themselves do not invariably lead to problems. The resources or personal assets and coping abilities that people can bring to bear on their situation must also be taken into account. When we apply this perspective to Mozart, we can recognise resources in a number of domains, and these are listed in Table 1. These suggest that he had psychological and social assets that might be expected to increase personal resilience in the face of difficulties in life.

For example, Mozart had an extraordinarily successful childhood, both in terms of creative activity and family structure. From the age of six he was the focus of his parents' devotion, and the central asset of the family. Although this cosseted background made the transition to maturity difficult (Steptoe 1996b), it is likely to have had a strong influence on the development of self-esteem. High levels of self-esteem are valuable, particularly when the individual experiences emotional losses or other events, since they help protect against feelings of worthlessness and guilt.

Table 1. Mozart's personal characteristics and psychosocial resources

Early life factors	Stable family background
	Successul childhood
Psychological makeup	High self-esteem
	Optimistic outlook
Social resources	Loving relationship with Constanze
	Numerous friends
Spiritual resources	Freemasonry
	Enlightenment beliefs
Creative resources	Composition and performance

At the level of personality, there is evidence that Mozart had an optimistic orientation on life. Optimism describes a complex matrix of beliefs concerning the way the world is organised, and the causal explanations people have for negative experiences. The evidence comes from empirical work on Mozart's explanatory style that I have carried out in conjunction with Martin Seligman and Karen Reivich.

Explanatory style describes the causal inferences that people make when accounting for bad events, and research on the topic originally emerged from attempts to understand cognitive aspects of depression. Seligman has argued that explanatory style is composed of three dimensions: whether people see the causes of bad events as stable and long-lasting or as temporary, as global and universal or as specific, and as internal and due to them, or as external (Petersen and Seligman 1984). It has been found is that pessimism is characterised by internal attributions ("the event was my fault"), that it is global ("it is going to undermine everything I do") and that it reflects a stable state of affairs ("it's going to go on like this forever"). Optimists on the other hand attribute negative events to outside and external circumstances, and consider them temporary or one-off occurrences. The importance of this feature of cognitive makeup is that it is related to risk of depression, to lack of success and low achievement in many walks of life from sport to business and politics, and even to poor physical health (Petersen et al. 1996).

Seligman and colleagues developed a technique known as the Content Analysis of Verbatim Explanations (CAVE). This is a method for analysing written or spoken explanations in terms of the three dimensions of explanatory style, and has been shown to correlate well with more direct measures (Schulman et al. 1989). We applied the CAVE method to explanations of negative events made by Mozart in his correspondence. The results suggested that Mozart had a rather optimistic cognitive style. In the present day, most people score between 11 and 12 on the scale of explanatory style, with higher ratings of 14 or 15 from depressed people. The rating we obtained from Mozart in his maturity was less than eight, indicating that he was much more optimistic than the average (Steptoe et al. 1993).

It is important to recognise that this technique is not concerned with overt expressions either of depressed mood or of cheerfulness. Both of these might easily be feigned or disguised in written correspondence, so their occurrence cannot be taken as a reliable indicator of mental state. The patterns identified are almost automatic processes of thought, and thus are much less susceptible to bias. An example of this pattern comes in a letter from 1778, and concerns the reception of the "Paris" symphony (K 297) at a concert in Paris on 18 June. Mozart was asked by the impresario to replace the slow movement for the second performance of the symphony. For a young composer to be told that one whole section of a recently completed major work was unsatisfactory and needed to be replaced might have seriously undermined his confidence. A pessimistic person might have believed that the criticism was correct, that his work was indeed poor, and only served to confirm what most people probably thought about his compositions. Mozart's response is quite different. He explained the impresario's opinion as being due to the fact that "the audience forgot to clap their hands as loud and to shout as much as they did at the end of the first and last movements." That is, he regarded the criticism as being due to an external, specific and temporary state of affairs.

Apart from his personality, Mozart had favourable resources in other domains (see Table 1). There is a substantial body of research which indicates that social resources are important both for the emotional support they provide in times of crisis, and for the material assistance (financial and other services) that may be available. Mozart was not an isolated man, but enjoyed a large number of close personal relationships with his family, friends and colleagues. In this respect, he was different from many highly creative individuals who are socially isolated and lack personal ties. He was particularly involved with his family by marriage, having regular contacts with his wife's sisters and their husbands. His friends came from many walks of life, ranging from fellow musicians and performers, successful merchants from the commercial world, to younger members of the nobility. These friends provided companionship, professional contacts, and financial support when necessary.

Friendship may be closely linked with the composer's spiritual resources, which were centred around Freemasonry and the Enlightenment. These beliefs had a complex role in Mozart's life, and in the lives of other cultivated people of the late eighteenth century. For the composer, they came to replace Catholicism as systems by which to live, while also providing him with contacts in elevated sectors of society from which he might otherwise be excluded by reason of his relatively lowly birth.

Finally, I would argue that the creative process itself provides psychological protection from adversity. For the creator who is confident in the value of his or her work, the awareness of this capability may serve to provide a reminder of self-worth. It seems likely that Mozart maintained his equilibrium partly through the sense of achievement and self-satisfaction derived from completing his compositions so successfully. He took pleasure in astonishing audiences, and the sense of exultation he experienced when performing can still be sensed in his words and music. His awareness of his own talent was an important, and presumably sometimes irritating, facet of his personality. It may have provided an important resource or consolation when he was set about with other difficulties. I believe that similar processes may operate for many creative individuals when they experience difficulties or emotional upset in their lives.

References

Amabile TM, Collins MA, Conti R et al. (1996) *Creativity in Context: Update to the Social Psychology of Creativity.* Boulder, CO: Westview Press.

Anderson TH (1978) Becoming sane with psychobiography. *The Historian* **41**: 1–20.

Baxandall M (1972). *Painting and Experience in Fifteenth Century Italy.* Oxford: Oxford University Press.

Ericsson KA (ed.) (1996) *The Road to Excellence: The Acquisition of Expert Performance in the Arts, Sciences, Sports, and Games.* Mahwah, NJ: Erlbaum.

Hitschmann E (1956) Some psychoanalytic aspects of biography. *International Journal of Psychoanalysis* **37**: 265–9.

Howe MJA (1999). *Genius Explained.* Cambridge: Cambridge University Press.

Lykken DT, Bouchard TJ, McGue M et al. (1992) Emergenesis: genetic traits that do not run in families. *American Psychologist* **47**: 1565–77.

Miller AI (1996) *Insights of Genius: Imagery and Creativity in Science and Art.* New York: Springer-Verlag.

Petersen C & Seligman MEP (1984) Causal explanations as a risk factor for depression: theory and evidence. *Psychological Review* **91**: 347–74.

Petersen C, Maier SF & Seligman MEP (1996) *Learned Helplessness.* New York: Oxford University Press.

Rubin PL & Wright P (1999). *Renaissance Florence: The Art of the 1470s.* London: National Gallery Publications.

Schulman P, Castellan C & Seligman MEP (1989) Assessing explanatory style: the content analysis of verbatim explanations and the Attributional Style Questionnaire. *Behaviour Research and Therapy* **27**: 505–12.

Steptoe A (1996a) *Mozart: Everyman – EMI Music Companion.* London: David Campbell.

Steptoe A (1996b) Mozart's personality and creativity. In: Sadie S (ed.). *Wolfgang Amadè Mozart.* Oxford: Oxford University Press.

Steptoe A (ed.) (1998a) *Genius and the Mind.* Oxford: Oxford University Press.

Steptoe A (1998b). Mozart: resilience under stress. In: Steptoe A (ed.). *Genius and the Mind: Studies of Creativity and Temperament.* Oxford: Oxford University Press.

Steptoe A, Reivich K & Seligman MEP (1993) Mozart's optimism: a study of explanatory style. *The Psychologist* **6**: 69–71.

Sternberg RJ (ed.) (1999) *Handbook of Creativity.* New York: Cambridge University Press.

52 Art and mental illness

Anthony Storr

By "Art" I mean the arts in general; painting, sculpture, music, literature and so on. Although the arts can provide the most exciting, uplifting, and profound experiences which we encounter during our lives, we sometimes take them for granted. But why the arts exist at all is a puzzle. For the most part, they do not serve any obvious biological purpose; that is, they do not feed us, protect us against danger, or encourage reproduction. It is certainly possible to argue that accurate draughtsmanship increases the artist's perceptual grasp of the external world. Perhaps this is why palaeolithic artists often drew animals: it may have helped them to hunt better. But most forms of art are not obviously adaptive in the biological sense. It is, for example, difficult to find a biological reason for the existence of music. Yet even very ancient, preliterate cultures display some form of music, and so we must assume that music has some positive function for human beings. I suggest some possible answers in my book *Music and the Mind* (Storr 1993).

All the arts originate from the imagination. The term imagination and the words "image", "imagine", "imaginative", are used in at least three different ways. We speak of a mental image as a picture in the mind's eye. We also use the term "imagination" as misperception, delusion, or fabrication; i.e. "it's just her imagination". In the present connection, I am using "imagination" in a third sense; as meaning creative invention; the ability to think of things which other people have not thought of, or cannot think of (Strawson 1974).

Freud, who had a lively appreciation of the visual arts and literature, found himself in a dilemma when attempting to give an account of imagination in psychoanalytic terms. This is because he could not conceive of imagination as adaptive. For Freud, imaginative activity was always escapist; fabrication, delusion – the second meaning to which I have just referred – "it's just her imagination". As late as 1917, Freud wrote:

> "An artist is once more in rudiments an introvert, not far removed from neurosis. He is oppressed by excessively powerful instinctual needs. He desires to win honour, power, wealth, fame and the love of women; but he lacks the means for achieving these satisfactions. Consequently, like any other unsatisfied man, he turns away from reality and transfers all his interest, and his libido too, to the wishful constructions of his life of fantasy, whence the path might lead to neurosis."
>
> (Freud 1917: 376)

So, for Freud, imaginative activity was a danger signal; an indication that the person who employed it was dissatisfied with, or out of touch with, reality. In another passage, he considers the nature of fantasy:

> "We may lay it down that a happy person never fantasies, only an unsatisfied one. The motive forces of fantasies are unsatisfied wishes, and every single fantasy is the fulfilment of a wish, a correction of an unsatisfying reality."
>
> (Freud 1908: 146)

Today, much of what Freud wrote is discredited, but the idea that well-adapted human beings don't engage in much imaginative activity, because they are so well and accurately adjusted to reality, lives on in disguised form in current psychiatric concepts of so-called "normality". Normality is implicit rather than defined by psychiatry; but in our culture, I imagine that a normal person would be equable, industrious, generous, polite, kind, stable in mood, politically neutral, religiously tolerant, financially reliable, abstemious, heterosexual, and a good parent. Such a person would also be excruciatingly dull. DSM-IV does not describe lack of imagination or stolid acquiescence in the status quo as abnormal, because such traits demonstrate "adjustment to reality", which is supposed to be a good thing. But when we describe someone as "lacking in imagination" we are criticising him, not praising him.

What Freud and those who attempt to define normality don't realise is that our biological adaptation to the external world is by way of incomplete or partial adaptation. By this I mean that human beings are the most successful species just because they are creative and inventive; but creativity is a by-product of *not* being precisely in tune with external reality.

Imagine a creature who is accurately adjusted to the environment in which it lives. Aeons of evolution have programmed exact responses to all normal environmental challenges. All its biological requirements, for food, reproduction, sleep, warmth, and companionship are met without difficulty. Who could ask for anything more? There would be no reason for such a creature to be inventive or to engage in imaginative activity. That is not the human condition.

Julian Barnes, in his novel *A History of the World in 10½ Chapters*, paints a picture of Heaven in which every wish is satisfied. Meals are always delicious, and you don't put on weight. Your sexual needs are satisfied; your golf game improves out of all recognition. He rightly concludes that, sooner or later, all human beings would so tire of this perfection that they would ask for another form of death (Barnes 1989). Being dissatisfied, and therefore engaging in fantasy, is part of being human. Freud is quite right in thinking that creativity is spurred by dissatisfaction; but he seems not to have realised that we are born to be dissatisfied. Buddhism teaches that the human condition is intrinsically unsatisfactory. Christianity assumes that we are all afflicted with "original sin". We are all misfits; there is something wrong with all of us. It always turns out that the people one assumes to be normal are the people one doesn't know very well.

Imaginative fantasy is a wonderful part of childhood. The little boy who wants to be a train driver transforms a stool into a train, and pushes it round the room making train-like noises. His fantasy is, in Freud's terminology, a fulfilment of a wish; a correction of the unsatisfying reality that he is not actually driving a real train. But we don't regard such a fantasy as turning away from reality or as likely to lead to neurosis. We welcome it as a sign of a lively imagination, and marvel at the fact that even tiny children can enter into games of make-believe which they enjoy, but which they know to be only "pretend". We should be right in thinking that there was something wrong with a child who could not engage in fantasy play.

But Freud not only treated art as escapist fantasy, but also accused artists of remaining in a childish state of immaturity.

> "The growing child, when he stops playing, gives up nothing but the link with real objects; instead of playing, he now fantasies. He builds castles in the air and creates what are called daydreams."
>
> (Freud 1908: 145)

> "The creative writer does the same as the child at play. He creates a world of fantasy which he takes very seriously – that is which he invests with large amounts of emotion – while separating it sharply from reality."
>
> (Freud 1908: 144)

Freud supposed that, as people grow up, they cease to play, but fantasize instead. But he also has a poor opinion of adult fantasies.

"If fantasies become over-luxuriant and over-powerful, the conditions are laid for an onset of neurosis or psychosis. Fantasies, moreover, are the immediate mental precursors of the distressing symptoms complained of by our patients. Here a broad by-path branches off into pathology."

(Freud 1908: 148)

Yet fantasies are also the source of creative discovery. Einstein linked thinking with childhood play by defining it as "free play with concepts". Einstein's fantasy of how the universe might appear to an observer travelling at near the speed of light enabled him to formulate the special theory of relativity. Freud's notion that really mature, well-adjusted people should not need fantasy is nonsense. But that is because mature, well-adjusted people in Freud's sense of the word do not exist.

It is certainly arguable that we need the arts because we find external reality unsatisfying. I'll take music as an example, because that is the art closest to my heart. Why do we need music, and why are we so deeply moved by a profound work of music?

Consider Mozart's String Quintet in G minor, K 516. This, like other works by Mozart in the same key, is a piece which, while expressing tragic emotion in tones of poignant beauty, at the same time makes sense out of tragedy by imposing coherent structural form upon it. Works of art are templates of how to deal with life. They reflect back to us what we all want to do; connect the prose and the passion, create order out of our unruly feelings, while at the same time giving them freedom of expression. If we were creatures governed by built-in instinctual patterns, the order would already have been imposed, and we should simply obey what Nature told us to do, with no need for imagination. As it is, we are always looking for order, for patterns which make sense; and we have to create these for ourselves because they are not given to us by Nature.

Our own lives may be incoherent and torn with conflict, but the creation of a work of art or a new scientific hypothesis makes at least temporary sense by forming a new pattern, or making a new whole out of previously discrete entities. Both science and the arts aim at creating new areas of order, and it is because we lack the sense of continuing order in ourselves that the discoveries of science and the formal beauties of the arts are so compellingly important to us. It is the nagging sense of incoherence and incompleteness within that drives artists and scientists to create new entities. The fact that a new unity can be created demonstrates that disharmony can be overcome, conflict resolved, and order imposed upon disorder.

The disputed relation between mental illness and creativity is not hard to resolve if the outline given above is correct. Human beings are less accurately adjusted to any one environment than are creatures with built-in programmes. Because of this, they are so constituted that they are never completely satisfied, always able to imagine something better. Necessity may be the mother of invention, but dissatisfaction is its father. If we were perfectly content with the world as it is, we should not be moved to make scientific discoveries, invent imaginary heavens, write novels, paint pictures, or compose music. Blissful happiness is not conducive to imaginative inventiveness.

Therefore, it is not surprising that some of the most inventive and creative of mankind should also be those who tend to be at odds with the world and with themselves. If one's own self and the world appear incoherent, the greater the pressure to seek coherence. In the field of pathology, we see this happening in people with schizophrenia, whose delusions are creative attempts to make sense out of their hallucinations and other bizarre sensory experiences. In the first edition of

Schizophrenia: The Facts (Tsuang 1982), Elizabeth Farr gives an account of her schizophrenic illness, which started in childhood with auditory and visual hallucinations. She writes: "In high school I became engrossed in religion, the occult, and the arts as a possible way to help explain what was going on. The central driving feature in my behaviour was to understand my experiences." She concluded that there must be "some unearthly or extra-dimensional power transmitting messages to me through some hidden speakers under the eaves of buildings. My logic was really quite intact; only the perceptions I had on which to build conclusions were unsound."

This is an example of creativity driven by puzzlement and confusion which ends in a delusional explanation. Many scientific theories have turned out in the same way – the phlogiston theory, for example. You will remember that phlogiston was an imaginary element that was supposed to separate from all combustible materials when they were burning. Phlogiston never existed. It was imaginary in the pejorative sense – a fabrication or delusion. Other theories have proved valid or, like Newton's theory of universal gravitation, have seemed unshakeably valid for centuries.

Manifest, severe mental illness precludes creative activity. Artists who become schizophrenic nearly always show deterioration in their drawings and paintings, which usually become stereotyped, repetitive, and dull. Manic patients may be brim full of new ideas, but are too restless to record them or elaborate upon them. Depression of any severity prevents the sufferer from engaging in any creative activity at all.

But liability to mental illness is a different story. A number of studies have confirmed the observation that writers, particularly poets, are prone to manic-depressive illness. And there is little doubt that schizotypal or schizoid personalities are commonly found among great abstract thinkers. In both groups, creative production may be functioning as a defence; that is, as a way of warding off or diminishing the threat of mental illness.

In his autobiography, Graham Greene wrote:

"Writing is a form of therapy; sometimes I wonder how all those who do not write, compose or paint can manage to escape the madness, the melancholia, the panic fear which is inherent in the human condition."

(Greene 1981: 211)

For those who are prone to depression, avoidance of the plunge into the abyss is a major undertaking. Those who have creative gifts are fortunate, because they can use their talents to gain recurrent fixes of public recognition which enhance their shaky self-esteem. Dickens and Balzac are both examples of writers liable to severe depression who kept it at bay by constant overwork. It is also true that the act of writing, by objectifying negative emotions, can enable the writer to control and overcome grief and despair. Writing is also a means of self-exploration; and a means of self-affirmation and self-expression for those who find such things difficult to achieve in ordinary life.

Let me briefly turn to the other great group of psychiatric disorders. People with schizophrenia mostly lose whatever creative powers they had when their illness becomes established. John Nash, the Princeton mathematician who won a Nobel prize in 1994, spent most of thirty years in mental institutions suffering from schizophrenia. He recovered: but the work in game theory for which he got the prize was completed before he became psychotic.

The near relatives of those with schizophrenia often show divergent and loosely associative styles of thought which resemble the "over-inclusive" thinking of sufferers, but which in normal people may indicate originality. A touch of so-called thought disorder may be fruitful.

One characteristic of people described as exhibiting schizoid or schizotypical personalities is their reduced capacity for close interpersonal relationships. Neither ICD-10 nor DSM-IV mention that an enhanced capacity for creative abstract thought sometimes goes hand-in-hand with this comparative isolation. Many of the greatest philosophers have had personalities in which the capacity for abstract thought has dominated them to the exclusion of human emotions like love. The list of philosophers who formed no close personal ties includes Descartes, Locke, Hobbes, Pascal, Spinoza, Kant, Leibniz, Schopenhauer, Nietzsche, Kierkegaard, and Wittgenstein. Newton, who might be described as a natural philosopher, was also a bachelor throughout his long life. Whatever passing relationships these thinkers had, none of them married, and most of them lived alone for the greater part of their lives. Einstein, who married twice, nevertheless described himself as "a loner, who never belonged with his whole heart to the state, his country, his circle of friends, or even his closer family, but who felt with regard to all those ties a never overcome sense of being a stranger with a need for solitude." (Einstein 1934: 26)

This suggests that some of the traits of personality described in psychiatric manuals as pathological are actually adaptive in the widest sense because they are necessary for man's greatest achievements in both science and the arts.

These examples bolster my conviction that we need to get rid of the medical model from our psychiatric diagnostic classifications, and replace it with something which takes more account of human variability. At present, we are labeling some of the most valuable human beings who have ever existed as pathological because they don't fit our implicit, dubious standards of "normality".

References

Barnes J (1990) *A History of the World in 10½ Chapters*. London: Picador.

Einstein A (1934) *Welthild*. Quoted in Fölsing A (1997) *Albert Einstein* (transl. Ewald Osers). London: Viking.

Freud S (1908) Creative writers and daydreaming. In: Jensen (ed.) (1959) *"Gradiva" and Other Works. The Standard Edition of the Complete Psychological Works of Sigmund Freud*, Vol. IX. London: Hogarth Press and Institute of Psycho-Analysis.

Freud S (1917) The paths to symptom-formation. In: Strachey J et al. (eds) (1963) *Introductory Lectures on Psycho-analysis. The Standard Edition of the Complete Psychological Works of Sigmund Freud*, Vol. XVI. London: Hogarth Press and Institute of Psycho-Analysis.

Greene G (1981) *Ways of Escape*. Harmondsworth: Penguin: 211.

Strawson P (1974) Imagination and perception. In: *Freedom and Resentment and Other Essays*. London: Methuen: 45.

Storr A (1993) *Music and the Mind*. London: Flamingo.

Tsuang MT (1982) *Schizophrenia: The Facts*. Oxford: Oxford University Press: 2–3.

Commentary on Chapters 51 and 52

John F Morgan

The erudite papers by Steptoe and Storr reproduced here as Chapters 51 and 52 were well received by the audience when they were first presented at the Royal Society of Medicine, Section of Psychiatry, meeting in May 2000, stimulating a broad discussion. The role of substance misuse in provoking and stifling creativity was considered, and found to be consistent with Storr's thesis that troubled souls may express their distress creatively through sublimation. But the panel rejected notions of "doors of perception" opened by alcohol and drugs. Many members of the audience noted the preponderance of jazz musicians who had struggled with alcohol and illicit drugs, but it was not felt that the drugs themselves had enhanced the creative quality of the artists concerned. Rather, as Storr contends, the integral dissatisfaction of the musician might on the one hand lead to creative fulfilment and on the other to self-medicated stupor. Doubts were expressed as to the artistic merits of some forms of contemporary art, perhaps most obviously when the art form itself fulfilled too direct a therapeutic function. But the accessibility of contemporary art forms was seen to outweigh the presumed artistic deficits. In the case of popular music, for example, the simplicity of that creative outlet to the general public was seen as an important avenue for self-expression which would otherwise be denied through more esoteric arts. The audience and the panel acknowledged the complexity in the relationship between art, creative expression and mental disorder.

Light is shed on the oversimplification of that complex relationship, with implications in understanding the stigmatisation of the mentally ill, when we examine the 18th century movement of Romanticism. The Romantic Movement swept across Western Europe in response to the rationalism and neo-classicism that preceded it. Steptoe's accurate representation of Bach's sobriety and work-ethic would not have appealed to the *Sturm und Drang* advocates of the 1770s. They revelled in concepts of transcendental inspiration, dejection and finally perceptual redemption through hallucination and fantasy. The origins of many of our current myths about creativity and madness can be traced to these roots. For example, Lady Caroline Lamb memorably stigmatised George Gordon Byron as "mad – bad – and dangerous to know." The archetypal Romantic poet, Byron was the product of childhood sexual abuse at the hands of his nurse, within a family system that tolerated the incest of his father, "Mad Jack", and a host of psychopathic familial role-models. No individual better encapsulates the Romantic notions of inspired genius, hovering on the brink of descent into lunacy, yet rising above his "madness" and "badness" to create *Don Juan*. That tale of unrestrained hunger, libidinous and gastronomic excess, reflects the artist himself. Lord Byron described himself as oscillating between "gorging like … a Boa snake" and leading the life of a "leguminouseating Ascetic." Byron's anorexia nervosa and bulimia have been well documented, and the epithet "mad – bad – and dangerous to know" crystallises both the promises and pitfalls in associating creativity and mental illness.

Romanticism posits madness and genius as two sides of the same coin. But genius itself is a form of stigmatisation and ultimately "un-understandable". Storr and Steptoe have cast light on creative genius expressed through the medium of art, engendering understanding. Storr defines the limitations of Byron's epithet, emphasising that mental illness itself is anathema to creativity. *Don Juan* is the work of a troubled and dissatisfied man, but not the result of mental illness per se. Rather, it is the *liability* to mental illness that may provide motivation towards artistic expression. It provides the fuel, but not the machinery. From a different perspective, Steptoe notes the reductionist folly of construing genius solely in terms of early childhood conflict, using the example of Wolfgang Amadeus Mozart. Mozart was abnormal for the strength, not the weakness, in the armour of his psyche. His creative output sprang from a peculiar combination of personal resilience, high selfesteem, and optimism. This puts paid to the Romantic notion of genius emerging from suffering. Instead, Steptoe demonstrates how Mozart could rise above his material disadvantages into the subliminal ether. Contrary to popular conceits, he reminds us that the expression of the creative impulse does not necessitate starving in a garret, that artists create despite, not because of, adversity. Thus he challenges the fallacy that sorrow and suffering are the *sine qua non* of artistic merit.

In associating mental illness too closely with genius, we risk glamorising the tragedy of psychological disease and adding to the stigma, with the best of intentions. The relationship between mental illness and creativity is complex. Neither is necessary or sufficient for the other. Disturbed minds may be more driven to create, but the quality of that creation may be worsened by the depth of the disturbance. Despite this, the high profile of some creative sufferers of mental illness can also disarm stigma by bringing the ubiquity of mental suffering out into the clear light of day. Spike Milligan, one of Britain's leading comic writers and performers, has been one of the few such figures to speak about his experiences of manic depression. In *Depression and How to Survive It*, co-authored with Anthony Clare, he addresses lay misconceptions about mental illness with greater conviction than a professional could carry. So it can be seen that examples of creative genius such as Spike can break down barriers and challenge the stigma, while too great an emphasis on links between genius and mental disorder may bolster the stigma. Navigating between this Scylla and Charybdis, we must attempt to drag the public's attitude towards the mentally ill kicking and screaming into the 21st Century.

In this regard, familiarity with mental illness through accessible role models may offer more than the examples of aloof, tortured genius of the Romantics' yesteryear. Comfort can be derived from knowing one is diagnosed with Churchill's melancholy or Milligan's mania. When creative individuals in the public eye can talk openly about their struggles with mental disorder, then the fear and loathing of mental illness expressed in a catalogue of tabloid headlines becomes not simply offensive, but quite preposterous. In conclusion, we need to render mental illness familiar, to discuss it *vis à vis* the accessible creativity of the entrepreneur, sportsman and politician, and to create an environment in which the mentally ill might safely enter into that discussion. When Members of Parliament can declare mental illness without fear of losing votes, then the battle will be won.

Reference

Milligan S & Clare A (1993) *Depression and How to Survive It*. London: Ebury Press.

Comment on creativity and mental disorder

Sidney Crown

The authors of Chapters 51 and 52 are academics and, in this area, I am merely a culture-freak and someone who finds all forms of creativity absorbing and mysterious, so I orientated my thoughts around the ideas suggested to me by the title of the chapter.

"Disorder"

What is "disorder" applied to human thought? Schizophrenia seems a clear candidate: thought "disorder". And manic depression, the other great psychosis? Disordered affect may lead to more generalised "disorder" and in some this seems compatible with creativity: witness Van Gogh. Is neurosis "disorder"? And ordinary human misery? Certainly, speaking as a psychotherapist who has treated many neurotic, miserable but creative persons, there seems an indefinable relationship between their disturbance and their creativity – so much so that I always discuss with such persons the possible negative effect of psychotherapy on their creativity. In the current exhibition at the National Gallery, "Seeing Salvation", Stanley Spencer, a truly creative artist, describes his mood while painting as "exaltation". Is exaltation a disorder?

Creativity

How creative does a person have to be to be "creative"? Benjamin Britten or the student prizewinner at the Royal Academy? Richard Branson or an entrepreneur with one really bright idea? In Italy, on a recent holiday, a writer on the Arts page tangled with "creativity" and decided he was left only with God and Michelangelo!

Can creativity be measured?

How? External criteria can be established in science and "evidence-based" medicine. But how to define a creative lawyer or a creative psychiatrist? What exactly do politicians and big business men mean by "creative accounting"? I always assume that means thinking that is suspect.

Creativity as impact

True creativity should, I suggest, have a significant impact on human affairs. In this sense Freud, despite the current flak around him, changed men's thinking about themselves. For me a contemporary imaginative figure, RD Laing, had the same impact. My thinking was never the same after reading *Divided Self*.

Collators and systematisers

Are these currently revered convergent thinkers creative? Is thinking about the classification of depression, or the nature of schizophrenia or autism creative? Will these assiduous collectors be remembered apart from the indexes of unread PhD theses?

Psychotic art

Is this creative? My feeling about the Guttman–Maclay collection is that it is weird, eccentric, eerie, creepy but not great art in any creative sense. I can remember little of the exhibition apart from the strange distorted bicycle which also seems to have been stolen by the artists of advertising!

Creativity, shock and permanence

At a recent exhibition of conceptual art at the Hayward Gallery, where I could see from the entrance that the floor was covered with strange objects, I stood by a radiator on the wall and looked with an open mind: was this an exhibit? With some difficulty I decided it probably wasn't! Conceptual art, from Duchamp's celebrated urinal to Tracy Emin's Turner Prize entry of her dishevelled, unmade bed complete with soiled tampons, Warhol's soup cans, Damien Hirst's split animals, full frontals of Gilbert & George's penises. Interesting, but permanent? Remembered in 20 years? I doubt it.

Comment based upon a study of biographies of 453 exceptionally creative men

Felix Post

Geniuses are unusual human beings, and thus statistically abnormal. Since the Romantic Period, they have also been widely regarded as mentally abnormal and prone to insanity. However, Juda (1949) conclusively demonstrated that the prevalence of severe mental illnesses (psychoses) was not significantly raised in German men of the highest mental ability in comparison with the general population. Since then, controversy has continued concerning the role of less serious psychopathology (personality deviations and neuroses) in people who have produced original and culturally valuable work. Only a minority of investigators have held that geniuses were extraordinarily gifted people with strong personalities, which enabled them to get their productions accepted, usually during their lifetime, as original and contributing to cultural advance. Certainly, a few had exhibited psychiatric symptoms, but if they had done so, only the form and content of their work might have been affected. However, it was claimed that their creativity originated in their strong and healthy personalities. Nevertheless, the great majority of investigators remained convinced that creativity developed out of psychopathological problems. This majority has been criticised by the minority (as summarised by Kessel 1989) for having ignored the considerable number of mentally healthy people who were exceptionally gifted.

My retirement from clinical duties more than 20 years ago gave me ample time to try and settle this controversy through discovering the prevalence of various mental abnormalities in a large sample of prominent creative members of several professions, by working through biographies since the 1840s, written after the subjects' deaths. Before that too few searching and critical biographies were available. My sample was restricted by the availability of biographies in English, French and German which dealt adequately with the subject's family, childhood and personality, as reported by others, as well as their physical and psychic disorders. I investigated 51 statesmen and national leaders (politicians); 53 scientific investigators, mathematicians and inventors (scientists); 57 composers; 75 painters, sculptors and architects (artists); 50 philosophers, theologians, historians, and economists (expounding writers or intellectuals); and 39 poets, 76 novelists and 52 dramatists (creative writers). Only a few of my 453 subjects, such as Einstein, Helmholtz, Schumann, Wagner, Monet, Picasso, Nietzsche, Wittgenstein, Heine, Wordsworth, Dickens, Proust, Wilde and Shaw, might be called geniuses, but all my other subjects were important enough to have their biographies written, often long after their deaths. Early on in my enquiry I had to give up famous women, as too few biographies were available. My findings must be accepted with caution because I was the sole investigator coding the facts reported by the biographers, even though I often consulted earlier biographies as well as the latest ones.

Some of the more important findings

Starting with physical health, no serious illnesses had been suffered until shortly before their deaths by three quarters of politicians and scientists, or by two thirds of composers. Far fewer members of the other professions, and only 19% of the dramatists, had escaped unscathed. On average composers had the longest lives, 76 years, while creative writers on average had died by 65. The much greater susceptibility to various illnesses found in these kinds of writers foreshadowed the main finding of this investigation: compared with the others, mood disorders and their consequences were also strikingly more common in poets, novelists and dramatists.

Almost all subjects demonstrated their outstanding abilities from childhood or adolescence onwards, though a considerable minority did not shine at school. All were very ambitious and driven, showing great industry and perseverance, first in learning and then in practising their skills. Even those with the most disorderly lives, on account of bohemianism, alcoholism or sexual overactivity, were most industrious and conscientious in their creative work. Contrary to tradition, only a few were lonely giants, admired for their achievements but disliked on account of being unapproachable, haughty, brusque or given to boring monologues. The vast majority were highly sociable. Even those who did not shine with brilliant conversation had long lasting and close friendships, and tended to be helpful and generous towards their colleagues; they were often described as magnetic or charismatic personalities. Many, but by no means all, worked in seclusion. Severely deviant personality traits, which affected their lives adversely, were registered more frequently than in the general population only in poets and novelists. However, only a single estimate of the general prevalence of less handicapping personality deviations is available. A postal survey yielded only 29% admitting to abnormal traits, but this seems almost certainly an underestimate.

Far more of my highly creative subjects exhibited mild, but pathological, deviations in personality or character; only 38% of scientists, 25% of politicians and composers, and fewer than 18% of artists, intellectuals and creative writers had no biographical data pointing to deviations from normal. The cluster of traits which might be called schizoform, because it often precedes schizophrenia, was rarely schizoid or paranoid-fanatic in type (mainly found in various dictators), but more often schizotypal: vague in manner of talking, neglectful in dress and personal hygiene, regarded as odd by others, and sometimes subject to trance-like states and paranormal experiences. As might be expected, these traits were commonest in intellectuals (one third). So-called dramatic traits were registered in well over half of dramatists and novelists, and in over a third of politicians and artists, but these were rarely the antisocial kind (only petty dishonesty and thieving), more often narcissistic or histrionic behaviour, and outbursts of temper. The most frequent abnormal characteristics were anxious and depressed moods, often with obsessional tendencies. These had affected more than three quarters of the artistic professions, most markedly poets, novelists and dramatists, but were also found in just under half the scientists and politicians. Altogether the high prevalence of these less seriously handicapping traits was striking, as was the frequency with which subjects had been affected by more than one type of such disability.

The 90% marriage rate of scientists and politicians was probably similar to that of other middle-class men of their period. By contrast, nearly half the artists and poets had remained single. Apart from politicians, lifelong virginity was claimed by creative men several times more frequently than by men in general, while an unusual number of sexual relationships was found in dramatists and novelists, who also had the highest proportions of disrupted marriages, more often than in men in general. Homo- and bisexuality were above levels estimated for the urban male population only in the case of poets and dramatists, and caused tragedies in only a few.

The lifetime prevalence of severe mental illnesses (psychoses) was not elevated in comparison with that of people in general, with the exception of depressive, manic and manic-depressive illnesses in poets, intellectuals and novelists. There were no instances of typical schizophrenia, as had also been shown by Andreasen (1987) in her study of living American writers. Old age mental deterioration was half as frequent as in old people in general, and moreover only relatively mild or doubtful.

The classical neuroses with hysterical, somatic, phobic or obsessional symptoms were, in contrast to other conditions, no more frequent in creative writers than in the other groups or, as far as statistics are available, in the general population. The situation was totally different in the case of non-psychotic mood disorders (without severe changes in conduct, loss of weight and delusional beliefs). Brief anxious or depressive reactions to stressful life events were understandably found to have occurred in half the politicians, in over a third of composers, novelists and dramatists, though less often in artists. More long lasting anxious-depressive episodes and chronic depressions, which nowadays would be recognised as requiring treatment, and which are, therefore, called "clinical depressions", had afflicted up to half the creative writers, but only a quarter to a third of all the others. A similar high incidence of clinical depressions has been found by Andreasen (1987), Jamison (1993) and Ludwig (1995). Suicide rates were much higher than recorded internationally in creative men with the exception of politicians, composers and intellectuals. Suicides were commonest in poets, and attempted suicides in novelists.

In many ways depressive tendencies were related to alcoholism and drug misuse. Earlier estimates of the prevalence of substance misuse are unreliable especially because psychoactive drugs were freely available "over the counter". However, alcoholism was certainly below present day levels only in scientists and intellectuals, and reached 42% in dramatists.

Finally, turning to family background, there are numerous well publicised accounts of how geniuses had to struggle against childhood deprivations and the hostile attitudes of their parents. In fact, as was also reported by Ludwig (1995), the great majority of parents had supported their sons in the choice of career, often making considerable sacrifices. Childhood had only rarely been unhealthy or unhappy. Moreover, the great majority of families had been comfortably off over several generations, and had more frequently risen rather than declined in status. Quite a number of earlier family members or siblings had been specifically gifted or even exceptionally creative. In contradicting earlier reports, both Andreasen's (1987) and the present investigation found no excess of schizophrenia in families, but writers had twice as many psychiatrically sick (mainly depressive and alcoholic) relatives than the others. Replicating Andreasen, depressive tendencies, greatest talent, and to a slighter extent creativity, only tended to cluster together in the family histories of creative writers, thus suggesting genetic linkages.

Conclusions

The results of this investigation have shown that a third of innovative scientists and a quarter of importantly originative politicians, artists, composers and intellectuals had only been affected by minor psychological deviations or had been completely mentally healthy. Creativity can, therefore, be brought forth from outstanding ability without any contribution from morbid psychopathology. Also, almost all kinds of psychiatric disorders occurred with the same frequency as in the general population with the exception of emotional disorders and related alcohol and psychosexual problems. These latter were far more prevalent in poets, novelists and dramatists. There is thus strong evidence for anxious-depressive-obsessional psychopathology playing a role in the creativity of writers.

The prevalence of affective disorders and of depressive personalities in ordinary people is only very imperfectly known, but it seems very likely that depressive conditions and personalities are far more frequent in creative writers, and to a lesser extent also in all other exceptionally creative people. In every case the prevalence of deviant personality traits, especially of the anxious-depressive-obsessional variety, was much higher than seems to be likely in the general population, though here again statistical information is lacking. Thus, the case for invoking morbid psychopathological factors in the creativity of scientists, politicians, composers and artists is much weaker than that for intellectuals and creative writers.

In spite of their psychological burdens, all the subjects in this study had been able through outstanding industry, meticulousness and perseverance to produce works and get them accepted as cultural advances, usually by their contemporaries, but always by posterity. Their fame was due to their ambitious drive and ability to enter supportive social circles. All these qualities add up to what is called "ego strength". As was probably first pointed out by Eysenck (1995), geniuses show the paradoxical combination of psychiatric abnormalities with great ego strength, when more commonly neuroticism is associated with a weak ego.

Many successful creative people have expressed fear that if they submitted to treatment for their depression and alcoholism they might lose the sources of their inspiration. On only anecdotal evidence so far, feelings of well being and productivity are increased, but whether the quality of work suffers remains to be investigated.

References

Andreasen NC (1987) Creativity and mental illness: prevalence rates in writers and their first degree relatives. *American Journal of Psychiatry* **144**: 1288–92.

Eysenck HJ (1995) *Genius: The Natural History of Creativity.* Cambridge: Cambridge University Press.

Jamison KR (1993) *Touched with Fire.* New York: Free Press.

Juda A (1949) The relationship between highest mental capacity and psychic abnormalities. *American Journal of Psychiatry* **106**: 296–304.

Kessel N (1989) Genius and mental disorder: a history of ideas concerning their conjunction. In: Murray P (ed.). *Genius: The History of an Idea.* Oxford: Blackwell.

Ludwig AM (1995) *The Price of Greatness.* New York: Guilford Press.

Plate 1

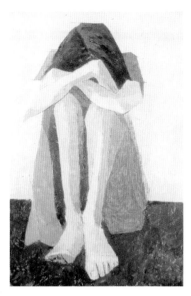

Marion Patrick, *Depression.* 1960s

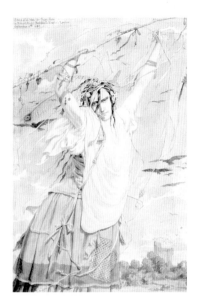

Richard Dadd, *Crazy Jane.* 1855

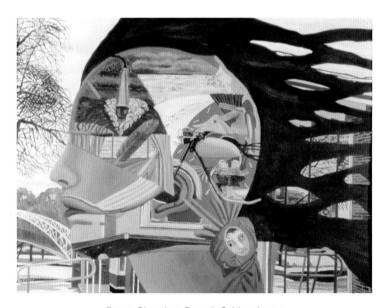

Bryan Charnley, *Broach Schizophrene.*

Plate 2

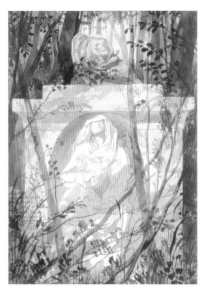

Richard Dadd, *Sketch to Illustrate the Passions. Grief or Sorrow.* 1854

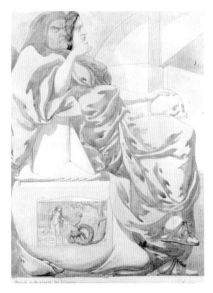

Richard Dadd, *Sketch to Illustrate the Passions. Deceipt or Duplicity.* 1854

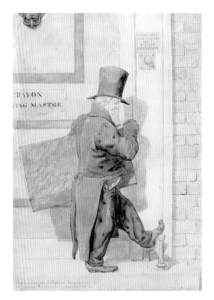

Richard Dadd, *Sketch to Illustrate the Passions. Insignificance or Self Contempt.* 1854

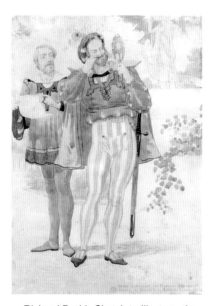

Richard Dadd, *Sketch to Illustrate the Passions. Self Conceit or Vanity.* 1854

Plate 3

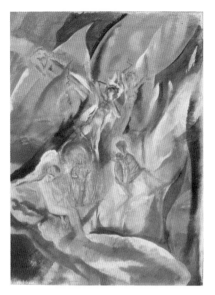

Charles Sims, *Crowds of Small Souls in Flame. c.* 1926–28

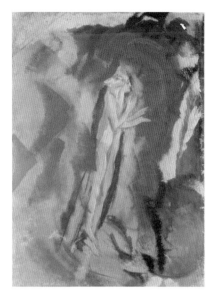

Charles Sims, *A Spiritual Idea. c.* 1926–28

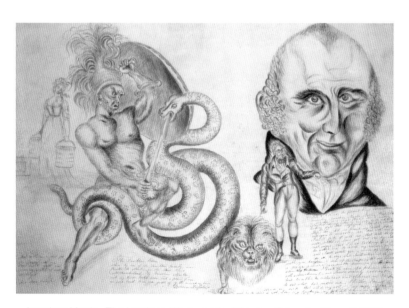

Jonathan Martin, *The Lambton Worm, and a Likeness Taken by Himself.* 1829

Plate 4

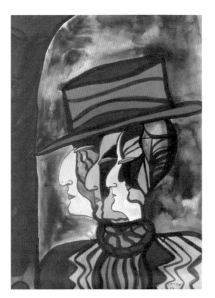

Stanley Lench, *Lord Clark of Saltwood 1.*
1977

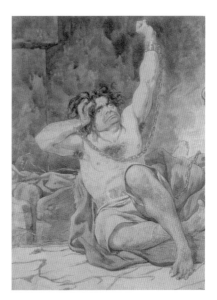

Richard Dadd, *Sketch to Illustrate the
Passions. Agony – Raving Madness.* 1854

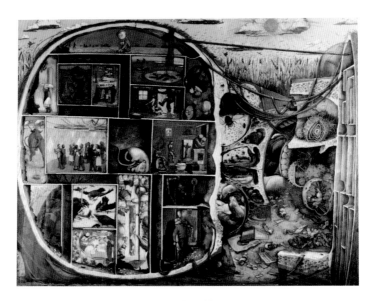

William Kurelek, *The Maze. c.* 1953

Plate 5

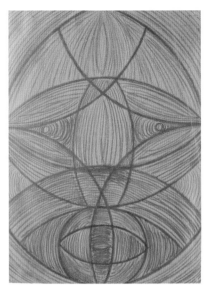

Vaslav Nijinsky, *A Mask. c.* 1919

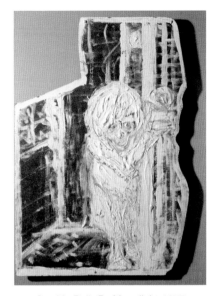

Cynthia Pell, *By Moonlight.* 1977

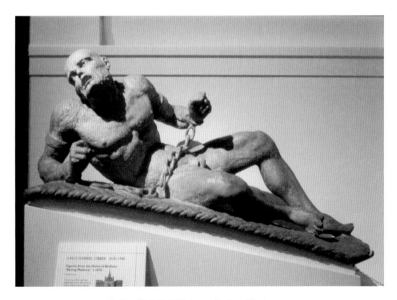

Caius Gabriel Cibber, *Raving Madness.*

Plate 6

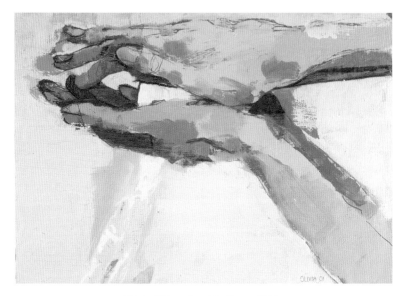

Olivia Gillow, *Craddle Soap*. 2001

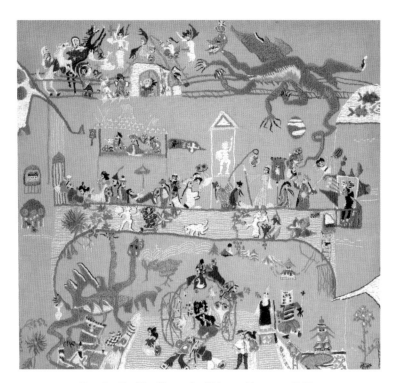

Dorothy H., *The Story of a Chinese Emperor*. 1958

Plate 7

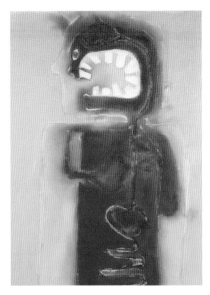

Elise Warriner, *The Anger Within.* 1993

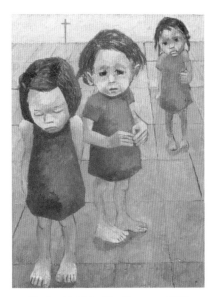

Marion Patrick, *The Cross. c.* 1967

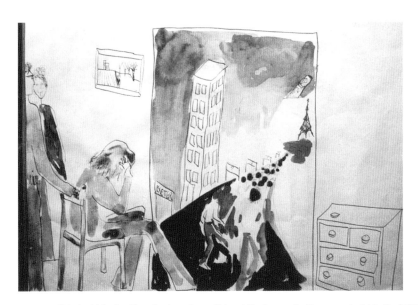

Anonymous artist, *Let Me Be.* Frontispiece from Crisp AH, *Anorexia Nervosa: Let Me Be* (1980), reproduced with permission from Psychology Press.

Plate 8

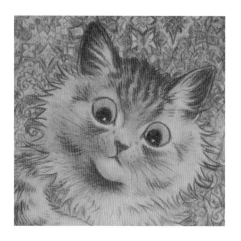

Louis Wain, *Ginger Cat.* 1931

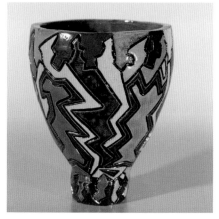

Bibi Herrera, *Electric.*

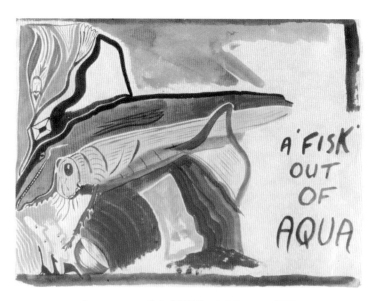

Anonymous artist, *A 'Fisk' out of Aqua. c.* 1950

Part 8

Spirituality and mental illness

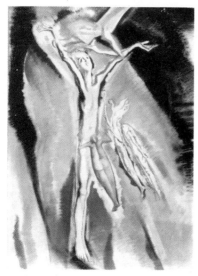

Charles Sims, *Aspiration, c.* 1926–28

53 The Christian perspective

Ian Ainsworth-Smith

> *"For I am under the same accusation with my Saviour*
> *For they said, he is besides himself.*
> *For the officers of the peace are at variance with me*
> *And the watchman smites me with his staff.*
> *For Silly Fellow! Silly Fellow! is against me*
> *And belongeth neither to me nor to my family.*
> *For I am in twelve Hardships,*
> *But he that was born of a virgin shall deliver me out of all."*
>
> *Words*, Christopher Smart
> (a Bethlem patient in the 18th century)

I am certainly grateful, humbled and delighted to be asked to address the subject in this chapter. I would say at the outset that my questions remain questions, and if the questions are explored further as a result of this chapter I shall be well content. I recently had the opportunity of setting a question for a diploma of pastoral studies, and I settled on the proposition "Experts give answers; pastors identify questions. Discuss." I am so pleased that there is now more dialogue about the areas of mental health and spirituality in which much of my professional life have been spent than in the living memory of most of us. You may also know that the Bethlem and Maudsley Hospital chaplaincy has a built-in research fellowship, aptly named after Bishop John Robinson of *Honest to God* fame, on mental health and spirituality; and indeed the Royal College of Psychiatrists has now developed its own division of spirituality.

What I offer in this paper are some reflections by a working chaplain, of how issues of spirituality and mental health have impinged on me over the years. As a preliminary I would of course want to enter a caveat about assumptions, which can easily turn into prejudices. I would also wish to highlight the danger of mutual horror stories being told about the worst aspects of psychiatry and religion simply to address stereotypes to attack. I have sat in Christian settings where comments have been made such as "The psychiatrists say . . .", over-definitively. I have sometimes wanted to challenge that by asking for clarification. Assumptions persist. I was recently interviewed by a television researcher who could not quite believe the chaplain she was talking to was a sceptic or at most a reverent agnostic about demonic possession. One ward round I attended in the psychiatric unit I remember well: I found myself adopting a sceptic position about the possibility of a particular patient needing an exorcism. The psychiatric team were quite prepared to entertain that possibility. As you will know, that area has been much debated in the religious world. Different views are held. I am certainly committed to a bilinguality of understanding: there are two languages that one can speak. I thought that for the patient in question you could only make sense of her distress in terms of an organic psychiatric illness. It was not necessary to postulate the demonic. The psychiatrist and I had a friendly and professional disagreement on that.

My starting point for any discussion of spirituality and mental disorder would be that religious and spiritual behaviour, like any other, can be described in psychological or psychodynamic terms. But that doesn't necessarily explain what happens. We also need to understand that this is an area which generates very powerful feelings. Feelings can be set up in carers by religious material they may not feel properly competent to understand. Some material brought by the religious patient needs to be accepted as it is and not necessarily interpreted. The interpretation can make it worse – an important point to remember in practice. I can think of one particular patient with an eating disorder, a former Catholic nun, whose therapist insisted on interpreting her frequent request for reception of Holy Communion, and indeed her anxiety if she didn't receive it, as a displaced wish for oral sex! Need one say that material of this nature needed to be handled with considerable care and discernment, and that interpretation was not a good enough way of dealing with it. I also recall one severely ill woman, who in the last resort had nothing else to fall back on except a construction of religious language and ideation which was certainly bizarre and theologically unorthodox. However, there were good reasons in this woman's story why this should have been the case. When she was young the only place she felt safe was in church. Although she had abandoned formal religion, I certainly thought that under pressure she metaphorically "went to church" and could only use religious language. Her therapist's constant interpretation of her religious material, which said more about the therapist at this point, meant that the area was dynamite. Other than just accepting the material, her interpretations, which were probably accurate, made this borderline personality patient "much sicker".

I would like to attempt a few simple definitions. I would certainly want to make a working definition and distinction between the religious, the cultural and the spiritual, and I have depicted these in three circles, not co-terminous but overlapping. A religious system gives us a way of understanding the world outside and beyond our own experience. A religious system will typically have books, literature and rituals, and designated people inside the tradition to try and help people explain it. It will have rituals which will help in a crisis, especially the crises of death and bereavement, of partnering and of welcoming a new life into the community.

The religious position today is very complicated. We may not necessarily have the same religious traditions with which we grew up. We may move religious traditions. Therapists may not be in the same religious tradition at all as the patient. Certainly, under pressure, it will be very easy when one is seeing the worst manifestations, simply to describe religion as a manifestation of neurotic guilt. And I have sometimes sat in staff meetings and thought that was a very apt description. But that may not be the whole story. As I have tried to indicate, a religious language might provide the only source available of meaning and connectedness. Religious language isn't sacred in itself, and certainly those of us who are pastors reckon we have a job, not necessarily to make someone speak religious language, but to help them use that language in a way that connects rather then disconnects with reality.

Our culture is a series of messages received as we grow up and mature, about how we are expected to behave. I think that many research studies clearly suggest that we have indeed been fully acclimatised to our culture very early on, possibly around the age of five. What is crucial, of course, is that the culture gives us a cue about how we behave in a crisis, and we have become increasingly aware that much of what appears to be or could be seen as a manifestation of mental illness might be a displaced experience of culture. We are aware that there is a high risk that people may be committed to mental hospitals or receive psychiatric care because of a failure to understand their culture. But culture and religion as I have tried to indicate are always very closely connected. A religious label by itself won't necessarily give us the whole story, and it may well be that somebody of no religion at all will be profoundly affected by a culture. Paul Halmos, many years ago, in a book called *Faith of the Counsellors*, which influenced many of us, pointed out quite rightly, I think, that many of the assumptions that counsellors and psychotherapists make are indeed the assumptions of Protestant Christianity – an emphasis, for example, on individual achievement and on understanding and enlightenment, which when we look at them are really quite culturally based.

Spirituality is maybe the most difficult commodity of all to describe. It is quite simply how in a crisis we make sense of our past and our present and our future. Spiritual distress is being much more talked about and much more researched now. Certainly 20 years ago I think we would have thought of it in terms of psychological distress or in terms of religious material. As people abandon more and more formal religious structures it may mean that the language that we have for expressing spiritual distress may be less available to us but every bit as important. I recently read a report of a study undertaken in a palliative care unit, which suggested very strongly that the highest level of reported distress among the patients apart from physical symptom control was quite simply spiritual distress. How did you make sense of it? Certainly from the Christian tradition we would want to take two things seriously, I think. The first is to say that every individual is unique and that no single person is a replica of another; that means that distress can only be described in very individual terms. But it also means that nobody functions in isolation. We are part of a community; we are part of a family. And distress can't just be understood in individual terms. We well know that there is a risk that a person with mental illness may indeed be the recipient of projections, if you like: other people's expectations, other people's fears that they have to carry. Indeed the words of Christopher Smart that I used to begin this article are very clear. Interestingly for me, he does indeed associate the burden he is asked to carry, the burden of his illness, with the sufferings of Jesus.

For those of us who have taken the psychodynamic understanding of human behaviour seriously, whose own lives and ministering have been deeply affected by the process of counselling and psychotherapy (and I hope informed by it), it is something on which we would never wish to go back. But I think there are questions which should be shared out of this discussion, having accepted fully the very unpleasant record of religion on occasions, quite simply to stir up neurotic guilt. By neurotic guilt I mean a constant linking in with the past, a belief that one is fully responsible for one's present condition and indeed there is no rescue from it. Interestingly I think that can often be seen in terms of omnipotence actually turned inside out. Guilt is a crippling experience, but at some level it may also be the only way that one may have of remaining in control of one's memories or indeed of one's experience. We are reminded from the Christian gospels that unpleasant symptoms, if you like, which are described there as devils, are quite easily removed. What is much more difficult is what you put in their place. All of that is, I am quite sure, true, but the other dimension is that of spiritual distress, and I have tried to link some of the indicators of spiritual distress in the diagram (Figure 1). They are things which I think are fairly self-explanatory: constant suffering where there seems to be no end and no relief.

There is something about memories which don't go away. I would want to draw a distinction between the guilt we have been talking about and appropriate remorse. I suggest that the need to say "Sorry" and to have "Sorry" said back, far from being demeaning, is in fact extremely important, and I suspect that it may be a dimension which has been lost from therapy and counselling. What do we do if actions in which

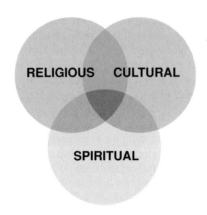

Some indicators of Spiritual Distress

1. Sense of meaningless, hopelessness
2. Intense suffering
3. Remoteness - unable to trust
   break with background

4. Anger - God, religion / clergy
5. Sense of guilt/shame
6. "Ethical" concerns
7. Unresolved feelings about death

Figure 1. Perceiving spiritual need.

we have been involved really do still remain troubling, and we know indeed that other people have been affected by them. Of course actions do have consequences. I remember one man who was in the throes of a clinical depression, who was deeply troubled by his wartime experience, when the ship where he was a crew member went through a group of survivors in the water and wasn't able to pick them up. He wasn't directly responsible but he felt terrible and very very bad about it. It was difficult to deal with that solely in terms of his depression, real as it was; there was more to be said than that. He did need to have some way of saying "Sorry" and of trying to make reparation. Indeed that would be not a criticism but a critique. One might want to say that some systems of therapy don't necessarily help if they constantly try to understand without helping us understand as well that actions do indeed have consequences; that words like forgiveness and reconciliation may have a place. The danger is that they may be misused. You can't reconcile until you have confronted the experience, and sometimes the person concerned as well, and forgiveness is a long process. Spiritual distress is sometimes best described by John Betjeman's night club hostess in *Sun and Fun*, where she says quite simply

> *"I'm dying now and done for;*
> *What on earth was all the fun for.*
> *For I'm old and ill*
> *And terrified."*

You can't necessarily put a psychiatric label on that experience. I would certainly wish to make a working distinction between depression and appropriate sadness. I think being sad is part of the human experience, and I hope that I would be treated, if I needed it, in a system that would allow me to be sad, and against a religious or spiritual tradition that would equally let me be sad and let me fail. I am quite sure Freud was right when he said that the experiences of sadness and happiness were really not far apart. A spiritual dimension might also be able to offer me something about the ability to hope and to be able to look forward. The built-in risks of some systems of therapy is that they are so heavily focused on the past without any possibility that there may be a future dimension as well. I think we will all of us be honest enough to say that we have seen people who should certainly be kept a long way away from anything that was remotely religious, and the other, rare, people for whom the psychiatric systems have little to offer. I think we need to be very humble indeed about what we offer and to know quite simply that we are individuals. What is going to help one person may not help somebody else and may be deeply oppressive. One hopes that the best thing about a religious tradition is that in the most significant sense it does teach us how to be humble, to know our limitations; because I think that it is when we know our limitations that we are best able to help each other and the people in our care to look beyond their present situation.

Overcoming stigma must involve, too, hearing the voice of the stigmatised, hearing the voice of the people who suffered, and again that will be at the heart of any Christian experience, to say that you can't learn about suffering from the sidelines. Christians are quite clear, if we are to use the theological shorthand, that God is present in the suffering as well as anything that happens afterwards. It quite simply doesn't fix that easily.

Maybe the best way to end would be with the words of somebody I have known for many years, who certainly had her treatment in the psychiatric system and at times has been helped by it and at times has struggled with it, and she said quite simply "It was the moment when I could begin to hope that transformed me." The parents of a young man who has been a service user for a long time, whom I have known for a while, happened to find out that I was writing on this topic, and they asked me to leave you with this illustration. I think their son is extremely unwell and he certainly is in the grip of a long-term psychiatric illness. Their comment was interesting. They certainly wouldn't describe themselves as formal believers. However, they began to wonder about how well their son was being heard when they talked about his well-developed spiritual dimension at a meeting with the psychiatrist (and I am sure that is true because I think that has kept him going even in the darkest bits of his illness), and somebody said "Oh, he'll grow out of that". And they said that was when they suspected that people weren't really understanding him, because in fact, as with all things spiritual, religious language can be used in an immature way. It can be the language of dependence, but it can also be that language and that dimension of life that takes us outside ourselves as well.

Reference

Halmos P (1966) *The Faith of the Counsellors: A Study in the Theory and Practice of Social Case Work and Psychotherapy.* New York: Schochen Books.

54 A Jewish approach to spirituality and mental illness

Julia Neuberger

First, it is important to stress that Jews do not necessarily understand the term "spirituality" as Christians do. Although there is a strong pietistic streak in Judaism, particularly amongst the very orthodox chassidim (descendants of 18th century East European mystics), the nature of spirituality for most Jews most of the time is in carrying out with devotion (*kavvanah*, which means devoted intent) the daily prayers, the ordinary rituals, the mundane tasks of everyday life, most of which have a blessing attached to them to give one a sense of God's presence in the world.

That sense of regularity, of the everyday nature of religious devotion, is extremely important when people are suffering from some form of mental illness. For many people who are in that state, their lives feel as if they are fragmenting, as if order is disappearing, as if nothing has any shape any longer, or, even more profoundly, any purpose. The very act of imposing order by carrying out the mundane, by saying the three times daily prayers, by engaging with the community, can be very helpful. A form of order is imposed upon disorder, without the sense of drugs numbing one's awareness. The performance of ritual, however hard to explain, gives people – albeit inexpressibly – a sense of purpose.

So one important insight into Jewish spirituality for people who are suffering from mental illness (and plenty of others besides) is the need for ritual and structure, for attending services regularly (whenever possible) and being included in the congregation as an equal, celebrating the festivals and fasting on fast days (not easy if one is taking medication), enjoying the progression of the Jewish year, season by season, festival by festival. At best, Jewish communities are welcoming to those with mental health problems, and include them in. That very inclusion gives people a sense of belonging, which itself allows for a structure which imposes order. The need for expressing longing and needs, doubts and disquiet, in prayer which is part of communal activity then becomes easier to handle, and the genuine spiritual longing and spiritual doubt which is part of that then becomes "normal", dealable with, and part of everyone's religious journey.

So someone with mental illness can share, be part of the community, be included in, and express his/her doubts and worries, agonisings and distress, in prayer, and no one should worry about it. But it is not always like this.

Jewish communities, like many other communities, can be hostile to people with mental illness and find them threatening. They know, very often, they should be welcoming and understanding. But their reaction is one of fear, one of seeing "the other", one of distress at the distress they perceive. That is despite well attested incidences of mental illness in the Hebrew Bible and Jewish literature. Chassidic (18–19th century Eastern European) literature is full of references to mental distress, and the Psalms recount the psalmist's (maybe David, who became King) own mental agony.

King Saul got moody and depressed, and became violent, and he needed David's music to calm him, though he would often then turn against him in a rage. Hannah, mother of Samuel, wept uncontrollably and lost her grip in the Temple, and was thought by the priest to be drunk when perhaps she was hallucinating. Some think that part of Job's suffering was a form of mental breakdown, and others regard the whole of the book of Lamentations as the expression of deep despair.

But all this demonstrates to us that the authors of the Hebrew Bible and later Jewish literature knew intimately what it was to experience mental illness. Depression, anxiety, despair, paranoid delusions, manic activity – they knew it all and it is all there. The Psalms (17, 22, 23, 25, 39, 40, 69, 90, 102, 103, 116 and 147) express the longings of someone who is suffering, and the Ethics of the Fathers teach us not to judge others until you find yourself in the same position (Avot 2:4), as if to suggest we may all experience mental illness, and we cannot judge how it feels until we feel it ourselves.

Nevertheless, stigma is there. It ranges from the stigma of a suicide in the family (despite the understanding that suicide is the product of illness) to the concern about a genetically transmitted predisposition to depression (as yet unproven). Even now, many Jewish people find it hard to talk about mental illness in the family, whilst they rejoice in going over physical symptoms in great detail.

And yet, at best, Jewish communities welcome those with mental illness. People are genuinely concerned about the well-being of their fellow congregants, and the community itself can act as a surrogate for families with whom some who have a long history of mental illness have lost touch. I have witnessed great tenderness in communal organisations shown toward people with Alzheimer's, whose inclusion in communal activities has been heartwarming. Drawing people in to Passover celebrations communally, or Jewish New Year, or the Day of Atonement, is commonplace, and understanding of the way ritual provides a form of healing in itself is growing.

Spirituality is therefore recognised, though different, within the community, and Jewish organisations and congregations try to be inclusive, and to draw in those who are suffering. But there is far more that could be done. Communal meals, in a religious atmosphere at sabbath and festivals, are an obvious way to draw people in. Encouraging people to speak at social gatherings after services about experiences of mental ill health is another. Recognising the religious questing and spiritual striving is another. Pastoral visits by rabbis and members of congregations where illness is acute is yet another. But the key lies in recognising that many who suffer mental ill-health are deeply religious people, with unmet spiritual needs. Communities, and their leaders, need to acknowledge that fact and encourage those people to explore their spirituality in safe surroundings, using a liturgy, such as the Psalms, that already recognises mental and emotional anguish.

55 The Muslim perspective: Every illness has a cure

Mawlana Sikander Khan Pathan

Bismilla-hir-Rahmaa-nir-Raheem
  In the Name of Allah the Most Kind the Most Merciful

Every illness has a cure

Praise be to Allah, Knower of all ailments and their hidden cures. May peace and salutations be upon His first prophet Adam, His final prophet Muhammad and all the prophets that came in between Amen! (Amen!).

Muslims like so many others believe in a creator. We believe that we were sent into this world as vicegerent of Allah. The Holy Quran informs us that man and jinn were created for the worship of Allah. After death we shall all be resurrected on the Day of Judgment and we shall be judged according to our deeds. Therefore our principle of life is:

> *"He Alone has the keys of the unseen treasures, of which no one knows except Him. He knows whatever is in the land and in the sea; there is not a single leaf that falls without His knowledge, there is neither a grain in the darkness of the earth nor any thing fresh or dry which has not been recorded in a Clear Book."*

> Quran 6.59 (Translator Malik)

It further says in the Quran:

> *"And Hold fast the rope of Allah, all together, and do not be divided"*

> Quran 3.103

Medication

There are many Ahadith (traditions of Prophet Muhammad peace be upon him (pbuh)) which encourage Muslims to seek medical treatment. Some of them are mentioned below:

Abu Hurayrah narrates that The Prophet pbuh said:

> *"There is no disease that Allah has created, except that He also has created its remedy."*

> Bukhari 7.582

Usamah ibn Shuraik narrated:

> *"... 'O Allah's Messenger! Should we seek medical treatment for our illnesses?' He replied: 'Yes, you should seek medical treatment, because Allah, the Exalted, has let no disease exist without providing for its cure, except for one ailment, namely, old age'."*

> Tirmidhi

Taking proper care of one's health is considered by the Prophet Muhammad pbuh to be the right of the body (Bukhari as-Sawm 55, an-Nikah 89, Muslim as-siyyam 183, 193, Nisai).

The Prophet not only instructed sick people to take medicine, but he himself invited expert physicians for this purpose (Development of Hospitals p.50; As-Suyuti's Medicine of the Prophet, p.125).

Imaan and Tawakkul

From this brief beginning one would gather that Imaan (faith) and Tawakkul (trust) have to be the uttermost important part of a Muslim's belief. Hence, problems, illnesses or troubles of life, should be very easy to cope with. But, since this material world has been classed as Darul Asbaab (a world of means) it is necessary to take medication for one's illness. In most cases Muftis would give a ruling of suicide for one who died in the event of not taking medicine. We all would be required by Shariah (Islamic Law) to have trust in Allah but search for the cure, which would be classed as the highest grade of Tawakkul – Trust in Allah.

Dr Shehzadi Munir, a retired psychiatrist, says:

"I found it very easy to practice on religious people because you direct their emotions to a certain pillar and the best pillar to have faith in is Allah – God, the Maker of the Universe."

To stop a person falling in the trap of worry and anxiety we have been advised that:

"Imaan (Faith) is between fear and Hope!"

Mishkat

Is it a Punishment?

One cannot stipulate that he is a sinner, hence he is being punished;

"O My servants who have transgressed against their souls do not despair of Allah's mercy, for Allah forgives all sins. Indeed it is He who is the Forgiving, the Merciful."

Quran 39.53

Some people believe that we are born sinners and therefore religion is to blame for the psychological condition of the patient. Islam teaches that man is born pure from sin; it is only later in life that he does good and becomes better or does evil and becomes worse.

What is the position of a mentally ill patient in Islam?

Islamic Law rules that the insane are excused, they will have no reckoning and all their sins will be forgiven.

"Allah burdens not an individual more than his capability"

Quran 2.286

Mufti Shafi comments on the above verse that:

"A person's actions can be divided into two categories, voluntary and involuntary. They will be reckoned for the voluntary actions but the involuntary ones are excused."

Ma aarifiul Quran 2.286

Islam is very compassionate and understanding towards human nature; hence we have been told from the very outset that:

"Mankind has been created weak"

Quran 4.28

In other words, if one does indulge in abomination, one should not become disorientated, but rise above the situation and turn to his Lord in repentance, for indeed He is Al-Gaffar (Most Forgiving) Ar-Rahman (Most Merciful).

"The repenter from sins is like one who has no sin at all"

Mishkat

Islam never ceases to encourage repentance for those who transgress!

A sinner is not allowed to mention the name of the committed sin (when seeking forgiveness) because in doing so he will torment the heart, which is forbidden. This teaches us that Islam is very understanding towards sinners, let alone the mentally ill.

In this day of modern medicine, man has discovered that mental illness is mostly a pathological, genetic or organic illness. It can also be a reactionary affect to socio-cultural dilemmas like divorce, separation, etc.

"Sometimes mental illness in patients has a cultural influence hence, an ill patient of England would sometimes see Isa (Jesus) pbuh, an African would see spirits but the Asian would see Jinn's, magicians etc."

Dr S Munir

Why the suffering?

When a person is in pain or suffering either he is a good person and his place in Jannah (Heaven) is elevated or else he is a sinner whose sins will be forgiven through this illness.

Abu Hurayrah has narrated from Prophet Muhammad pbuh that:

"Whenever a Muslim is afflicted by illness, continuous pain, anxiety, grief, injury or by a thorn with which he is pricked, Allah causes this to be an atonement for his sins."

Mishkat

Abu Saeed Khudri and Abu Hurayrah narrate that the Prophet pbuh said:

"No fatigue, disease, sorrow, sadness, hurt, or distress befalls a Muslim, even if it were the prick he receives from a thorn, but that Allah expiates some of his sins for that."

Bukhari.7.545

Patients' rights

God, The Lord of Honour and Glory, will say on the Day of Judgement:

"Son of Adam, I was sick and you did not visit me."

The man will say:

"My Lord, how could I visit You and You are the Lord of the universe!"

God will say:

"Did you not know My servant so and so was sick and you did not visit him? Did you not realise that if you had visited him, you would have found Me with him?"

Development of Hospitals p.42, Muslim Al-Birr, 25

Abu Musa Ashari narrates that the Prophet (pbuh) said:

"Feed the hungry, visit the sick, and set free the captives."

Bukhari 7.552

Amulets and pendants

There is a misunderstanding in some communities that Islam discourages medical treatment and classes psychiatric illness as the spell of Devils and associates it with evil so they try out different Taweez (amulets and pendants). This is a thing which can be found in some communities who have been heavily influenced by their family traditions and cultures.

The Prophet pbuh used amulets but when needed he always took medicine.
Abu Said Khudri narrates that The Prophet pbuh said:

"Once when the Holy Prophet (upon whom be peace) fell ill, Gabriel came and asked: O Muhammad, are you ill? The Holy Prophet answered in the affirmative. Gabriel said: I blow on you in the name of Allah from everything that troubles you and from the evil of every soul and the evil look of every envier. May Allah restore You to health. I blow on you in His name."

Muslim Aishah narrates that:

"Whenever Allah's Apostle paid a visit to a patient, or a patient was brought to him, he used to invoke Allah, saying, 'Take away the disease, O the Lord of the people! Cure him as You are the One Who cures there is no cure but Yours, a cure that leaves no disease.'"

Bukhari 5.579

Aishah narrates that:

"During the Prophet's fatal illness, he used to recite the Mu'auwidhaat (Surah Al-Falaq and Surah An-Naas / Quran chapters 113 and 114) and then blow his breath over his body. When his illness was aggravated, I used to recite those two Surahs (chapters), blow my breath over him and make him rub his body with his own hand for its blessings. (Ma'mar asked Az-Zuhri: How did the Prophet used to blow? Az-Zuhri said: He used to blow on his hands and then passed them over his face.)"

Bukhari 7.631

Abdul Aziz narrates that:

"Thabit and I went to Anas bin Malik. Thabit said, 'O Abu Hamza! I am sick.' On that Anas said, 'Shall I treat you with the Ruqya (Amulet) of Allah's Apostle?' Thabit said, 'Yes.' Anas recited, 'O Allah! The Lord of the people, the Remover of trouble! (Please) cure (Heal) (this patient), for You are the Healer. None brings about healing but You; a healing that will leave behind no ailment.'"

Bukhari 7.638

The Prophets' Sunnah (Tradition):

Anas ibn Malik narrates that:

"A woman who had a defect in her brain, said: Allah's Messenger, I want to talk to you. He said: Mother of so and so, choose on which side of the road you would like to stand and talk, so that I may fulfill your need. He stood with her on the sidewalk until she spoke to her heart's content."

Muslim 1081

This shows that the Prophet pbuh never discriminated between the sane or insane. As long as this woman conversed with him patiently he continued to listen.

"Anas used to tell of the Prophet (peace be upon him) that he would visit the sick."

Tirmidhi 1529

Don't discriminate!

"The prophet in his visits did not discriminate against ailing people. He even visited sick non-Muslims."

Bukhari Tafseer Surah 59

Traditions of the early Muslims

During the Islamic period attempts were made by the Muslims to provide appropriate facilities and assistance to sick people.

"The ten years (13/634–23/644) under the rule of the second Caliph, Umar ibn al-Khattab, saw many public welfare works in the Islamic State. The Caliph was so concerned for the welfare of ailing people that he accompanied a team of physicians with the army proceeding towards Persia."

Development of Hospitals p.58

Ibn Tulun Hospital

"Ibn Tulun the governor of Cairo 259/872 established a hospital on the pattern of the hospital in Baghdad. In addition, various wards were constructed for eye diseases, orthopaedic and surgical cases. Ibn Tulun took a special interest in the welfare of the patients and he used to inspect the progress of the patients personally every Friday. In this Hospital he had also made a separate section for the treatment of the insane."

Development of Hospitals p.63, Tib al Arab Translation of Arabian Medicine by E.G. Brown by N.A.A. Wasti p.448

Benjamin of Tudela, a Jewish historian, who visited Baghdad in 556/1160 found at least sixty medical institutions there and wrote regarding Sultan Salah al-Din.

"All are well provided for from the king's stores with spices and other necessaries. Every patient who claims assistance is fed at the king's expense until his cure is complete. There is another large building called Darul Maraphtan in which are locked up all those insane persons who are met with during the hot season, every one of whom is secured by iron chains until his reason returns when he is allowed to return home; they are regularly examined by the king's officers appointed for this purpose and when they are found to be possessed of their reason again they are immediately liberated. All this is

done by the king in pure charity towards all those who come to Baghdad either ill or insane, for the king is a pious man and his intention is excellent in this respect."

Development of Hospitals p.68, C. Elgood, *A Medical History of Persia*, p.172

Bimaristan al-Salihani Ayyubi:

"The Sultan Salah al-Din Ayyubi converted a palace in Cairo into a hospital in 577/1181. On its walls the entire Quran was written. Ibn Jubayr describes the hospital in these words:

'This hospital is one of the prides of Salah al-Din. This is a magnificent and beautiful palace. The rooms are most elegant; in each room beds are spread, on which mattresses and pillows are placed in an orderly manner. There is a separate room for the dispensing of medicine and for this purpose chemists and compounders have been appointed. For lunatics, there are separate houses, which include a vast courtyard.'"

Juju Sedan, Tarkio al Tamaddun al-Islami, V.111 p.188, quoted in Tib al Arab, p.451, Development of Hospitals p.67

First European mental hospital

It is interesting to note that the Brothers of St John built the first European mental hospital in the 15th Century CE at Valencia in Spain. This European institution was based on a similar institution in Cairo and modelled on the Bimaristan of Baghdad (which was built in 136–158/754–775). The same brothers were later summoned to France by Marie de Medici to to build psychiatric hospitals at Charenton and the Charite at Senlis.

(Development of Hospitals p.70, S.H.Z.Naaqui, Islam and Development of Science, *Nigerian Journal of Islam*, V. i, p.5, (1971–72).

Conclusion

We believe that each illness has a cure but it is unto man to research and find the cure. Let us pray to Allah that He strengthens our faith for the peace and tranquility that are such vital ingredients for us being an ideal society.

The advice of the Prophet Muhammad pbuh

"Allah, The Most Merciful, has mercy on the merciful therefore, be merciful upon the dwellers of the earth. He will have mercy upon you Who is in the heavens."

Hadith

Amr ibn Maymun al-Awdi narrates that: Allah's Messenger (peace be upon him) said to a man in the course of an exhortation:

"Grasp five things before five others: your youth before your decrepitude, your health before your illness, your riches before your poverty, your leisure before your work, and your Life before your death."

Tirmidhi 1337

A message of the Holy Quran

Whoever kills a human being, not in lieu of another human being nor because of mischief on earth, it is as if He has killed all mankind: and if he saves a human life, it is as if he has saved the lives of all mankind.

Quran 5:33

Commentaries on Part 8

Commentary I

Andrew Powell

There is a pressing need for psychiatrists and mental health workers to pay more attention to the spiritual concerns of their patients. We know this to be true, because our service users are telling us that we are out of touch with what they are asking of us. A recent survey by the Mental Health Foundation (1998) showed that more than half of service users hold their religious and spiritual beliefs to be important in helping them cope with mental illness. Unfortunately, the survey also showed that these service users did not feel free, as they would wish, to discuss their beliefs with the psychiatrist.

In many parts of the world, a widening divide between science and religion has accompanied the advance of science. Psychiatrists-in-training are taught a model of mental functioning which aims to integrate the "hows" of neuroscience with the "whys" of psychology. This alone is a formidable task, so it is perhaps not surprising that spiritual concerns get handed over to someone else, often the hospital chaplain. Certainly, the word "soul" does not figure in the mental state examination, nor in the curriculum of most training schemes in psychiatry.

At this point, it might be useful to make the distinction between spirituality and religion. The priest is authorised to proclaim spiritual truth according to the doctrinal point of view. For all the big questions, there will be an established teaching – heaven and hell are a case in point. This by no means excludes an understanding of how religious symbols reflect archetypal human psychology, with the attendant longing for reassurance, security and forgiveness. Yet priests are identified as being different, set apart from the rest of us. The benediction they bestow in the name of the Almighty is confidently asserted, whatever private doubts and difficulties they may be having.

For the many people who have no deep commitment to a religious faith, the priest comes and goes at times of ritual blessing (marriage) and in the face of the unknown (death). Other times, the materialist society of today offers new gods, and large numbers of people now make window-gazing in the new shopping mall their preferred form of Sunday worship.

Spirituality, on the other hand, can be everybody's concern, whether or not they belong to a religious denomination. No belief in a scriptural God is required; rather, it is the intuition of the presence of the sacred and, most importantly, that sense of being part of a much greater whole, or unity. As Lao Tse wrote 2,500 years ago, "The Tao that can be told is not the eternal Tao. The name that can be named is not the eternal name ..." This is why we can speak of the soul, which we instinctively do when talking of matters spiritual, without worrying too much about how we should define it.

Why do mental health professionals so often discourage the conversation from taking a spiritual turn, even unawares? We have not been encouraged to trust our intuition and we are more at home with facts. But spirituality cannot be discussed with patients on the basis of fact; instead, what is called for is dialogue. The big questions include: "Why we were born in the first place, why must we suffer illness, mental and physical, what is the nature of our relationship to God and, not least, what happens when we die?"

How should the mental health professional respond? Sometimes it seems judicious to re-frame these questions within the framework of psychopathology. Therapeutically speaking, there is a bottomless pit to be filled; by 1990, depression had been identified as the fourth most important determinant of the global burden of disease and the largest determinant of disability in the world (Murray and Lopez 1997). Notably, within five years of Prozac coming on the market in 1989, over 10 million prescriptions had been issued worldwide.

Can such an epidemic of depression really be due to better diagnosis, or is it that we are looking at the emergence of a terrible malaise, which reflects a profound sense of loss of meaning and purpose in life? It is said that animals know pain and humans know suffering. To suffer means to know that you are in pain through the faculty of self-awareness, and the keenest form of suffering, perhaps its only true form, is to feel that the pain you suffer serves no purpose. Worse still, suffering is not just of the here-and-now, but of the past and the (anticipated) future too.

If the big existential and spiritual questions are to be taken seriously and not discounted as epiphenomena of depressive illness, what else avails? Where it is appropriate, the psychiatrist can ask the priest for help. Chapters 53–55 contribute Christian, Jewish and Muslim perspectives. In Chapter 53 Ian Ainsworth-Smith, who is both a clergyman and psychotherapist, draws our attention to the complex overlap of psychotherapy and spirituality. Clumsy or ill-advised interpretations can have a powerfully detrimental effect; but bad psychotherapy is being illustrated here. The therapist is imposing a meaning on the hapless patient instead of facilitating the symbol as a vehicle of communication to be understood psychodynamically, spiritually or both.

Elsewhere, a request for deliverance is cited that was not felt to be appropriate. Those of us who have worked in this area might on other occasions be rather glad to find a psychiatric team that would countenance the possibility of such an intervention, if truly consonant with the patient's wishes and beliefs. In my experience, spirit release in mental illness is not so much a theological matter as a pragmatic approach to be undertaken with care and mindful of the risk, just as any other treatment may carry side effects.

"Neurotic" versus "true" guilt usually says more about a person's history of emotional abuse than about religion and/or spirituality per se. Religion misapplied may indeed inculcate a sense of enduring unworthiness; so can a harsh and unloving parent. On the other hand, the inculcation of values of the soul, for example, the love of truth and honesty, compassion and respect for others, peacefulness and sovereignty over the self, are the rightful concern of both Church and family. Guilt can then be a healthy, inward spur to spiritual growth and social maturation.

In Chapter 54 on the Jewish faith Rabbi Neuberger emphasises spirituality in action, expressed day by day in the prayers, rituals and opportunities for sharing within the Jewish community. Communities and cultures that provide a strong sense of social identity can protect against breakdown through the group support offered in times of crisis and hardship. Neurosis is characterised by estrangement and alienation from kith and kin; this is why the therapeutic group can be a powerful instrument for healing and restoration of the self in such cases. There is, however, a caveat. When the individual cannot be accommodated within the group norm, rejection can at times be uncompromising and without mercy. The primary concern of the group is to protect itself "for the greater good". The fate of the individual is of lesser importance and so eccentric, antisocial or psychotic behaviour gets short shrift.

This highlights once again the difference between religion and spirituality, and equally so in the case of Islam. Religion is that which binds us (Latin *re-ligare*) not only to the Divine but also to each other through the observance of shared tradition and received wisdom. In Chapter 55 by Mawlana Sikander Khan Pathan, a compassionate and inclusive view of mental illness is articulated from the Islamic perspective. Yet Islam, meaning submission to the will of Allah, is both a religion and a way of life. Precepts and injunctions govern every aspect of conduct – private and public.

When a person needs psychiatric help and is accompanied by evidence of a caring religious community, the support of that community is invaluable both during and following treatment (aside from the problem area of cults). But what is the psychiatrist to do when a patient without a framework of faith tentatively raises those big and crucial questions?

Once the psychiatrist braves the use of the word "soul" by trusting to intuition (since it is no good looking to empirical science for a definition), the discussion may take an unexpected and surprisingly productive turn. We find that for a change we don't have to know the answers. We do have to share in the questions. Yet the big questions no longer seem unapproachable or unmanageable. Contact with the patient deepens and the skew of the transference recedes, since both doctor and patient are patently fellow travellers on the path of life. The psychiatrist still has special skills to offer the other, but can also provide the opportunity for the patient to discover his/her own truth, one that may turn out to have the potential to transform breakdown into breakthrough.

References

Mental Health Foundation, London (1998) *Knowing our own Minds*.
Murray CJL & Lopez AD (1997) Alternate projections of mortality and disability by cause 1990–2020: global burden of disease study. *Lancet* **349**: 1498–504.

Commentary II

Peter Fenwick

The major difficulty highlighted by Chapters 53–55 is the implicit, and sometimes explicit, assumption that our current scientific world view is complete. The genesis of this scientific view was in the 17th century at the time of the Enlightenment, when Galileo argued for a universe constructed of matter and energy (although since Einstein we only think of energy), and having two sets of qualities: primary and secondary. Primary qualities were those of weight, mass acceleration, etc., which can be represented mathematically, and secondary qualities were subjective; redness, love, beauty etc. Galileo argued that science should deal with primary qualities only. Subjective quallities were to be ignored. Our current Western science is still a primary quality science. We assume an objective, outside world composed of dead matter, with subjectivity arising from a very special part of this world, the brain. Thus whatever theories we construct, either about brain function or the nature of the world, have the fatal flaw of this subject/object split. The result is that any therapies based on this concept of human understanding miss the target. Psychoanalytical and counselling methods, based on a rational framework and limited to brain function and culture, cannot extend beyond into the spiritual domain. This is why a psychoanalytical interpretation is so very inadequate when it comes to understanding and explaining spiritual experience. This is well illustrated in Chapter 53 by Ian Ainsworth-Smith, which describes a religious nun who has her desire for communion and spiritual nourishment interpreted by a therapist as a displacement of a desire for oral sex.

Surveys show that mystical experiences are very common in the population (Hay and Morisy 1978). Thirty percent of people report having stood in awe, at some time in their lives, of a spiritual power greater than themselves. About 10% of normal people have deeper, transcendental experiences in which they become surrounded by light and see the structure of the universe as being composed of universal love.

In psychiatry the transcendent is frequently misinterpreted as the pathological. In a rational science the experiences of those who, in an altered mental state, see through the structure of the universe to the spiritual domain beyond can only be attributed to a malfunctioning brain. And yet these experiences are normal in the sense that they are very widespread. They also indicate that, if taken at face value, the world is underpinned by a spiritual reality and that the foundation of the universe is universal love. These statements are of course quite nonsensical when interpreted from the viewpoint of the dead matter universe of Galileo.

Ian Ainsworth-Smith points to the importance of culture, and more particularly to the culture of the therapist, stressing that many of the assumptions which underpin the counselling schools are those of Protestant Christianity. Gardner (1983) quotes the following incident to show the importance of culture when discussing the nature of miracles:

"When modern missionaries left some gospel books behind in Ethiopia and returned many years later, they not only found a flourishing church but a community of believers among whom miracles like those mentioned in the new testament happened every day – because there had been no missionaries to teach that such things were not to be taken literally."

This raises the question of how much of our experience is negated because it is not permitted by scientific missionaries who deny the reality of spiritual experience. A survey into belief in parapsychology makes this point strongly (Table 1).

The closer you are to the scientific centre, the more strongly you hold to the scientific beliefs.

The post-modern view is that there are any number of sciences, that these sciences arise within their own culture, and that scientific truths are value-laden from the culture in which they arise. The idea that the scientist is uncovering facts about a universal truth is simplistic; rather science is constructing a world view predetermined by its culture, and this is particularly true of views relating to mental illness.

Spiritual experiences have not been widely studied by science, because they are seen only as pathological, due to the implicit assumptions of a Western scientific world

Table 1. American survey into belief in parapsychology

General public	68%
Professors	57%
American Association for the Advancement of Science	30%
National Academy of Science	4%

view. One set of spiritual experiences which have been looked at are near-death experiences (Fenwick and Fenwick 1995). We have just completed a study of near-death experiences in a coronary care unit (Parnia et al. 2001). We found that the experiences appeared to arise when the heart had stopped, brain systems involved in the maintenance of consciousness had been disrupted, and the patients were deeply unconscious. Near-death experiences suggest a series of steps which the individual takes during the dying process. In brief, the entrance of the person into the light which is composed of pure consciousness, joy and love, is the first step. Usually the person will return without progressing further, but in the deepest experiences that have been reported to us the person goes further, loses his bodily form and becomes pure energy. There is then the possibility of fusing with universal consciousness and the recognition that the universe is a unity. These experiences are also highly moral and indicate that the experiencer is responsible for everything that he has done in his life, although there is no judgement apart from that of the individual himself, who is able to compare his actions with those he would now make when surrounded by perfect love.

Quite clearly these kind of experiences are not a generally acknowledged or accepted part of our culture and certainly are attributable only to pathology by our science. Many of the people who had these experiences were initially frightened to discuss them for fear of being considered and stigmatised as mad. General questionnaire surveys suggest that about 10% of the population are reported to have experiences like this. But these people function perfectly normally in the community both before and after the experience, and on any diagnostic criteria are certainly not mentally ill.

In Western scientific culture, which is based on the subject–object split and the dead matter universe, it is very difficult to consider spiritual values without them being labelled pathological. Until the limitations imposed by a rational science are understood, spiritual experience will continue to be unrecognised and undervalued.

References

Fenwick P & Fenwick E (1995) *The Truth in the Light.* London: Headline.

Gardner R (1983) Miracles of healing in Anglo-Celtic Northumbria as recorded by the venerable Bede and his contemporaries: a reappraisal in the light of twentieth century experience. *British Medical Journal* (Clin Res Ed) **287**: 6409.

Hay D & Morisy A (1978). Reports of ecstatic, paranormal or religious experience in Great Britain and the United States – a comparison of trends. *Journal for the Scientific Study of Religion* **17**: 255–68.

Parnia S, Waller DG, Yeates R & Fenwick P (2001) A qualitative and quantitative study of the incidence, features and aetiology of near death experiences in cardiac arrest survivors. *Resuscitation* **48**: 149–56.

Part 9

Some strategies to tackle stigmatisation and discrimination

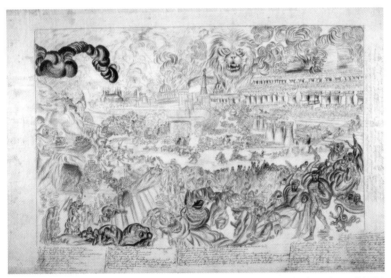

Jonathan Martin, *London's Overthrow*, ?1830

56 The destigmatising effect of listening to the patient

Sally Mitchison

Someone who is stigmatised by society and by his or her inner equivalent of "society" becomes painfully self-conscious. The patient with a psychiatric disorder feels marked out in the eyes of others and exposed as shamefully lacking in courage, stamina, will power, self-control and other adult qualities. The emotions that accompany psychiatric disorders: pain, fear, loneliness, anger, envy and despair are hard to acknowledge and articulate because of this sense of shame. Fear often results in disability, which shame covers and hides, leading to secondary handicap. Even as this is happening the sufferer knows that the hidden disability may be hard for others to perceive; this feeds envy and anger. For some there is a muddled, maybe hopeless sense of trouble now where trouble has been before.

The recent emphasis in the UK on mental health as a national priority (the National Service Framework: Department of Health 1999) is welcome and may help to reduce the stigma attached to psychiatric disorder. Access to appropriate treatments and advice and support in crisis are rightly emphasised as achievable goals. But this is separate from what happens when the patient meets the doctor or nurse. Not enough has been said about the importance of this interaction and the destigmatising effect of listening to the patient. Listening is not as simple a process as some imagine. In this chapter I shall examine its component parts and comment on the value of dialogue, understanding and naming.

Listening

The first thing to say about listening is that the setting must be right. A professional setting is to be preferred because although a patient's home may be comfortingly familiar it is rarely sufficiently private and may reflect back to the patient the painful reality of tasks not completed and hopes unfulfilled. This can make it more difficult to talk, and without talk there can be no listening. Talk often needs to be actively encouraged with sufficient, uninterrupted time set aside for it. Psychiatrists are usually aware of this and commonly set aside a full hour for each new patient (but sometimes forget to leave their bleeps elsewhere). Talk demands continuity, and while psychiatrists and nurses understand the importance of the patient seeing the same person each time, they may overlook the importance of the same room and, where possible, the same day of the week and time.

For talk to be productive, the speaker should feel listened to. Good listening involves close but discreet observation, undivided attention and indications of such attention. Such indications vary from culture to culture. In mainstream UK society careful, attentive listening to personal material is not best conveyed by neutral silence on the part of the listener. Instead, our dominant cultural code for good interpersonal listening includes a posture and body language that mirrors the other person, small body movements such as the occasional nod, non-intrusive vocalisations – "uh huh" and "mmm" – and the occasional last word or phrase of the speaker quietly repeated to encourage further comment. Not all sub-cultures within the UK have the same code, though, and it is important to be aware of those that are based on either more or less active responding.

The crucial thing is for the patient to feel heard. So active listening may involve translating feelings into words. The listener may need to acknowledge the feelings that are being expressed or to make simple interpretations ("I guess you must have felt ..."). Once difficult or terrifying feelings can be expressed in words they lose some of their force. The listener's acknowledgment of them conveys a sense that they are, to a degree, normal and universal. This almost always brings some relief. It also helps if the speaker can take back and acknowledge feelings that have hitherto been repudiated or projected onto others. Active listening can tactfully promote this ("I wonder whether it wasn't just your wife/son/mother who felt ..."). Although acknowledging denied feelings is often painful immediately afterwards, it is enabling because it promotes an increased sense of self and mastery.

Feeling properly listened to is a containing experience and one that many patients do not have in their personal lives. Sometimes this is all that a patient wants. It may be difficult for nurses and, more so, for doctors to appreciate when they are being called upon simply to listen: to be there rather than do something about what they are hearing. Most assessment procedures involve a careful cascade of questions, a systematic enquiry into a patient's inner life and social world. But the problem about this is that though the professional ends up with answers the patient may not feel heard. The skill here is to create the opportunity for the patient to talk without imposing too much in the way of structure. Many patients cannot simply come out with what troubles them and may need some initial chat or enquiry before getting started. Once the patient is able to embark properly on his account the doctor or nurse must have the confidence simply to let the talk flow without impediment. Contrary to common expectation, with the assistance of the active listening techniques that have already been mentioned most patients can communicate the heart of their complaint in some twenty or thirty minutes. If the patient cannot talk freely, grinds to a halt or talks exclusively in distancing, intellectualised discourse the doctor or nurse must then intervene and enquire not about the content of the patient's talk but about the process ("It seems very difficult for you to talk about this to me", "Is it too upsetting to go on?", "You seem to be talking about things in the abstract").

Understanding

Feeling fully listened to depends on feeling understood. And understanding is another active process. The doctor or nurse has to be able to relate to and make sense of the patient's experience. This does not require the doctor or nurse to have had the same experience – indeed, similar life experiences can lead one to presume that one knows what it must be like instead of enquiring with an open mind. Cultivating an open mind is not easy. Often doctors and nurses feel under pressure to reach a diagnostic formulation, clarify risk factors and define a care plan. But these need to be based on understanding rather than substitute for it. Patients usually read non-verbal cues from their doctor or nurse quite skilfully though not necessarily consciously. They can distinguish times when they have been understood from others when the professional has been operating in a more active, managerial role. At times the patient's anxiety, shame and fear blend with the professional's own anxiety about establishing a diagnosis and assessing risk. This may result in an interrogation rather than an interview and lead more to a shared sense of worry than of understanding and being understood.

The professional needs to be able to make sense of the patient's experiences and symptoms. This requires an explanatory model. The best understanding seems to come when the model used is consciously selected from a range of possible models. These could be tried on for size. ("I wonder if you think there is a link between feeling so low and imagining people are all looking at you when you go out" or "Some people get quite angry when they lose someone close" or "Do you think your own childhood experiences have some bearing on how you feel when your children are not with you?"). No one model explains everything. It is often helpful to combine different models of human behaviour and of the mind so as to increase one's understanding of the vast range of human experience and response that patients bring to their doctors and nurses. Symptoms can be construed as signifying illness or as reflecting a transition. Or they might be understood as a response to an existential dilemma, an impossible situation or the ordinary, relentless recurrence of those aspects of the human condition that test us all: death, decay, disease, disappointment and discord.

I have found it helpful in understanding patients to hold in mind Erikson's "crises of the healthy personality" – dilemmas faced at different stages of the maturational process (Erikson 1980). He delineates these as stages of childhood characterised by a series of issues:

- Trust versus mistrust
- Autonomy versus shame and doubt
- Initiative versus guilt
- Industry versus inferiority
- Identity versus identity diffusion

and then, at different stages of adulthood:

- Intimacy and solidarity versus isolation
- Generativity versus self-absorption

and finally:

- Integrity versus despair.

The value of Erikson's description of these life stage issues lies in his emphasis on their universality. John Bowlby also made a valuable contribution to our understanding of the shared experience of adult relatedness with his emphasis on the universal importance of attachment relationships not just in childhood but continuing on in adult life (Bowlby 1988). He corrected a tendency to disparage such relationships as an unhealthy dependency and construed them instead as necessary connections both to contemporary intimates and to important figures in childhood.

In addition to these and other psychological models, understanding can be increased by cultivating political and social awareness. While it is important to develop the capacity to empathise with what has been called "the woes that man doth suffer from" it is critical to appreciate the difference made to these woes by a steady, adequate income, a good education and a sense of social entitlement. Many patients have experienced none of these. Most doctors and nurses appreciate that psychiatric distress is inevitably increased by poverty and debt. But it is hard for middle-class professionals to appreciate some of the realities of many patients' lives: the sheer grind and constant juggling of life on social security benefits, the vigilance and diplomacy necessary to survive on many council estates, the practical difficulties and wasted time and effort of shoddy housing, and the impingement and sheer stress of crowded households or neighbours living close at hand.

An appreciation of each patient's circumstances, social world and life experiences as well as a careful enquiry about symptoms is not, though, sufficient in itself for the patient to feel understood. It needs to be complemented by an understanding of the meaning of all of these for that particular individual. To grasp this the nurse or doctor has to take account of that individual's unique inner world. This really is the key to understanding and feeling understood. It may not be necessary for the professional to explore the patient's inner world in detail; what matters is a shared interest in this inner world, peopled by figures from the patient's family of origin, enriched by memory and metaphor and perturbed by unwanted affect, desires and aversions. It finds expression in quirks of character, in choice of partner, in dreams and in the particular nature of a patient's symptoms.

Naming

Patients know – though not always consciously – that their symptoms are particular to them. What they fear is that they could be unique to them. How they feel about this ranges from distressing self-consciousness to terror that they may be going mad. This is where the destigmatising, humanising power of naming comes in to play. Just as it helps to feel understood, it is usually a great relief for our symptoms to be named and ascribed to a known disorder. Patients who fear they have some personal fault that marks them out as different from "normal" people can be greatly comforted to hear that they have a recognised illness or condition. The importance of reaching a diagnosis or diagnostic formulation goes beyond reassurance and comfort for the patient, of course, but it is more important than doctors and nurses sometimes realise to share this with the patient. This is best done collaboratively, establishing first what the patient believes to be wrong and then, in the case of diagnoses, such as schizophrenia, that may feel frightening, by citing the evidence and approaching the subject clearly but still tentatively ("these voices and the sense you describe of having special powers could possibly indicate an episode of schizophrenia"). Psychiatrists, nurses and psychologists are trained in different ways and may work from different models. This sometimes means that they give different diagnostic formulations, emphasising different aspects of a disorder. It is worth allowing enough time for patients to discuss what they may have been told previously and, where necessary, to explore any confusion or uncertainty that may therefore arise.

A proportion of patients feel sufficiently helped by being properly listened to that no treatment or further appointments are needed. They cease to feel shamefully stigmatised by their symptoms and find they can get these into proper proportion and find the resources to tackle them. This form of enablement is far preferable to trailing back and forwards to out-patient appointments. But for it to happen the patient must first be listened to skilfully and sensitively.

Conclusion

If they are to develop their skills and sensitivity, doctors and nurses need encouragement, training and support as well as adequate time with their patients. Personal therapy for the professional – and we all have personal issues that could do with being attended to – helps to develop sensitivity. Clinical supervision – not to be confused with line management – can elicit new skills and strengthen existing ones. The components of good listening that I have discussed in this chapter can all be communicated and learned. The only prerequisites are commitment and an open attitude.

References

Bowlby J (1988) *A Secure Base: Clinical Applications of Attachment Theory.* Bristol: Tavistock/Routledge.

Erikson EH (1959) *Identity and the Life Cycle* (republished 1980). New York: Norton.

Department of Health (1999) *National Service Framework for Mental Health.* London: HMSO.

57 Solutions to stigma: Sharing knowledge with the patient

Peter D White

"Knowledge itself is power" (Bacon 1597)

Self-knowledge and power

Sir Francis Bacon's whole life was spent in the pursuit of knowledge not only in the sciences, but also in politics, the law and as a courtier to King James of England. As his quote above makes plain, he was acutely aware of the importance of knowledge. Knowledge of something gives us the power to change or influence it. The corollary is that a lack of adequate knowledge of a problem may lead to the wrong solution. How much more important is this when it comes to understanding our own ill health?

Equality and secrecy

The most consistent complaint of patients about doctors is that doctors can't or won't communicate properly with their patients. Thus patients feel uncertain, frustrated, and left out of the inner circle of the health system they have entered. In such circumstances patients commonly fear or imagine the worst. Self-blaming explanations of illness are common, particularly when suffering from a mental health problem. The patient is cast into the role of victim, with the all-knowing doctor, or professional, the only person with the power to help. With popular understanding of mental illnesses so ignorant and unsympathetic, is it any wonder that sufferers feel the double jeopardy of both stigma and the illness itself? Although the Access to Health Records Act 1990 gives patients the rights to see their medical records (so long as their treating doctor does not think it would damage their health), few patients exercise this right.

The need for a diagnosis and the dangers of labelling

Patients need a diagnosis for several reasons (Sharpe 1998). It gives a name to a malady that allows acknowledgement of the genuine nature of their suffering. Giving fear a name reduces uncertainty, thus diminishing its threat. A diagnosis enables patients to start to make sense of what has gone wrong, so that they can put it right. A diagnosis is a passport of explanation and normalisation, which can be shared with family, friends and employers. Finally, a diagnosis allows a patient to receive the treatment, support and financial benefits to which they are entitled.

Ethical and sociological concerns have been raised about the stigmatising effects of psychiatric diagnostic labels, even when the diagnoses are valid (Shackle 1985). One of my patients once wrote to me: "It is bad enough to be ill. To have a psychiatric label attached to me as well simply adds insult to injury." Against this must be set the debilitating effects of the uncertainty and fear of being kept in the dark, by not being told what is wrong.

There are particular concerns when a patient is given a diagnosis such as schizophrenia, which may have serious implications regarding prognosis and disability. Clafferty et al. (2000) asked 211 consultant psychiatrists their views about whether they would tell patients with schizophrenia their diagnosis: 59% said they would tell their patients the diagnosis after the first episode, 89% after a second episode of illness; 15% would never use the term "schizophrenia" when giving the diagnosis.

"Schizophrenics" do not exist

If we label someone by their illness, this categorises them by that label alone, and society indelibly links the illness with the person. Doctors and other mental health professionals are as guilty of this as anybody else. Thus we talk about our patients as schizophrenic, manic-depressive, neurotic, etc. The media follow our lead more colloquially, writing headlines and talking about "schizos" and "loonies" (see Chapter 27 in this book). Professionals should never use this language, and instead talk about "Mr AB, who is currently suffering from schizophrenia".

"You've having a nervous breakdown"

No doctor would tell a patient "you're having a *physical breakdown*". Why should psychiatric illnesses be any different? Surveys of the general public show that they have a reasonably sophisticated view of mental health, being able to differentiate not only different diagnoses, but even different causes (see Chapter 3 in this book). The phrase "nervous breakdown" was first used (Great Britain and Ireland Post Office 1911) to describe what is now colloquially referred to as "repetitive strain injury", a chronic pain in the arm which has little to do with depressive illness. The phrase "nervous breakdown" has little useful meaning now. Talk of "mental illness" and "psychiatric disorder" does little more to improve understanding or knowledge. This is hardly surprising, since these descriptions include everything from Alzheimer's disease to zoophobia. Separating "mental illness" from the rest of medicine in this way continues the Cartesian dualistic fallacy that human beings are made up of separate and divisible minds and bodies. Whereas the reality is that every week marks publication of yet another study elucidating the physiological and sometimes pathological processes of the brain that cause us to think, sense and feel in the way that we do. Professionals should instead use specific diagnoses (e.g. depressive illness, schizophrenia) to initiate the process of explaining the illness to patients and their families. Where the diagnosis is uncertain it is most sensible to say so.

Writing letters to patients

Thomas investigated his patients' interest in receiving a letter from him following a psychiatric outpatient visit (Thomas 1998). Of 79 patients, 61% said they would like to receive a letter. When comparing those wanting a letter with those who didn't, there was no significant difference in age, gender, duration of illness, social class or marital status. People with a diagnosis of schizophrenia were less likely to request a letter (25%), compared to patients with other diagnoses (70%). Thomas wrote the letters directly to his patients, with a copy sent to the general practitioner, making a real effort to avoid technical jargon. At 18 months follow-up, 91% of patients contacted had found the letters helpful and 87% found them easy to understand. Two thirds of patients showed their letters to others. A fifth of patients used the letters as aide-mémoires. Others reported that it helped them to see their problems more clearly. Two patients found the letters positively unhelpful.

Goddard et al. (1997) compared showing a clinical summary to patients in two groups: those attending a general psychiatric clinic and those suffering from a somatisation disorder. Of 30 patients with somatisation disorder, 93% thought it was a good idea to read the summary and 87% thought that it had provided helpful information. However, 57% of patients with somatisation disorders reported increased concerns about undiagnosed illnesses as a result of reading their clinical summary, compared to 27% of patients attending a general psychiatric clinic.

A personal experience of writing to patients

In the last twelve years as a consultant adult psychiatrist, I have sent copies of every letter I write about a patient to the patient themselves, unless they specifically ask me not to. This amounts to approximately 1,000 new patient assessments and at least 7,500 follow-up letters. I have found this practice has significant advantages for both my patient and myself. The patient has a written account of the assessment and the advice given. We do not know whether this aids compliance, but it is unlikely to have a negative influence. The patient learns that they can trust what the professional says to them verbally, since a written account is (hopefully) the same. This encourages and improves the professional–patient relationship. It also gives a message to the patient that they have some responsibility themselves for what they do about their illness, such as complying with medication or abstaining from alcohol.

Other advantages have included correction of factual errors in my initial history, although these are usually of minor importance. Patients have a written record about detailed advice regarding, for instance, medications which allows me to tell my patients how to alter their dose regime over time, depending on side effects. When a general practitioner hasn't received a copy of my letter, the patient is able to provide them with a copy. I encourage patients to take a copy of the letter along with them the next time they see their general practitioner. This also enables a patient to discuss the plan of treatment with their general practitioner. The general practitioner or referrer knows that the patient has received exactly the same information as they have, which may enhance their own communication with their patient.

Warnings and adverse effects of letter writing

Particular care needs to be taken over recording sensitive knowledge, such as childhood traumas and abuse. Other sensitive knowledge objected to by my patients in the past include a past history of significant substance misuse, time spent in prison and difficulties in a marital relationship. To avoid inappropriate information being put in the letter, I usually ask my patients how they would like me to record sensitive information, and whether there is any information that they would like excluded. Phrases such as "Ms XX had a traumatic childhood" are usually acceptable. Very often the general practitioner is already aware of the history and therefore this isn't an issue.

A few patients have expressed concern about the wrong person opening the letter. All envelopes are addressed "Personal & Confidential" to try to avoid this problem. It is particularly important that addresses are kept up-to-date and are checked by a reliable secretary. In the last ten years only three of my patients have specifically asked for letters not to be sent to them. Another patient has asked for the letters to be sent to an alternative address rather than their home address.

Out of the 1,000 new patients assessed, only three patients have particularly objected to the content or opinions in my assessment letters. All three patients suffered from personality difficulties and decided not to attend my clinic any more. I have learnt that such diagnoses need to be explained very carefully and recorded in a letter without the use of any words that could possibly be interpreted as pejorative. Two patients have asked me to revise my letters and send the revision to their general practitioner or referrer. The revisions requested have been of such a nature that I have been able to comply. However, it is sometimes important to explain to a patient the difference between a factual account of their illness or previous lives from my own clinical interpretation provided in a diagnosis and explanations of how they came to be ill.

The final consideration is cost. There is a small administrative cost and the extra cost of postage. This may be offset by the reduced costs of fewer complaints, which are likely to be diminished by better communication.

Contra-indications to writing to patients

There may be occasions when a patient cannot understand or read a letter, which might cause confusion or uncertainty. Examples would include illiteracy, severe learning disability and dementia. Occasionally one might be concerned about inappropriate use of the letter, to a patient's later regret, such as during acute mania when a patient might inappropriately share a letter with others. Particular care should be taken when writing to a patient involved in a childcare dispute when the other party is living at the same address. There will be occasions when a doctor might give confidential advice to a third party that is not shared with their patient. An example would be giving advice to a partner of someone suffering from severe morbid jealousy with a history of violent actions or threats. Other examples can be found in the practice of forensic psychiatry, such as when a psychiatrist is giving advice to a court.

Letter writing in other branches of medicine

Some psychotherapists and family therapists find it helpful to write a formulation of a client's difficulties to the client at some stage in the therapy. Writing letters to patients, or their parents, is also becoming established in other areas of medicine such as paediatrics (Essex 1998), genetic counselling (Hallowell 1998), breast screening services (Lewars 1998), gastroenterology (Eaden et al. 1998) and elderly medicine (Coni 1998). Hallowell found that 93% of 40 patients commented that his letters aided their understanding and/or recall of information. The letters were also shown to other clinicians to aid further care and support. Coni reported that 79% of 35 patients found letters "very helpful" and a further 18% found them "helpful". Eaden et al. sent a copy of their letter to the general practitioner to their patients, and found this as successful as sending a letter directly to the patient, although they urged caution about generating anxiety in patients with "serious" diseases. They were particularly cautious about introducing new information.

Third-party information

The best way to avoid the problem of third-party consent to sharing information is to interview the family together in the same room, which is my normal practice. The large majority of people find this helpful, particularly if it is made clear that they can have part of the interview with me alone. Occasionally I will remind the patient that they can see me alone if it becomes clear that they are having difficulty recounting a difficult and personal part of the history: this is usually unnecessary. My own experience is that close family members know only too well the personal and more sensitive parts of a patient's history and illness.

Medico-legal, insurance company and employer's reports

The other area of concern to patients regards financial matters, such as supplying reports to insurance companies or employers. I find this is usually resolved by sending a draft letter to the patient to correct any factual errors and to make sure that they give written consent to my sending the letter. In these circumstances, a patient will often ask for a slightly different emphasis in the words used, which I can usually incorporate without changing the factual accuracy of my report. It is important to clarify that it is the patient's decision as to whether the letter is sent or not.

When a doctor is asked to provide a report for a third party which is confidential, this has to be respected. Examples include independent medicolegal reports, or reports for insurance companies, when the doctor is not caring for the person. My own experience is that it is usually in the interests of all parties if such reports are shared with the person they most concern, particularly when the report includes suggestions about further investigations or treatment. I usually recommend to the addressee that a copy of the whole or the relevant part of the report is sent on to their client or their doctor.

How to write to a patient

Wyatt (2000) has described the ways in which doctors might provide information for patients. He comments that very few patients are adequately informed about their health, health care and choices, and suggests that we should be more responsible in informing them. He helpfully describes the important principles of effective letter-writing for patients. They include placing the most important information first or last, writing short sentences and short words, focusing on the specific experience of the patient, cutting out irrelevant information, and appropriate use of headings to aid clarification, amongst other things.

Does letter writing help reduce stigma?

We don't presently know whether writing to patients in this way reduces a patient's sense of shame and stigma. However, there is evidence that patients generally appreciate a closer involvement in making decisions and like to know what doctors have recorded about them. My personal experience is that the large majority of patients appreciate this service and there are few adverse effects. Avoiding jargon and generalities aids comprehension, and I find it useful to spend the first few minutes of the second consultation asking for corrections and clarifying misunderstandings. At its least effective, it cannot be harmful to reduce the sense of secrecy, which sometimes surrounds doctors' communications and their medical records. After all, the illness belongs to our patients, not ourselves.

Use of leaflets and videos about a condition

I specialise in the assessment of treatment of patients with chronic fatigue and provide a leaflet for "sufferers, their carers, families, and friends". Although this has been received positively, this doesn't have the same impact as a copy of my initial assessment. Being a leaflet about an illness in general means that there are topics covered by the leaflet of no relevance to a particular patient. The same criticism applies to videotapes, although they have the major advantage of using other media than the written word.

References

Bacon F (1597) Of Heresies. In: *Religious Meditations*.

Clafferty RA, McCabe E & Brown KW (2000) Telling patients with schizophrenia their diagnosis: patients should be informed about their illness. *British Medical Journal* **321**: 384–5.

Coni N (1998) Summary letters may be especially appropriate after emergency admissions. *British Medical Journal* **316**: 1831.

Eaden JA, Ward B & Mayberry JF (1998) Letters should be used carefully. *British Medical Journal* **316**: 1831.

Essex C (1998) Consultants could give patients a letter summarising their consultation. *British Medical Journal* **316**: 706.

Goddard N, Bernadt M & Wessley S (1997) Showing medical records: comparison of general psychiatric patients with somatisation disorder patients. *Psychiatric Bulletin* **21**:, 489–91.

Great Britain and Ireland Post Office (1911) *Departmental Committee on Telegraphists' Cramp Report*. London: His Majesty's Stationery Office.

Hallowell N (1998) Providing letters to patients: patients find summary letters useful. *British Medical Journal* **316**: 1830.

Lewars MD (1998) GPs can be given copies of letters sent to patients. *British Medical Journal* **316**: 1831.

Shackle EM (1985) Psychiatric diagnosis as an ethical problem. *Journal of Medical Ethics* **11**: 132–4.

Sharpe M (1998) Doctors' diagnoses and patients' perceptions: lessons from chronic fatigue syndrome. *General Hospital Psychiatry* **20**: 335–8.

Thomas P (1998) Writing letters to patients. *Psychiatric Bulletin* **22**: 542–5.

Wyatt JC (2000) Information for patients. *Journal of the Royal Society of Medicine* **93**: 467–71.

58 Decreasing employment discrimination against people who have experienced mental health problems in a mental health trust

Rachel Perkins and Duncan Selbie

Introduction

The importance of work in enhancing and maintaining the mental health and quality of life of people who experience mental health problems has been widely documented (Bennett 1975; Rowland and Perkins 1988; Shepherd 1989; Nehring et al. 1993; Warner 1994; Pozner et al. 1996). Yet it remains the case that employment opportunities for such people remain scarce: the 2002 Labour Force Survey showed that 79% of those with significant mental health problems were unemployed.

For many people with mental health problems the only barrier to open employment is the prejudice of employers. Others have more disabling problems that impede their work performance. In the UK, such people have traditionally been excluded from the open labour market and directed toward hospital-based industrial units or community sheltered workshops. In contrast, in the USA, there is good evidence that, with help and support, many people with serious mental health problems can sustain open employment (Bond et al. 1997, 2001). In the UK this model has been developed for those with learning difficulties, but less often for people with mental health problems.

There are a variety of reasons why mental health services might usefully include in their workforce people who have experienced mental health problems (Mowbray 1997). As a result, it is now commonplace in many areas of the USA for mental health services themselves to employ people who experience such difficulties (Mowbray et al. 1997). By contrast, in the UK there is a tendency to look exclusively to employers outside the health arena to provide work for those with mental health problems, a tendency that can be seen in the survey of employers conducted by Manning and White (1995).

Ensuring that people who have experienced mental health difficulties can be accommodated within the workforce can actively enhance the quality of mental health services offered. Recognition of the value of personal experience has a long history. In the late 18th century at Bisetre Hospital in France it was the policy to select staff from among recovered and convalescing patients. Pinel described such people as best placed to understand the needs of patients as a result of what they themselves had experienced. The employment within mental health services of people who have themselves experienced mental health problems increases the skill mix of staff and can act as an important role model for both clients and staff.

The NHS is also desperately short of most major staff groups, especially nurses, and heavily reliant on agency staff. Reducing the barriers to employment of people with experience of mental health problems can serve to partially address these difficulties.

Mental health services are major employers. If other employers are to be encouraged to offer jobs to people who experience mental health problems, then it is important that mental health services lead by example. Given the expertise present in mental health services, they are well placed to take a lead in demonstrating what 'reasonable adjustments' (Disability Discrimination Act of 1995) might be necessary in employing those with psychiatric problems.

The South West London and St George's Mental Health NHS Trust User Employment Programme*

The aim of the Trust's User Employment Programme is to increase access to employment within a mental health service for people who have experienced mental health problems. The programme has three components:

1. A supported employment programme

This programme offers people who are disabled by mental health problems support and help to gain and sustain employment in existing posts within the Trust. Posts are advertised in the usual way, but in addition the Trust's Vacancy Bulletin is circulated to people with mental health problems who have expressed an interest in working within the Trust and to local mental health employment projects. Person specifications specify that "personal experience of mental health problems", in addition to all the other qualifications, experience and personal attributes required for the post, is desirable, and the "equal opportunities statement" on advertisements encourages applications from people who have experienced mental health problems (see below). Job packs contain information about the programme so that people with mental health problems can seek its support if they wish. If an interview panel want to offer a post to a suitably qualified applicant who has experienced mental health difficulties, but feel that the person may require help/support to perform the job, the person can gain support from the programme. Existing staff who develop mental health problems may also make use of the support offered by the programme to return to work and sustain their employment.

In all cases, the expectations and standards to which individuals are expected to perform remain the same as for all recruits. The only difference is the support offered. The type of support offered to employees can be seen in Box 1; however, support and advice are also offered to managers. In line with research in the area (Bond et al. 1997; Crowther et al. 2001) support is available without limit of time. When they are settled into work some people cease to need support but, given the fluctuating nature of many mental health problems, some require assistance over longer periods. All support is tailored to the needs of the individual concerned and typically adopts a "problem-solving" approach (see Perkins et al. 2001), although practical assistance is also offered where necessary.

*Formerly known as the Pathfinder User Employment Programme.

Box 1. Support offered to employees (see Perkins et al. 2001)

Assistance in the recruitment process, for example:
- Information about the requirements of jobs and the support available
- Assistance in completing application forms
- Interview practice and assistance in preparing for interview
- General support and encouragement

Assistance in the transition to work, for example:
- Specialist advice about welfare benefits
- Identification of workplace mentors
- Assistance with the practicalities of starting work
- Help to consider the pros and cons of disclosing mental health problems to colleagues at work
- General support and encouragement

Ongoing support to retain employment, for example:
- Help with difficulties that arise at work
- Assistance with problems outside work that might interfere with work performance (including assistance to access other services)
- Working out ways in which a person might cope with specific symptoms in a work context
- Assistance with career development
- General support and encouragement

---

2. Decreasing employment discrimination throughout the Trust

Many people who have experienced mental health problems do not require special support in employment. However, they may continue to experience discrimination because of their psychiatric history (Read and Baker 1996) and may as a consequence have given up applying for jobs.

Therefore, in an attempt to decrease such employment discrimination throughout the Trust, and in line with the requirements of the 1995 Disability Discrimination Act, a Charter for the employment of people who have experienced mental health problems was adopted.* This Charter recognises that the absence of employment is detrimental to mental health, that prospective employees may be subject to discrimination in recruitment as a consequence of their mental health problems and that, in a mental health service, staff who have themselves experienced mental health problems have gained experience and expertise that may be valuable to others who experience similar difficulties.

The Charter:

- Specifies that mental health problems alone will not form a barrier to selection providing that the person fulfils the other requirements of the post.
- Recognises the positive contribution that personal experience of mental health problems can make to the service offered by the organisation. Person specifications for all clinical and client contact posts should be modified to include "personal experience of mental health problems" as desirable experience in addition to all other qualifications and qualities required for the post unless a specific case is made that a particular post should be exempt.
- Commits the Trust to monitoring progress in recruiting people who have experienced mental health problems, via an addition to existing confidential equal opportunities monitoring, and working towards a target of at least 25% of the workforce being people who have experienced mental health difficulties.
- Ensures that all Trust job advertisements carry an equal opportunities statement encouraging applications from people who have experienced mental health problems.

*Copies of the Charter are available from the first author.

The introduction of this Charter was accompanied by a programme of seminars across the Trust that gave people an opportunity to discuss their reservations and concerns about employing people with mental health difficulties.

3. Work preparation and work experience

There are a number of people with mental health problems who have never worked, are unsure about whether they are able to do so, or are uncertain about whether they wish to work in the mental health field. Therefore the programme has developed work preparation and work experience programmes. The work preparation programme is offered via a contract with the Employment Service, now Job Centre Plus, and offers a 10-week programme, four times per year, that provides work experience and assistance to find and apply for jobs. For those who need a longer period of work experience prior to applying for open employment, a six-month work experience and work preparation is also available from the programme.

Outcomes

The Supported Employment Programme

Between 1995 and 2001, 81 people who had experienced mental health problems were supported in employment within the Trust. Of these people, 15 were employed in positions requiring professional mental health qualifications, a further two supported employees have gone on to undertake training in one of the major mental health professions and two more had secured places on such courses. The remainder were employed in clinical and non-clinical positions not requiring professional qualifications or posts requiring secretarial/administrative qualifications. The mean age of these employees was 40.3 years, 58% were female, 74% were white European and 26% Black African/African Caribbean or Asian; 25% had a primary diagnosis of schizophrenia, 39% depression and 14% bipolar disorder. The majority had been admitted to hospital and they had been unemployed for a mean of 2.5 years prior to taking up employment within the Trust.

Six years after the start of the programme, 33 of these people continued to work within the Trust, receiving support. Of the 48 no longer requiring support from the programme, 20 continued to work in the Trust without support, 12 had moved on to employment outside the Trust and 4 had entered full-time education.

Because of concerns that sick leave among supported employees might be high, absence through sickness was monitored during 1998/99. Sickness absence for supported employees was 3.8% while that for all direct care staff within the Trust was considerably greater at 5.8%.

The Charter for the Employment of People who have Experienced Mental Health Problems

In the year in which this Charter was adopted (1997) confidential equal opportunities monitoring showed that 9% of those recruited had experienced mental health problems. By 1999 this had risen to 21% and by 2000 to 27%.

Work preparation and work experience

Between October 2001 and December 2002, 23 people took the 10-week work preparation course. The mean age of these people was 35.1 years, 70% were female, 59% were white European and 35% Black African/African Caribbean or Asian; 53%

had a primary diagnosis of schizophrenia, 23% depression and 18% bipolar disorder. The majority had been admitted to hospital and they had been unemployed for a mean of 2.8 years prior to taking up employment. Of these people, 12 (52%) gained open employment and a further 5 (22%) went on to mainstream education or training.

Between January and December 2002, 14 people undertook the longer, six-month, work experience programme. The mean age of these employees was 30.0 years, 69% were female, 62% were white European and 38% Black African/African Caribbean or Asian; 50% had a primary diagnosis of schizophrenia and 25% depression. They had been unemployed for a mean of 5.3 years prior to taking up employment. Seven people (50%) gained open employment and a further four (29%) entered mainstream education/training.

Discussion

The outcomes of the User Employment Project at South West London and St George's Mental Health Services NHS Trust indicate that people who have experienced mental health problems can be successfully employed within a mental health service in both supported and unsupported positions.

It is important to emphasise that in no instance were "special" posts created: everyone was employed in existing posts within the Trust. Supported employees were expected to perform the same work as those without mental health difficulties: the main "adjustment" made was the availability of support. In this context, it is important to note that much of the support provided – like help with problems that arise at work and assistance with career development, and the availability of a workplace mentor – might simply be described as good employment practice. It is possible that if such assistance was available to all staff, sickness rates could be reduced to the levels observed for supported employees.

Although the majority of supported employees were employed in positions that did not require professional mental health qualifications, the number of qualified mental health professionals provided with support has increased over recent years. In this context, support for existing employees who develop mental health problems may be particularly important.

The data presented here suggest that work preparation and work experience programmes typically serve a higher proportion of people with a diagnosis of schizophrenia who have been unemployed for longer periods of time. The success of these programmes in ensuring that at least 70% of these people enter open employment or mainstream education/training is therefore noteworthy.

Providing support in employment for people who have experienced mental health problems not only increased the skill mix of the workforce in terms of the experience and expertise that this personal experience endows. It has also resulted in the employment of a groups of non-professionally qualified staff who have a higher level of educational qualifications than might be usual in this group. Of the first 30 people recruited to posts that did not require professional qualifications (OT technician posts, heath care assistant positions etc.) 9 were graduates and a further 8 had other types of further education qualifications in subjects as diverse as counselling, art, computing, sports, secretarial, nursery nursing, printing and horticulture.

In addition to the supported employment programme, the steps taken throughout the organisation to decrease employment discrimination against people who have mental health problems have further increased work opportunities. Of recruits to posts throughout the organisation, 27% had experienced mental health problems and these recruits spanned all professionals and grades.

There have been some who have questioned the risks involved in employing people who have experienced mental health difficulties. In this context it must be stressed that a clear distinction has been drawn between mental health difficulties and a forensic history, where the usual Trust policies apply to all. There may, however, be some ways in which increasing access to employment has decreased risk. Many people who experience mental health problems feel obliged to deny such difficulties through fear of the discrimination and rejection that which may result from disclosure. It appears that decreasing employment discrimination has enabled more people to be open about their mental health difficulties, thus enabling appropriate support and help to be provided to circumvent potential difficulties.

The programme shows that mental health services can move beyond their traditional provider role. As major employers, such services can take a lead in reducing the discrimination and social exclusion experienced by those who have mental health difficulties. Since the establishment of the User Employment Programme at South West London and St George's Mental Health NHS Trust, similar initiatives have been established in a number of trusts, and the Department of Health have introduced guidance on the employment of people with mental health problems in the NHS (Department of Health 2002) to which people involved in the programme contributed. The expertise available within mental health services should place us in a good position to develop expertise in relation to the employment of people with mental health difficulties that might act as a model for other employers.

References

Bennett C (1975) Techniques of industrial therapy, ergotherapy and recreative methods. In: Auflange Z (ed). *Psychiatric den Gegenwart*, Vol 3, 2nd edn. Berlin: Springer-Verlag.

Bond GR, Drake RE, Meuser KT et al. (1997) An update on supported employment for people with severe mental illness. *Psychiatric Services* **48**: 335–45.

Bond GR, Becker DR, Drake RE et al. (2001) Implementing supported employment as an evidence based practice, *Psychiatric Services* **52**: 313–22.

Crowther RE, Marshall M, Bond GR & Huxley P (2001) Helping people with severe mental illness to obtain work: systematic review. *British Medical Journal* **322**: 204–8.

Department of Health (2002) *Mental Health and Employment in the NHS*. London: DoH Publications.

Manning C & White P (1995) Attitudes of employers to the mentally ill. *Psychiatric Bulletin* **19**: 541–3.

Mowbray CT, Moxley DP, Jasper CA & Howell LL (eds) (1997) *Consumers as Providers in Psychiatric Rehabilitation*. Columbia, MD: International Association of Psychosocial Rehabilitation Services.

Nehring J, Hill R & Poole L (1993) *Work, Empowerment and Community*. London: Research and Development in Psychiatry (now Sainsbury Centre for Mental Health).

Perkins R, Evenson E, Lucas S & Harding E (2001) What sort of "support" in employment? *A Life in the Day* **5**: 6–13.

Pozner A, Ng ML, Hammond J & Shepherd G (1996) *Working It Out*. Brighton: Pavilion.

Read J & Baker S (1996) *Not Just Sticks and Stones*. London: Mind.

Rowland LA & Perkins RE (1988) You can't eat, drink or make love eight hours a day: the value of work in psychiatry. *Health Trends* **20**: 75–9.

Shepherd G (1989) The value of work in the 1980s. *Psychiatric Bulletin* **13**: 231–3.

Warner R (1994) *Recovery from Schizophrenia*, 2nd edn. London: Routledge.

59 Mental illness in medical students and doctors: Fitness to practise

Rosemary Lethem

Introduction

Recent high-profile cases of professional malpractice have focused attention on the medical profession and its capacity for self-regulation in order to protect the public from incompetent or unfit doctors.

Mental illness is one of the main causes of lack of fitness to practise. Doctors are physically healthier but more prone to mental ill health than the general population.

Mental illnesses are recognised clinically. Adopting a broad spectrum and dualistic approach, medical students and doctors, like the population in general, may suffer from:

- **"Organic" mental illness**
  - Substance-related disorders (drugs and/or alcohol)
  - Cognitive decline
  - Secondary to physical disease (e.g. multiple sclerosis, AIDS)

- **Severe mental illness**
  - Schizophrenia
  - Major affective disorders

- **Other mental illnesses and related mental health problems**
  - Suicide
  - Deliberate self-harm
  - Mood disorders
  - Anxiety disorders
  - Somatoform disorders
  - Stress
  - Burn out

- **Behavioural disorders**
  - Eating disorders
  - Factitious disorders

- **Intrapsychic conflict**

Some illnesses, including mental illnesses, both in terms of their precipitation and their course, are known to be sensitive to adverse life events and related stress.

Certain illnesses and presentations are commoner at particular times. It is useful to think of the medical career as having its own "life cycle" with a number of stages, starting with apprenticeship as a student doctor, graduating to become a novice, before progressing to medical maturity and finally "winding down" in preparation for retirement (Wilhelm et al. 1997).

Many cases of impaired fitness to practise in medical students and doctors, at all stages in their medical careers, will present as inappropriate behaviour in a clinical setting, or through impaired performance (Wilhelm et al. 1997). Away from clinical settings, problems can present in a variety of ways. In clinical settings they may be noticed by peers, colleagues, lecturers and supervisors, or patients and their families. Unfit doctors may present to their own doctor or to medical administrators. There may be official complaints.

This chapter will discuss the concept of professional competence before discussing the mental illnesses and health problems to which medical students and doctors are vulnerable, the context within which they occur and an outline of some issues relating to prevention and management, particularly mechanisms for ensuring that the safety of the public is not compromised.

Competence to practise

In the UK the General Medical Council (GMC) is the regulatory body for the medical profession, under the Medical Act 1983. Doctors have a duty to meet the standards of competence, care and conduct set by the GMC. "Fitness to practice" is not defined. The Act allows investigative procedures where there is concern over possible "seriously impaired" fitness to practise, that is, such as to compromise the welfare of patients.

With the publication of *Good Medical Practice* in 1995, the GMC described for the first time the duties and responsibilities of doctors explicitly and set out the principles of good medical practice. Doctors were reminded that registration with the GMC gave them rights and privileges in return for which they must fulfil their obligations to the public. Patient care must be the first concern of every doctor.

Good Medical Practice states that "doctors must act when they believe that a colleague's conduct, performance or health is a threat to patients, if necessary by telling someone from the employing authority or from a regulating body" (GMC 1998a). Such action thus has become a professional obligation.

Doctors are most likely to maintain good practice when they work in properly functioning clinical teams (Irvine 1999). Effective teams have a sense of collective and personal responsibility for their professional performance, a no-blame culture and a commitment to understand and look after each other and their patients.

Mental illness in medical students

Student life

The pressures on students in general are acknowledged to have increased greatly in recent years (Rana et al. 1999). Reasons for this include the widening access to higher education, political pressure to include greater numbers of those who hitherto have been under-represented in higher education, increased financial pressures, societal shifts reflected in increased instability in family life, and decreasing accessibility of mental health service provision.

The proportion of students applying for higher education who indicate that they have a disability on mental health grounds has remained small at approximately 0.05%. However, there is broad agreement from university counselling services that the severity of emotional and behavioural disturbance amongst students is increasing (Rana et al. 1999). Student suicide is a not uncommon phenomenon. Serious psychiatric disorders such as schizophrenia, bipolar affective disorder and eating disorders are likely to present most acutely in the 16- to 25-year-old age group. Substance use and misuse is highly prevalent.

The Disability Discrimination Act (1996) has raised mental health related issues for institutions, by granting rights to training, education and employment to people with disabilities. Disability is defined as "a physical or mental impairment which has a substantial long-term effect on a person's ability to carry out normal day-to-day activities". Mental disability is not further defined. Mental illness is recognised on clinical grounds but there is debate over the status of stress disorders and fatigue. Reasonable adjustment to student life is expected, but "reasonableness" is context-dependent.

Medical student training

Undergraduate medical training must be completed within seven years. There is no facility for restricted registration with the GMC on the grounds of mental or other illness. Medical students face additional stresses due to the nature, length and intensity of their training. There are some sources of stress that are generic to medical students throughout the world: adjusting to medical training, including the realities of disease and dying patients; coping with the volume of material to be learned; confronting ethical dilemmas; balancing academic demands with life outside medicine; and delaying gratification of many wishes (Myers 1997).

The personality characteristics of medical students and doctors may constitute a source of stress. The selection processes of medical schools place a high degree of emphasis on academic success. They cannot be expected to predict future personality development. Competitive, successful individuals who deal poorly with emotional pressures by intellectualising or denial are often selected. Medical training tends to concentrate on "head" and "hands" skills at the expense of "heart", often leading to varying degrees of alienation and cynicism due to an "emotionally marasmic existence" (Coombs and Virshup 1994).

Nature and prevalence of mental disorders

Studies of utilisation of psychiatric services have shown that between 4% and 18% of medical students annually identified themselves as "impaired", with a further unknown number not seeking help. About half of help-seekers make only a single contact (Myers 1997).

Many medical students suffer from intrapsychic and interpersonal conflicts, for example delayed psychosocial and psychosexual development, sexual dysfunction, the sequelae of earlier sexual abuse, confusion over sexual orientation or being HIV-positive (Myers 1997).

Relationship problems amongst students and doctors are common (Myers 1997), frequently caused or exacerbated by their lifestyle. Lack of an intimate relationship or marital conflict are psychosocial causes of stress and may be precipitating factors in the onset of many mental illnesses. Common illnesses in medical students are:

- Substance-related disorders (especially involving alcohol and cannabis); see below
- Mood disorders (especially major depressive disorder) (up to 5%)
- Anxiety disorders (panic disorder, phobias, obsessive compulsive disorder, post-traumatic stress disorder, generalised anxiety disorder) (up to 7%)
- Adjustment disorders
- Eating disorders (anorexia nervosa and bulimia nervosa) (Myers 1997) (up to 10%)

Rarely, severe mental illnesses classified as psychoses in ICD-10 and characteristically involving loss of insight (schizophrenia and hypomania) may present in this age group. Suicide is a leading cause of death, along with accidents, amongst medical students, although it is a rare event. Figures collected from a questionnaire survey of American medical schools for the period 1989–94 demonstrated a lower rate than in earlier studies and than in the nation as a whole. Of 15 reported deaths, 9/13 had known psychiatric histories (Hays et al. 1996).

Substance-related disorders are rarely diagnosed in medical students, but many doctors subsequently treated for alcohol or drug dependency report that their pattern of overuse began during medical school or even earlier. Alcohol and "soft" drug use are endemic amongst medical students as socially sanctioned means of escape from the pressures of the training. A questionnaire study of the drinking behaviour of medical students from 13 British medical schools revealed that 23% of male students and 10% of female students reported drinking more than the recommended sensible limits in a typical week (Howse and Ghodse 1997). Older medical students may have an established disorder during medical school. Some medical schools have peer support programmes for students with substance-dependence problems (Myers 1997; Brookes 1995).

Prevention

Medical schools must be aware of selection pressures on would-be medical students and institute screening procedures to identify and deal with vulnerable applicants (Hays et al. 1996). As those with vulnerabilities generally become visible only as the course progresses, there should be health surveillance throughout (Brookes 1995). Medical students should be taught about suicide risk, with particular attention to drugs and alcohol (Hays et al. 1996). There should be greater emphasis throughout medical training on emotional and psychological development and practice (Wilhelm et al. 1997).

The responsibility for such teaching should not be left to psychiatrists or to the psychiatry module. There should be effective clinical role models at all stages of training (Wilhelm et al. 1997; Hays et al. 1996). Medical schools should have a variety of measures in place to integrate students into the life of the medical school and ensure effective support and counselling (for example, pairing with a more senior student, tutoring systems, social clubs, minority groupings) (Coombs and Virshup 1994). There should be rapid and easy access to counselling or health services.

Treatment

A biopsychosocial orientation is crucial when assessing and treating medical students (Myers 1997). There should be rapid and easy access to services (Myers 1997). In most cases, there will be a university health or counselling service with access to conventional general medical and psychiatric services. Alternatively students may consult their general practitioners. Students should not be assessed or treated by clinicians who are involved in their training (Myers 1997). Privacy and confidentiality must be respected (Myers 1997).

Students who develop serious mental illness should be managed along conventional lines. There will need to be careful supervision throughout the course and beyond, firstly, to ensure that patients are not put at risk, and secondly, to ensure that the student or new doctor remains able to cope.

Mental illness in doctors

Background

Doctors are a distinctive group in occupational health terms (Wrate and Baldwin 1997). They are more prone to anxiety/depression, suicide, and alcohol and substance misuse than comparable occupational groups, for example nurses, veterinarians, lawyers and accountants. None of these groups suffers the medical profession's twin afflictions of a comparatively high suicide rate and alcoholism with a remarkably low sickness absence rate.

Mental illness in doctors in general presents in the same way as elsewhere but is more often concealed. Many doctors are not registered with their own general practitioner and may prescribe for themselves or colleagues.

Doctors' working conditions create psychosocial stress and render them vulnerable to mental illness (Wrate and Baldwin 1997). These include excessive workloads, out-of-hours on-call duties extending throughout their careers, the relative inflexibility and competitiveness of medical career pathways, prolonged exposure to patients' pain and relatives' needs, unavailability of locum cover for sick leave, and ethos of stoicism and denial. "Presenteeism" is common: 80% of recently qualified doctors in one survey reported having worked through illness where they would have advised a friend or colleague to take time off (Baldwin et al. 1997). Doctors are deified and then blamed when, inevitably, solutions cannot be provided. Health service reforms have shifted power and control away from doctors, with consequent increase in stress.

Doctors fear loss of confidentiality and the stigma of mental ill health, particularly in career advancement and working relationships. Opportunities exist for unconventional behaviour such as self-medicating or prescribing.

There is currently a lack of rigour in the health surveillance of doctors. Outside the regular career structure, opportunities abound for anonymous locum work and unsupervised non-training posts. In private practice there are no constraints.

The nature of the problem and the type of intervention required tend to vary with the stage within the medical "life cycle". Amongst younger doctors, prevention and early intervention are important needs, whilst assessment and treatment take precedence in older doctors (Wilhelm et al. 1997).

Problems in young doctors

On graduating, young doctors acquire additional stress from sleep deprivation, overwork and disillusionment. Typical problems in the young doctor group (age 25–34) are adjustment to hospital life, anxiety and somatoform disorders, and alcohol and substance misuse.

The pre-registration year or intern year has been found repeatedly in surveys to be stressful. An Australian study (Hume and Wilhelm 1994) reported 8% of interns as seeking help during the year, with anxiety, depression and eating disorders as their main concerns, 3% had entertained (but not acted on) suicidal plans. Of the entire group, 72% had experienced significant episodes of anger. In another study, 79% of British house officers had experienced emotional distress, with over 50% of the females reported as becoming clinically depressed (Firth-Cozens 1990).

Problems in mid/late career

Mature doctors (age 35–55) commonly suffer from depression, alcohol and substance misuse/dependence and marital problems. In the older doctor (age 55+), common presentations are with depression, early physical and cognitive decline, alcohol dependence, and delusional disorder.

A random survey of doctors in which senior doctors were over-represented on the New South Wales Medical Register (Pullen et al. 1995) found that 26% had a condition warranting medical consultation, 18% had emotional disorders and 3%

alcohol problems. Almost a fifth reported mental problems. Under half had their own general practitioner.

According to the British Medical Association's Health Policy and Research Unit, up to a third of consultants and a half of GPs are currently showing signs of stress serious enough to affect their health and impair the quality of care to patients due to excessive workload and other factors (see Wrate and Baldwin 1997). Suicide rates are two to three times higher than in the general population.

Prevention

A BMA working party in 1998 reports that up to one in fifteen doctors have an addiction problem at some time in their career. The first step in seeking to improve the mental health of those in the medical profession must be to acknowledge and define the problem, before seeking to prevent the development of serious problems, at all stages in the training and career of doctors. In addition, the profession needs to have good systems for the detection, management and, occasionally, removal of doctors with mental health problems (Smith 1997).

From the earliest stages in the recruitment and training of doctors there should be greater emphasis on emotional wellbeing, including learning appropriate strategies to maintain psychological health and allow help-seeking behaviour. There should be more emphasis placed on developing communication time and anger management skills in the year after qualification. Psychiatrists are in a position to highlight issues with those responsible for the welfare of young doctors (Wilhelm et al. 1997).

The stigma of mental illness, both within and without the medical profession, remains highly resistant to change. Progress in this area is more likely to come from a change in emphasis to non-discrimination against those suffering from mental ill health, backed by legislation, in the same way as has been achieved in the area of race, physical disability and sexual orientation.

Effective occupational health schemes (including for general practitioners) should be available for screening, surveillance of vulnerable individuals and to encourage access for doctors with problems.

The Ritchie report, published in June 2000 following the inquiry into the work of Mr Rodney Ledward, has made wide-reaching recommendations to protect the public from unfit doctors. These include the assessment of all students starting medical courses and doctors changing jobs for their mental and physical suitability. Private health care should have the same standards of care as the NHS. How this might be achieved in practice has not yet been determined. The cultures of continuous professional development and revalidation, as proposed by the GMC, could be used to promote a sense of responsibility in doctors for their own wellbeing and that of colleagues. Working conditions should be improved. Coherent teamwork and good organisational practice are innovative and necessary developments to improve both quality of work and life for doctors (Firth-Cozens and Moss 1998).

Reduction in the stresses imposed by excessive workload currently experienced by senior British doctors would be achieved by implementing straightforward remedies: evaluating work demands and reviewing staffing levels, increasing the number of consultants, implementing the working time directive which caps hours at 48 per week, encouraging uptake of annual and study leave and organising properly trained locum cover. Consideration should be given to detecting and treating mental health problems in doctors who work as locums and in private health care.

The British Medical Association's Medical Students' Committee agreed at their annual conference that there should be random drug and drink tests performed on doctors and other health care workers, as in other professions, in order to protect the public and identify doctors with addiction problems at an early stage.

Management

Doctors willingly presenting should be referred, assessed and managed along conventional lines, although the nature of the medical profession is such that frequently this does not occur.

The situation commonly arises where it becomes apparent that a trainee or colleague is suffering from mental illness or a mental health problem but is either unaware of the need to seek treatment or unwilling to do so. Possible approaches in such situations are described by Brandon (1997). In the first instance the affected doctor should usually be approached in a sympathetic and private manner and encouraged to seek help in a conventional manner.

Many doctors are reluctant to consult their own GPs. There are a number of other support agencies which can be approached by the affected doctor, a close relative or a colleague. These include the Medical Council on Alcoholism, the National Alcohol Help Line, the National Association for Staff Support and the National Counselling Service for Sick Doctors. The last was set up in 1985 and deals with about 500 referrals annually, yet the majority of doctors are unaware of it (for details see Brandon 1997). In addition, many health regions have their own guidance and support units.

If these approaches are unsuccessful, formal procedures designed both to protect the public and to help the sick doctor may have to be invoked. It has been proposed that in each locality there should be a key individual nominated who will act as the first point of contact for doctors seeking advice (Nuffield Provincial Hospitals Trust 1996). He or she may be able to persuade the affected individual to seek help. Alternatively, the National Counselling Service for Sick Doctors (NCSSD) can be contacted, anonymously.

If further measures are required, at present the "three wise men" procedure can be invoked. (This is due to be revised to take account of new NHS structures.) The local medical community can convene a trio of "wise men" following the expression of concern about a colleague. If advice is rejected, action may be taken to protect patients. This may involve arranging suspension of the affected doctor and/or informing the GMC. The GMC itself may be approached directly and anonymously by any doctor wishing to discuss anxieties about a colleague. Formal notification of the GMC may result.

Formal measures to deal with seriously impaired doctors: the health procedures of the GMC

The GMC receives 2,500–3,000 enquiries each year from employers, patients and other doctors or from the police following criminal conviction (GMC 1998b). In 1997 the Fitness to Practice Policy Committee was established to co-ordinate policy in dealing with dysfunctional doctors. If the doctor in question seems to be seriously impaired because of ill health then the case will be referred to the health procedures, which have been in place since 1980. Almost all such cases involve mental illness or addiction.

Psychiatric presentations of sufficient severity to come to the attention of the GMC's health procedures or equivalent tend to be spread through the 20- to 40-year age group. Cases of drug self-administration tend to present in the 30- to 50-year age group and alcohol abuse slightly later. Problems in older doctors are likely to be under-reported. Many doctors have suffered from serious problems for years, often known to colleagues who have hesitated to take action. All information received by the GMC which suggests that a doctor is suffering from a health problem of any kind is considered by an appointed medical member of council known as the Screener for Health, who will decide whether there is evidence of a problem sufficiently serious to warrant formal action under the health procedures. Most doctors are willing to co-operate.

The health procedures are designed (i) to protect the public from doctors whose fitness to practise is seriously impaired on health grounds and (ii) to assist the doctors concerned in following a programme of medical supervision and rehabilitation. If further action is to be taken, the doctor is invited to agree to medical examination by at least two examiners chosen by the Screener. They are usually psychiatrists. Between 1980 and 1995, 606 doctors suffering from various impairments were asked to undergo examination (Table 1) (Kesteven et al. 1997).

Table 1. Impairment in doctors seen by GMC health screeners, 1980–1995

Impairing condition	Number	(%)
Alcohol only	168	(28)
Drugs only	104	(17)
Psychiatric illness only	147	(24)
Physical illness only	9	(1)
Illness involving two of the above	155	(26)
Illness involving three of the above	23	(4)
Total	606	(100)

If the examiners conclude that the doctor is fully fit to practise then the case will be closed. Otherwise they will make recommendations for the doctor's medical supervision and treatment, and perhaps to limit or prevent practice. If the doctor cooperates with this process, a system of monitoring is set up with the medical supervisor, who liaises with any consultant involved with treating or supervising the doctor. Supervision is likely to continue for a period of years, given that most doctors are suffering from relapsing conditions.

The outcome of the medical examinations conducted between 1980 and 1995 was as follows: 11% fit, 66% fit with limitations and 23% unfit (Kesteven et al. 1997). In 1997, 181 doctors were under supervision. Approximately 40–50 doctors are placed under or discharged from supervision annually (GMC 1998b).

Those few doctors unable or unwilling to cooperate with the voluntary procedures come under the jurisdiction of the Health Committee, referral to which can be made at any stage. In 1997, there were 39 doctors on its caseload. There were 4 new referrals, 13 doctors subject to conditional registration and 23 suspended (GMC 1998b).

The Medical (Professional Performance) Act 1995 enables the committee to impose indefinite suspension, once a doctor's registration has been suspended for a total period of not less than two years. By 1997 this power had been used in 13 cases (GMC 1998b).

The GMC has recently implemented wide-ranging reforms in its role as the regulator of the medical profession. Following legislation in 2002, a new Council was established on 1 July 2003, with 35 as opposed to 104 members. A new single complaints process will include "fitness to practise" cases. There is now available a pool of over 200 people who can be drawn upon to hear such cases. The same outcomes and sanctions continue to apply. Currently there is no backlog of cases waiting to be heard.

Conclusion

Mental illness generally in medical students and doctors is very common, and more so than in comparable professional groups and the general population. Of particular concern are the high rates of depression, suicide and addiction problems.

The reasons for this include the personality types of many doctors and medical students, selection pressures, neglect of emotional issues during training, stressful working conditions, and the expectations of society. The profession itself promotes concealment of mental health problems and inappropriate methods of treatment. Doctors are not empowered to take responsibility for their own health care.

There is growing awareness of these problems and considerable professional and public controversy over possible solutions. Although the duty of the medical profession is primarily to protect the welfare of patients, in recent years there has developed much greater concern over the identification, treatment and rehabilitation of sick doctors. However, it is clear that much more could and should be done to promote good mental health in practising doctors and the doctors of the future.

References

Baldwin PJ, Dodd M & Wrate RM (1997) Young doctors' health: how do working conditions affect attitudes, health and performance? *Social Science and Medicine* **45**: 34–40.

Brandon S (1997) Persuading the sick or impaired doctor to seek treatment. *Advances in Psychiatric Treatment* **3**: 305–11.

Brookes D (1995) The addicted doctor: caring professionals? [editorial]. *British Journal of Psychiatry* **168**: 149–53.

Coombs RH & Virshup BB (1994) Enhancing the psychological health of medical students: the student well-being committee. *Medical Education* **28**: 17–34.

Firth-Cozens J (1990) Sources of stress in women junior doctors. *British Medical Journal* **301**: 89–91.

Firth-Cozens J & Moss F (1998) Hours, sleep, teamwork, and stress. Sleep and teamwork matter as much as hours in reducing junior doctors' stress [editorial]. *British Medical Journal* **317**: 1335–6.

GMC (1998a) *Good Medical Practice*, 2nd edn. London: GMC.

GMC (1998b) *Annual Review (1998)*. London: GMC.

Hays LR, Cheever T & Patel P (1996) Medical student suicide, 1989–1994. *American Journal of Psychiatry* **153**: 553–5.

Howse K & Ghodse AH (1997) Hazardous drinking and its correlates among medical students. *Addiction Research* **4**: 355–66.

Hume F & Wilhelm K (1994) Career choice and experience of distress among interns. *Australian and New Zealand Journal of Psychiatry* **28**: 319–27.

Irvine D (1999) The performance of doctors: the new professionalism. *Lancet* **353**: 1174–7.

Kesteven S, Mann S & Sims A (1997) *Health Procedures of the General Medical Council (1997)*. 297–304.

Myers MF (1997) Management of medical students' health problems. *Advances in Psychiatric Treatment* **3**: 259–66.

Nuffield Provincial Hospitals Trust (1996) *Taking Care of Doctors' Health*. London: Nuffield Provincial Hospital Trust.

Pullen D, Lonie CE, Lyle DM et al. (1995) Medical care of doctors. *Medical Journal of Australia* **162**: 481–4.

Rana R, Smith E & Walkling J (1999) *Degrees of Disturbance: the New Agenda. The Impact of Increasing Levels of Psychological Disturbance Amongst Students in Higher Education. A Report from the Heads of University Counselling Services, Association for University and College Counselling*. Rugby: British Association of Counselling.

Smith R (1997) All doctors are problem doctors [editorial]. *British Medical Journal* **314**: 841–2.

Wilhelm K, Diamond M & Williams A (1997) Prevention and treatment of impairment in doctors. *Advances in Psychiatric Treatment* **3**: 267–74.

Wrate RM & Baldwin PJ (1997) Health of tomorrow's doctors: obstacles to appropriate health seeking. *Advances in Psychiatric Treatment* **3**: 290–6.

60 Stigmatisation of mentally ill medical students

Ruth White

In 1999 the General Medical Council published guidelines on the management of medical students' health and conduct. Within these guidelines they suggested that some physical and some psychiatric conditions might preclude acceptance for graduation as a doctor. Such conditions include depression, manic depression, psychosis, schizophrenia, anorexia nervosa, bulimia, and alcohol and drug abuse.

There are many publications reporting psychological ill health in medical students; in particular, anxiety and depression (usually measured on rating scales rather than standardised interviews). Many of the studies use the General Health Questionnaire. Firth (1986) found that 30–31% of medical students met the criteria of psychiatric caseness on the GHQ compared with 10% of a non-university peer group.

Anxiety

A recent survey of British medical students found that 39% had clinically significant levels of anxiety (Ashton and Kamali 1995). Clinically significant levels of anxiety were often reported in those studying for examinations, and also those whose anxiety stemmed from psychosexual problems. Other causes of anxiety included fear of failure, uncertainties about supervisors' expectations and uncertainties about performance.

In a longitudinal study of 173 Scottish medical students (Miller and Surtees 1991), 15 students were found to have high GHQ symptom levels throughout a six-month period; only one of these 15 students had sought professional help. Firth-Cozens (1987) suggested some degree of intolerance of psychiatric symptoms among the medical profession, and this may leave students reluctant to admit they are emotionally distressed. Tyrrell (1997) suggests that the climate in medical schools is changing and there is now interest in remedying stressful aspects of training and providing effective student support services.

Depression

There have been many studies of depression and suicidal ideation among students. In a four-year longitudinal study, Clark and Zeldow (1988) monitored depressive symptomology in a class of medical students. They found that at least 12% of the class scored above the threshold number of symptoms on the Beck Depression Inventory. They also concluded that the figure of 12% probably under-estimated the prevalence of depressive illness in the medical student population.

Alcohol and drug consumption

Ashton and Kamali (1995) report high rates of illicit drug use in medical students (49.2% used cannabis and 22% had tried other illicit drugs – this compares with figures in 1984 of 20.9% cannabis and 3.3% for other illicit drugs). They also report high levels of alcohol consumption (25.5% of those who drank alcohol exceeded recommended risk levels). Herzog et al. (1987) also found 17.5% of a 329 sample of medical students in Massachusetts to be at risk of substance disorders, of which approximately 6% were at high risk.

Other psychiatric conditions

There are no large studies of medical students who have developed serious psychotic illnesses during training. The rate of anorexia nervosa and other eating disorders is reported to be higher in female medical students than in the general population, but manic-depressive psychosis, schizophrenia and major depressive episodes are not reported to be found more frequently than in the general population. The latter conditions are those most likely to be cited by the GMC as to render the student unsuitable for graduation. It is, however, unlikely that a medical student with a psychotic illness would have experienced more than one or two episodes of illness during the training period, as most of these conditions do not have a particularly early onset (with average onset being in the early 20s). It is therefore quite difficult for a proper appraisal of the course of any such illness to be made prior to graduation. Furthermore, some of these illnesses run a relatively benign course, particularly with advances in treatment.

Of the many factors contributing to stigmatisation of medical students suffering from mental illness, the difficulty of the student's confidentiality being maintained must be included. This is often because students who are ill within their own medical school are frequently seen by psychiatrists attached to their medical school (although practices do sometimes include the facility for the student to be cared for out of area) and any medically serious incidents resulting from the illness, such as overdose or suicide attempts, may become the common currency of the hospital and of the student body. The recovery from psychiatric illness is made more difficult by peer-group knowledge of the illness and also by the attitudes of some doctors.

Discrimination at the beginning of a career may be particularly stressful, as the individual who has recovered from a mental ilness may find themselves justifying their medical history to an interview panel, despite such interviewing practice being strongly discouraged. On a more positive note, however, some Trusts have operated a positive discrimination policy for some years in respect of employment of people with mental illness or a history of mental illness.

References

Ashton CH & Kamali F (1995) Personality, lifestyles, alcohol and drug consumption in a sample of British medical students. *Medical Education* **29**: 187–92.

Clark DC & Zeldow C (1988) Vicissitudes of depressed mood during four years of medical school. *Journal of the American Medical Association* **260**: 1521–28.

Firth J (1986) Levels and sources of stress among medical students. *British Medical Journal* **292**: 1177–80.

Firth-Cozens J (1987) The stresses of medical training. In: Payne R & Firth-Cozens J (eds). *Stress in Health Professionals*. Chichester: Wiley.

Herzog DB, Borus JF, Hanbury P, Ott IL & Cercus A (1987) Substance use, eating behaviors and social impairment of medical students. *Journal of Medical Education* **62**: 651–7.

Miller P & Surtees PG (1991) Psychological symptoms and their course in 1st year medical students as assessed by the interval General Health Questionnaire. *British Journal of Psychiatry* **189**: 199–207.

Tyrrell J (1997) Mental health and student health professionals: a literature review. *British Journal of Occupational Therapy*, September **60**(9).

61 Law and stigma: Present, future and futuristic solutions

Jill Peay

Prohibition of discrimination

"The enjoyment of the rights and freedoms set forth in this Convention shall be secured without discrimination on any ground such as sex, race, colour, language, religion, political or other opinion, national or social origin, association with a national minority, property, birth or other status."

Article 14, European Convention on Human Rights

The relationship between legal provisions and stigma is both complex and paradoxical. Law can serve both to discriminate and to combat the urge to discriminate. Even the latter category of law can be stigmatising in its impact. Thus, the same legal instrument may embody conflicting objectives, as is illustrated by the European Convention on Human Rights (ECHR) cited above. Is mental disorder contained by implication in Article 14 (on the "prohibition of discrimination") within "other status"? At first sight, this would appear eminently defensible since enduring mental disability in its broadest sense is a status which one in five of us is likely to experience at some point in our lifetime. However, if it is included, it is paradoxical, for one need look no further than Article 5.1 (concerning the "right to liberty and security") to observe that although "Everyone has the right to liberty and security of person", persons of "unsound mind", together with alcoholics, drug addicts, vagrants and those suffering from infectious diseases, constitute an exception to this provision (under Article 5.1.(e)). What the law gives with one hand, it takes away with the other.

This chapter will first address how law might adopt a principled and overarching approach to de-stigmatising the relationship between law and mental health; secondly, it will reflect upon the more piecemeal and pragmatic approach which is most likely to be adopted in future legislation (and adopted probably only in part); third, it will briefly review some aspects of existing legislation which have been implemented to redress the stigma and discrimination that those with mental disorder currently experience; and finally, the chapter will reflect upon the intractable nature of addressing discrimination through law, when most relationships exist only in the shadow of the law, or in the context of a misperception of the law's ambit and requirements.

A principled approach

The relationship between law and discriminatory attitudes is potentially both circular and self-reinforcing. In the minds of the public, the very existence of law which is "special", in that it applies only to those suffering from mental disorder, might lead to an association between such disorders and the notion that people with mental disorder require exceptional powers to be applied to them because they in some way lack control over themselves. In turn, this can contribute to widespread perceptions that those with mental disorder pose a risk to others from their uncontrolled and uncontrollable actions. Indeed, research has demonstrated, at least amongst the American public (and there is no reason to assume that the populace of the UK has been immune to such shifts), that conceptions of mental illness frequently incorporate elements of violent behaviour, and do so more frequently now than they did in the 1950s (Link et al. 1999). Finally, such public misperception provides the basis for a political agenda whereby further discriminatory law is proposed to restrain the "dangerous mentally disordered" (see Eastman and Peay 1999; Home Office/Department of Health 1999).

Thus, if legislation is to address stigma it needs to finesse the paradoxical objectives of striving to normalise, without enhancing, by its mere presence, a net discriminatory effect in practice. This dilemma was confronted in the report of the Richardson Committee (Richardson 1999), the expert body set up by the Department of Health in 1998 to advise the Department on the scope of the necessary reforms to existing mental health legislation.

Richardson (1999) espoused the view that the principle of non-discrimination on grounds of mental ill health should lie at the heart of any reform of legislation. Further, the Report recognised that the current statute, namely, the Mental Health Act 1983 (MHA), was fundamentally discriminatory. One aspect of that discrimination was stark. People with a physical disorder could refuse medical treatment whatever the consequences of that refusal provided they had sufficient capacity to make that choice. By contrast, those with mental disorder could be compelled to accept treatment against their will even if they had made a capable decision to refuse. To permit, as does the MHA, the status of being a detained patient automatically to deprive one of the possibility of making capacitous and enforceable decisions about aspects of one's own mental health was fundamentally discriminatory and stigmatising.

To address this specific issue of discrimination, Richardson recommended the introduction of a capacity test to regulate decisions about the use of compulsory treatment. For those without the necessary capacity, the law should be there to provide for care and treatment in the absence of consent; for those with capacity, a refusal to undergo treatment should only be overridden where there was a real and serious risk to others (or possibly to themselves) and where the disorder could benefit from a compulsory health intervention. Although it might be argued (Zigmond and Holland 2000) that Richardson ducked the central issue, of pursuing parity between somatic (physical) and mental ill health through the introduction of an Incapacity Act encompassing both forms of disorder (whilst leaving risk takers and harm causers to be dealt with under the criminal justice system; see Matthews 1999; Bynoe and Holland 1999), it did make clear that in those areas where the law was to discriminate against the mentally disordered, it should do so only on clear and justifiable grounds (see Richardson 1999, paras 2.1–2.16).

Thus, at the heart of the Richardson proposals was the recognition that non-discrimination was tied up with patient autonomy; indeed, this central thrust of the Richardson proposals, that emphasis should be placed within a new statute on a patient's capacity, attracted overwhelming support amongst those consulted. Thus, Richardson recommended "wherever possible the principles governing mental health care should be the same as those which govern physical health" (para 2.15).

However, whilst the Richardson Committee had toyed with the notion of having a non-discrimination clause per se within the body of any new Act, they ultimately accepted that there was an inherent contradiction in elevating the principle of non-discrimination in a statute which would also permit the compulsion of individuals essentially on grounds of mental disorder. In this sense, they failed to solve the central dilemma outlined above. However, Richardson did recommend that the principle of non-discrimination be given considerable emphasis within the Code of Practice and that government be invited to address the issue of non-discrimination in relation to such specific areas as employment, travel, insurance, housing, education and the public representation of mental disorder (para 2.16).

A piecemeal approach

The government's response to the Richardson Committee's report was essentially negative (Peay 2000). They produced in turn first a Green Paper, then a White Paper and ultimately, the Draft Mental Health Bill 2000. These met with various degrees of hostility from practitioners and academics alike (see Peay 2003, Chapter 5), partly on the grounds that the various proposed criteria for the use of compulsion would have made it possible to place on a mental health section virtually anyone with a mental disorder. This would have had the effect of drawing the ambit of future legislation even more widely than the current MHA. Moreover, the proposals would have consigned both non-discrimination and patient autonomy to matters of guidance to be covered potentially, and only, in a Code of Practice. At the time of writing there is still no information about when a new Mental Health Act will be published, even though assurances were given to Parliament that one would be brought forward during the 2002–03 Parliamentary session.

Whilst the existing government proposals have given no reassurances about the need to address discrimination in legislation other than the MHA, for example in the areas of travel or insurance where discrimination may stem from having been detained under the MHA or having been subject to psychiatric ill health, two specific areas will serve to illustrate how the law has addressed or might address issues of unjustifiable discrimination and social exclusion – first, in relation to the right to vote (see Pedler 1999a), and second, in an area where the law remains in an unsatisfactory state, in respect of jury service (see Pedler 1999b).

It is notable that much of the fine detail of statutory discrimination persists not because it serves any useful purpose, but because time has not been devoted to its amendment or abolition. The right to vote is one good illustration where matters have been remedied. At present, under common law, the returning officer must be satisfied that a person offering themselves to vote is sufficiently compos mentis to discriminate between the candidates, to answer the statutory question "Are you the person whose name appears on the register of electors?" and to take the oath, if required so to do, in an intelligible manner. Whilst this is a capacity test which applies to us all, one wonders how rigorously it is enforced; my experience of voting has been one characterised by an exchange of grunts and the handing-over of my polling card. It is hard to know how the returning officer might know that I am compos mentis, or even whether I had read and understood the necessary literature so that I could "discriminate between the candidates".

Whilst forming a judgment under common law based on capacity is defensible (if largely ignored), real discrimination against the mentally disordered used to be embodied in statute law, where the legal entitlement to vote for detained patients had been rendered effectively meaningless by the need to register to vote when the electoral register was being complied. It used to be the case that detained patients could not use their hospital address as their residence, and, whilst health Service

Guidelines (1996) made plain that detained patients could register at their home address, those who had been detained for more than one year were effectively excluded. However, the Representation of the People Act 2000 has remedied this, making it possible for both detained patients and those resident in mental hospitals without detained status to be eligible to be registered to vote. Offenders detained subject to the MHA are, however, disenfranchised by s.2 of the 2000 Act, thereby placing them on the same footing as prisoners. Of course, eligibility to register to vote in theory and ensuring in practice that one's name appears on the register of electors are not the same thing; where patients are considered to lack the capacity to make decisions it is possible that staff will not facilitate their registration. If this were to happen, it would be regrettable – first because the threshold under common law for voting is so low (see above) and second because not only can a patient's capacity fluctuate, but the decision-making abilities required for different tasks will also vary.

Another area where people who are suffering (or who have suffered) from mental disorder may find themselves discriminated against, and which could be easily remedied, concerns jury service. Under s.1 of the Juries Act 1974 everyone between the ages of 18 and 70 who is on the electoral register (and this is not aproblematic, since it could constitute a form of indirect discrimination, see above) and who has been resident in the UK for at least five years, is liable to serve on jury unless they fall into one of the ineligible or disqualified categories. Ineligible means (1) the judiciary; (2) others concerned with the administration of justice, for example solicitors/barristers; (3) the clergy (and for these three categories it is a criminal offence to sit as a juror); and, finally, (4) mentally disordered persons. This last category is very broadly drawn and includes anyone who "suffers or has suffered from mental illness, psychopathic disorder, mental disorder, mental handicap or severe mental handicap and on account of that condition either (a) is resident in a hospital or other similar institution; or (b) regularly attends for treatment by a medical practitioner OR is under guardianship OR has been determined by a judge to be incapable, by reason of mental disorder, of managing and administering his/her property and affairs." As Pedler (1999b: at 148) questions, would (b) include those in receipt of anti-depressant medication or those who attended for quarterly appointments with a psychiatrist but who were not on medication? Again, the contrast with physical disability is pertinent. Here, it is now for the judge to determine whether, on account of disability, the person would not be capable of acting effectively as a juror (see s.9A of the Juries Act as amended by s.41 of the Criminal Justice and Public Order Act 1994). As Pedler points out, it would be simple enough to extend this recent positive presumption to mental as well as physical disability. However, the government has taken an entirely contrary line. For, whilst it makes sense in jurisprudential terms to persist with the first three categories of ineligibility, these are to be abandoned (see schedule 27 to the Criminal Justice Bill 2002). Yet, schedule 27 explicitly preserves the exclusion on eligibility on mentally disordered persons, thereby sustaining the very status-based discrimination so convincingly condemned by Pedler. Why is a case-by-case assessment by the judge deemed inappropriate?

A present and partial approach – positive rights

Attempts to combat discrimination on grounds of disability are embodied in the Disability Discrimination Act 1995. This Act makes "it unlawful to discriminate against disabled persons in connection with employment, the provision of goods, facilities and services or the disposal or management of premises"; it thus constitutes a positive attempt to protect those under a disability from discrimination. However, its definition of what constitutes a disability is narrowly drawn. Section 1(1) of the 1995 Act defines mental impairment as a disability where it has "a substantial and long term adverse effect on his ability to carry out normal day-to-day activities". Schedule 1 to the same Act further narrows the definition by including mental illness as a mental impairment only if the illness is a "clinically well-recognised illness" and where the adverse effect of the impairment has lasted or is likely to last for at least 12 months. This constitutes a marked contrast with the broad definitions used above where law is intended to exclude.

However, two recent employment law cases suggest there may be grounds for greater optimism. First, the Employment Appeal Tribunal held in the case of Goodwin v Patent Office (1999) that the "adverse effect" test could be satisfied even where a person was able to carry out day-to-day activities provided that the adverse effect was more than minor or trivial. Secondly, there is the case of Andrew Watkiss, reported in the *Guardian* (24 December 1999: 2). Watkiss had a history of schizophrenia; he argued that the John Laing Construction Group unlawfully discriminated against him in respect of their recruitment practises. They admitted that, in withdrawing their offer of appointment as Company Secretary on the "medical" grounds that the post would be too stressful for Mr Watkiss, they had unlawfully discriminated against him. Although the case does not set a legal precedent, since it was settled out-of-court rather than constituting a finding of the tribunal, the company's admission of culpability was written into the tribunal record. Moreover, whilst the level of compensation was kept confidential, it will most likely have been substantial as it would have included damages for injury to feelings and loss of future earnings. Employers should accordingly be on notice that people must be treated on their merits and not on the basis of stereotypical and stigmatising views; in turn, this positive message should encourage people with a disability to apply for jobs for which they are appropriately qualified, and not be deterred by the prospect of unfair treatment.

Finally, the European legal dimension may become increasingly important. The Treaty of Amsterdam 1997 embodies disability rights and, with the passage of the Human Rights Act 1998, which serves to incorporate parts of the ECHR into domestic legislation, a range of further avenues for redress will open up to those discriminated against on grounds of mental disorder (Fennell 1999). Moreover, whilst the ECHR is largely about protecting procedural rather than substantive rights, it might provide one method for challenging the treatment of patients with capacity detained under s.3 of the MHA (that is, those whose detention has not been authorised by a criminal court) since such treatment might constitute "inhumane or degrading treatment" under Article 3 of the ECHR. Indeed, Fennell (1999) has questioned whether enforced treatment in the community might constitute a violation of the right to family life under Article 8, thereby throwing the government's plans for a community treatment order into potential confusion.

Discrimination, law and stigma

There are three paradoxes at the heart of the relationship between law, mental health and stigma. First, where legislative provisions apply only to those suffering from mental disorder, even if those provisions include elements designed to protect the fundamental rights and freedoms of those with mental disorder (as does the MHA), they are fundamentally discriminatory. In the minds of the public, the very existence of special law can be stigmatising. Secondly, many laws discriminate in their fine detail either directly or indirectly against those suffering from mental disorder. However, this fine detailed discrimination probably does not stigmatise generally, since few people would be aware of the existence of these laws. It is only those individuals whose lives are touched who are stigmatised. Third, law can be internally contradictory. The Human Rights Act 1998, whilst trumpeting the arrival of non-discriminatory practices with its "Delphic words", in fact permits widespread discrimination against the mentally disordered because it adopts the broad and archaic language of the ECHR. Indeed, the government's wide-ranging proposals on dangerous severe personality disorder (Home Office/Department of Health 1999) would probably not be contrary to the ECHR, because the latter permits the detention of those suffering from "unsound mind" provided that they are deprived of their liberty in accordance with a procedure prescribed in law and provided that there is a means to challenge the lawfulness of that detention by a court (Article 5.4). Finally, it is noteworthy that a major report of the US Surgeon General (US Public Health Service 1999) which extensively addresses the roots of stigma, has very little to say about the role of law reform in this task. Perhaps this merely reflects an acceptance that whilst law might encourage people to be fair in their treatment of others, and may provide redress for those subject to unfair discrimination, the fundamentals of fair treatment lie in our attitudes towards others. Law may overtly attempt to rectify any imbalance, but its very presence may be as much counterproductive as beneficial.

References

Bynoe I & Holland A (1999) Law as a clinical tool: practising within and outwith the Law. In: Eastman N & Peay J (eds). *Law without Enforcement – Integrating Mental Health and Justice*. Oxford: Hart Publishing.

Eastman N & Peay J (eds) (1999) *Law without Enforcement – Integrating Mental Health and Justice*. Oxford: Hart Publishing.

Fennell P (1999) The third way in mental health policy: negative rights, positive rights, and the Convention. *Journal of Law and Society* 26: 103–27.

Goodwin v Patent Office (1999) *Industrial Cases Reports* 302.

Health Service Guidelines (1996) *Electoral Registration of Patients Detained under the Mental Health Act 1983*. HSG(96)43, 24 June. Department of Health.

Home Office/Department of Health (1999) *Managing Dangerous People with Severe Personality Disorder – Proposals for Policy Development*. London: HMSO.

Link B, Phelan J, Bresnahan M et al. (1999) Public conceptions of mental illness: labels, causes, dangerousness, and social distance. *American Journal of Public Health* 89: 1328–33.

Matthews E (1999) Mental and physical illness – an unsustainable separation? In: Eastman N & Peay J (eds). *Law without Enforcement – Integrating Mental Health and Justice*. Oxford: Hart Publishing.

Peay J (2000) Reform of the Mental Health Act 1983 – squandering an opportunity? *Journal of Mental Health Law* 2: 5–15.

Peay J (2003) *Decisions and Dilemmas: Working with Mental Health Law*. Oxford: Hart Publishing.

Pedler M (1999a) Citizens' rights? – Mental health and voting. *Journal of Mental Health Law* 1: 105–10.

Pedler M (1999b) Jury service and mental health. *Journal of Mental Health Law* 1: 148–9.

Richardson G (1999) *Review of the Mental Health Act 1983*. Report of the Expert Committee. London: Department of Health.

US Public Health Service (1999) *Mental Health: A Report of the Surgeon General*.

Zigmond A & Holland A (2000) Unethical mental health law; history repeats itself. *Journal of Mental Health Law* 2: 49–56.

62 The World Psychiatric Association global programme against stigma and discrimination because of schizophrenia

Norman Sartorius

The stigma attached to mental illness is pervasive. Mental illness is considered untreatable and treatments used in mental health services are seen as inefficient and dangerous. Mental hospitals are viewed with horror, and staff working in psychiatric services are portrayed as being mentally abnormal, incompetent, corrupt or evil. Medicaments that are proposed for the treatment of mental illness are viewed with profound suspicion and their use and side effects monitored with much more zeal than other drugs. Stigmatisation does not stop at the person who has a mental illness: it spreads to the family and remains present across generations.

The stigma attached to mental illnesses is the main obstacle to the provision of mental health care. It affects the priority which is given to the development of mental health services and makes the discipline less attractive than others to the medical graduate in search of a career. It prevents timely contact of the person suffering from a mental illness with mental health services and makes rehabilitation exceedingly difficult. It has a negative impact on the geographical placement of mental health services and reduces the availability of research funding for psychiatry.

It is for this the reason that the World Psychiatric Association (WPA) has made the fight against stigma and discrimination due to schizophrenia one of its institutional projects and given it a high priority. Schizophrenia was selected as the main target for the programme because it is the most stigmatised of all mental illness. It is expected, however, that the experience gained in the programme will be helpful in the development of programmes that deal with all mental illness and indeed with other stigmatised illnesses.

The programme was started in late 1996 and its launch coincided with the XI World Congress of Psychiatry in 1999. There are several features of the programme which make it unique:

1. The programme is built on the basis of information received from patients and their families. This information is combined with results of surveys of attitudes to mental illness and persons suffering from it. The surveys cover segments of the general population or its representative samples.
2. The programme is multi-centric and international. Nineteen countries are participating now and others are likely to join in the near future. The first, pilot site was in the province of Alberta, Canada. Soon after that the programme was initiated in Spain and Austria. In the third group of participating countries are centres in Egypt, Germany, Greece, India and Italy. Groups in Brazil, Chile, the

Czech Republic, Japan, Kenya, Morocco, Poland, Romania, Slovakia, the UK and the USA joined the programme next.

3. The programme has a fixed sequence of steps (developed on the basis of experience gained in the pilot phase) but it is flexible in terms of timing the steps.

4. The programme is cumulative: the experience of the first set of centres is put at the disposal of the newcomers, whose experience in turn will be added to the materials for the next group of centres so that each of the groups joining the programme can examine the experience obtained and use or adapt the products of the programme from the different countries.

5. The programme is multi-sectoral. In addition to mental health workers and other representatives of the health sector, it seeks to involve organisations of families and people suffering from mental illness, government authorities, various community organisations, industry, educational institutions, the media and the legislators.

The programme has a governing structure composed of a Steering Committee which coordinates and links the Working Groups developing the material for its use, the centres in which the work is done and the agencies supporting it,[1] for example the societies of psychiatrists in the countries concerned. The materials produced so far include a set of guidelines for the conduct of the programme, a description of schizophrenia in which the features of the illness and its treatment that are of particular importance for the creation or maintenance of stigma are given particular emphasis, a set of descriptions of programmes undertaken in the past to fight stigma, a "toolbox" containing materials developed in this programme and elsewhere (e.g. videotapes, posters, etc.), and annual reports of the work done so far in the centres participating in the WPA programme. Papers in scientific journals as well as a training manual and a bibliography are also available.

The strategy of relying, in the selection of targets, on reports from families and patients and on first establishing the feasibility of projects resulted in differences in the focus of action and in the type of interventions in the centres. The Canadian centre, for example, has youngsters aged 15–17 and staff of emergency health centres as target groups of the programme; in India the staff of primary health care facilities was addressed with a series of educational activities; in Spain, the targets in the beginning of the programme were psychiatrists and other mental health service personnel; in Austria the general public was addressed through a media campaign; and in Italy shopkeepers in the area of the project were among the first groups whose attitudes were addressed. In each instance the programme does not intend to stop after the first target group has been reached; instead, work with population groups rather than with the total population serves to test the project teams' structure and organisation and to allow tailoring the interventions to a particular group rather than applying blunderbuss educational approaches, which have been shown to be of little cost-effectivenes and can even have negative results. It is expected that the teams will add targets to their programme, in accordance with their resources and the experience gained in the beginning of their work.

The work in a centre is usually started by a small group that takes the initiative and composes a larger group in which there are representatives of the health care system,

[1]   Steering Committee: J Arboleda Flores, A Okasha (President), JJ Lopez Ibor, N Sartorius (Scientific Director), C Stefanis, N N Wig. Chairmen of the Working Groups: W Fleischhacker, H Haefner, J Leff, R Warner. Members of the Working Groups are from 22 countries.

the social sector, business and industry, family and patient organisations, the clergy, the media, and other key members of the community. The groups have a working character, members taking on different tasks and reporting back to the group, which meets at regular intervals.

An evaluation of the effects of the programme, carried out a year after it began, has been undertaken in Canada, the first of the centres to start work. The results have been encouraging: there was a clear change of attitude in the target groups and several of the measures that were developed for application in the programme have been instituted. The experience gained in the work with emergency services helped to develop proposals for the work of these services that have been formally introduced in the country as a whole and the materials produced in the course of the work with the adolescent groups have been used in Canada and in other countries with success. Other centres have undertaken an evaluation of their results, and these are being published.

The WPA programme against stigma and discrimination because of schizophrenia has created a website (openthedoors.com) that is frequented by many, probably witnessing the interest that individuals and organisations worldwide have in developing programmes dealing with stigma – this undoubtedly most difficult obstacle to the improvement of care for people suffering from mental illness and to a better quality of their life and of the life of their families.

63 Mind's Respect Campaign – an overview

Melba Wilson

Context

The Respect Campaign ran from 1997 to 2001. Its central mission was to reduce discrimination on mental health grounds, including multiple discrimination. It was a broad-based campaign around a single theme.

Broad-based campaigns, with a number of targets, can:

- take account of the complexity of what actually creates change: for instance, new law alone, if not accompanied by pressure for changes in local practice, is ineffective in areas where policy is largely delegated to local commissioners/practitioners. Choosing several targets – if change really is dependent on all of them – can make change deeper and more lasting. Mind's Stress on Women Campaign is an example: by targeting Government, parliament, professional bodies, the media and local services, there was a cumulative effect, which shifted both policy and practice (Sayce 1996);
- facilitate an entrepreneurial approach, enabling people locally and nationally to link into the campaign in a variety of ways and to develop new, creative ideas.

The Respect Campaign

The aims of the Respect Campaign were to "increase opportunities for users of mental health services to be part of communities, workplaces, families, social circles – and to reduce the rejections that keep so many people trapped on the social margins."

The peg for the campaign was to promote "a fair deal":

- in the public eye
- in working life
- as citizens

In the public eye

The goal was that by 1999, Mind aimed to have created a measurable shift in media coverage, with less "mad axeman" and stereotyped coverage, and more examples which illuminate the different realities of people's lives. Mind also aimed to have implemented an effective schools education programme.

In working life

The goal was that by 1999, Mind aimed to have increased knowledge amongst employers of "reasonable adjustments" in the workplace and good practice generally for people with mental health problems, to have informed the public that disability discrimination law includes mental health service users, and to have built the basis of a strategy to increase the employment rates for service users. (Note that "reasonable adjustment" is the term used in the Disability Discrimination Act (DDA), 1995, for flexible working hours, additional support at work and other adaptations to improve access to work for people defined as "disabled" under the Act.)

As citizens

The goal was that by 1999, Mind aimed to have succeeded in extending anti-discrimination law, through lobbying and test cases; and to have publicised the realities of discrimination to the general public.

Some of the achievements were:

- *A fair deal in working life* – including work on Employment.
  This resulted in:
  (a) The publication of *How to Survive Working Life*, a training pack for employers and information booklet for employees (May 2000).
  (b) Setting up Work Net – to promote employment opportunities for people with mental health problems.
- *A fair deal as citizens* – incorporating:
  (i) The Arts initiative – September/October 1999 (posters and postcards were distributed nationally through regional offices, Diverse Minds and Mindlink.)
  (ii) Older People – which included a Debate of the Age contribution (1999/2000).
  (iii) Mental Health Act Review work, which resulted in the publication of *Mind the Law*, Mind's authoritative response to the government's consultation on the Mental Health Act Review (1999); and work with other mental health organisations – including formation of the Mental Health Alliance – to influence new legislation.
  (iv) Social Inclusion (Phase 1) – including publication of a comprehensive report *Creating Accepting Communities*, on the social exclusion of people with mental health problems (November 1999).
  (v) Social Inclusion (Phase 2) – Developing and promoting good practice – based on the *Creating Accepting Communities* report (April 2000) and ongoing.
- *A fair deal in the public eye* – incorporating:
  The Campaign to Complain – about mental health in the media. This was launched in November 1999.

Impact

It has been noted that campaigning is a difficult activity to evaluate because (a) reliable indicators of progress are often hard to find and (b) social change is typically caused by a complete set of inter-related events and a direct causal link between campaign actions and a change in the policy or practice of the target is often difficult to establish (Lattimer 1994). There are, however, some parameters to which we can look in the Respect Campaign to at least begin to contextualise its impact.

Tangible changes

The impact of a campaign can be gauged on the basis of the tangible gains or activity associated with it (e.g. the number of events held nationally, locally and regionally, number of mentions/stories in the media, number of enquiries, etc.) These are largely to do with issues of visibility – for Mind, for raising and providing information on the issue.

Examples of the Respect Campaign's success in this area include:

- The launch of *Not Just Sticks and Stones* (1996 – stigma and discrimination); *Tall Stories in the Backyard* (1997 – nimbyism), and *Raised Voices* (1997 – issues for black and minority ethnic communities) – all of which generated high-profile national, regional and local attention and media coverage on the multiplicity of stigma and discrimination faced by a range of mental health service users.
- The Arts Project – produced posters and postcards and a Year 2000 calendar which were widely distributed and informative and served to raise the profile of Mind and the needs of people with mental health problems in general. In Mind's Northern Region, for example, the police commissioned their own reprint of the languages poster to go up in police stations. The project work also promoted positive aspects of mental health.
- The Campaign to Complain has attracted more than 300 groups and individuals on to the network and has issued alerts aimed at countering stigma and discrimination in the media.
- In Mind Cymru there was wide media coverage for "Ten Tips for Employers" on discrimination at work, increased work on mental health awareness addressing race and culture, as well as rural issues.
- The Education Pack was launched in September 1999 and achieved national media coverage. Copies were sent to named teachers in 4000 schools, and by agreement with the Qualifications and Curriculum Authority to 220 schools involved in piloting NVQ Health and Social Care. Publicity material was sent to all other schools in England.
- A related collaboration took place with the Health Education Authority to run the "Stigma Partnership" aimed at addressing issues of stigma and discrimination around mental health issues which are prevalent amongst the 16 to 24 age group.

In this context, Liz Sayce (formerly Mind's Policy Director) has noted that "the campaign has succeeded in its ambition to use a relatively small amount of money – £30,000 – to spearhead change and harness energies to a common purpose", and that its first year revealed "a huge wealth of activity at local and national level".

Intangible change

The other aspect on which a campaign's success or failure can be judged is more *intangible* – the extent to which public opinion is changed, the degree to which the public policy agenda is changed, and the degree to which alliances shift and partnerships emerge.

Though the intangibles may be less overt, and more within the realm of subjectivity, there is evidence, nevertheless, to suggest that the Respect Campaign's impact can again be felt. Examples of this include:

- Increased links with the disability movement, which in turn helps to ensure that mental health is considered a natural part of that agenda.
- The Creating Accepting Communities Inquiry and its effect in raising issues of social exclusion/inclusion (and thereby awareness of the impact on people with mental health problems) across a wide range of constituencies – including the statutory sector, business, religious groups and government.
- Influencing and working with psychiatric professionals, e.g. the Royal College of Psychiatrists' Changing Minds Campaign, launched in October 1998.

- Likewise collaboration with the World Psychiatric Association's educational programme to reduce the stigma and discrimination faced by people with a diagnosis of schizophrenia was also an aspect.
- The Campaign to Complain, it can be argued, has contributed to greater awareness about how common the incidence of people being in mental distress is. It has helped to foster the view that it is no longer acceptable to use (or at the very least that there should be a degree of discomfort about using) negative or disparaging terms in the media. Mind's press office, for example, complained about the title of a Channel 4 series "Psychos", and was consulted about an advertising campaign associated with it. In the longer term, such input can be expected to impact favourably on public opinion, through more positive portrayals of people with mental health problems.
- Mental Health Act Review – Mind's response to this review and the associated consultations, networking (both at a grassroots and Parliamentary level), as well as raising the issues regarding compulsory treatment in the community at ministerial level has served to broaden the public policy agenda. To a large extent, the stance we have taken in our work around the review has helped to create a climate in which those who would argue *for* compulsory treatment can no longer do so on the basis that it is the obvious solution. It can be argued that we have extended the parameters of the debate to ensure that the needs of people with mental health problems (even if some of those people are "difficult") nevertheless should be taken into account in a real and meaningful way; and in such a way that their human rights are not disregarded or violated.
- The Mind Inquiry – with its theme of "Creating Accepting Communities", has also served to broaden public understanding of the complexities of social exclusion/inclusion for people with mental health problems. The Inquiry has also helped to change the focus from merely being one of *exclusion* to that of *inclusion*.
- The Fair Deal in Working Life Employment Project tackles stigma and discrimination on the economic front – with the publication of a training pack to educate employers about good practice and the setting up of a net – work to foster employment opportunities for people with mental health problems.
- Yellow Card – work aimed at highlighting side effects of medication from a user perspective (First report 1998; Second report with a focus on black and ethnic communities, 2001).
- Creating Accepting Communities (Phase II of the Respect Campaign): Social Inclusion. The Cyber Café Project involved creating a sustainable model of community development, working between local agencies in the London Borough of Merton. Outcomes included 52 mental health service users and 11 staff trained in IT skills, improved access to further education for mental health service users, and ongoing partnership working between agencies.

References

Sayce L (1996) Campaigning for change. In: Abel K et al. (eds). *Planning Community Mental Health Services for Women.* London: Routledge.

Lattimer M (1994) *The Campaigning Handbook.* Directory of Social Change.

64 Introduction to The Royal College of Psychiatrist's Campaign

Arthur Crisp

The Royal College of Psychiatrists has embarked upon a 5-year long Campaign to combat the stigmatisation of people with mental illnesses. The Campaign was launched in October 1998 after a year of planning, coupled with a survey of public opinions concerning people with any of the six mental illness categories being addressed (anxiety disorders, depression, schizophrenia, dementia, eating disorders, and drug and alcohol addiction/misuse). The results of this survey are outlined in Chapter 3 of this book and have also been published in the medical press (Crisp et al. 2000). They have provided for us a baseline of reported opinions concerning the mentally ill. A repeat survey, using the same methodology and instruments, was conducted in July 2003. When these data are available, comparisons will be made with the 1998 profiles. We are not expecting any great changes in reported public opinions at this point, even though several nationwide campaigns, apart from our own, are currently afoot. If there are any changes, interpretation of them will be difficult!

We are aware that even temporarily changing public attitudes fuelled by traditional fears, often reinforced by the media, often also against a background of avoidance of personal contact with people known to have or to have had a mental illness, is especially difficult.

During this last five years a range of Campaign instruments has been produced. The contributions that follow give an indication of these. They are held within the Campaign toolkit (see the appendix to this chapter) on www.changingminds.co.uk. Advertisement of this site on London Underground tube cards during July 2002 temporarily increased the hit rate six-fold. It remained at two-fold the pre-advertisement level after the cards had been taken down. We regard it as being of paramount importance to keep the website address in the public eye, and are continuing to try to fund further and more widespread advertisement of it. It is also designed to attract an optimal number of people browsing the Internet for related topics. The site is intended as the Campaign's legacy and will be maintained by the College for the future.

We believe that pursuit of goals such as underwrite our present campaign, to reduce stigmatisation of people with mental illnesses and consequent discrimination against them, needs to endure. Only then may appropriate public attitude changes develop within current and future generations. The Royal College of Psychiatrists aims to continue to play its part in this process.

References

Crisp AH, Gelder MG, Rix S, Meltzer HI & Rowlands OJ (2000) Stigmatisation of people with mental illnesses. *British Journal of Psychiatry* 177: 4–7.

Appendix: Changing Minds Campaign – Toolkit

Changing Minds – Every Family in the Land is a five-year campaign co-ordinated by the Royal College of Psychiatrists. Launched in 1998, it aims to increase public and professional understanding of mental health problems and reduce the stigma and discrimination associated with them. The Campaign is focusing on six of the most common mental health problems:

- Anxiety – affects more than 1 person in 10
- Depression – affects 1 person in 4
- Schizophrenia – affects 1 person in 100
- Dementia – affects 1 person in 5 over 80
- Alcohol and drug addiction – affects about 1 person in 3
- Eating disorders – affects 1 person in 50

Websites

(i) Campaign websites

www.changingminds.co.uk
The Changing Minds Campaign website, with information about the Campaign and all its materials.

www.stigma.org/everyfamily
80-author, 200,000-word, electronic book, "Every Family in the Land". An in-depth study of the stigmatisation of people with mental illnesses.

(ii) Other recommended websites

Information about other recommended websites on mental health and stigma. Available on www.changingminds.co.uk.

Videos

Campaign videos

(i) *Stigma* Campaign video (9 minutes). The origins and nature of the stigma of mental illness. A useful tool for those interested in stigma and for educational events. Aimed at mental health professionals and the general public. VHS video copies available at £5 from leaflets@rcpsych.ac.uk.

(ii) *1 in 4*. A two-minute film, originally made for showing in cinemas, using challenging images to question our preconceptions about mental illness. Aimed at young people aged 15–25. VHS video copies available at £5 from leaflets@rcpsych.ac.uk

Materials to download from the campaign websites

(i) General information available on www.changingminds.co.uk

Information about mental disorders. Seven illustrated leaflets, challenging people's attitudes towards those suffering from anxiety, depression, anorexia and bulimia, schizophrenia, Alzheimer's disease, or drug and alcohol addiction. Aimed at the general public.

Stigmatising suicide – Can our attitudes help prevent it? Report on the ethical issues relating to suicide, our attitudes towards people who are suicidal, and what we can do to help.

Creativity and mental disorder. A 37-page illustrated report, discussing the relationship between creativity and mental disorder.

Personality disorder and its treatment. Article about personality disorder and the ethics of treatment.

Opinion survey. National survey of public attitudes, carried out for the Campaign by the Office for National Statistics, 1998. The results showed that stigmatising attitudes were common. A full analysis of the survey, published in the *British Journal of Psychiatry* 2000; **177**: 4–7 can be downloaded.

References to published articles. The Campaign has promoted research and discussion about stigma in the medical press. A list of references to over 70 published articles is available.

Declaration of Intent. Numerous individuals, organisations and voluntary groups have backed the Changing Minds Campaign by signing our Declaration of Intent. Signatures continue to be invited. Available on www.changingminds.co.uk.

(ii) General research and information available on www.stigma.org/everyfamily

Every Family in the Land. Internet book about the stigmatisation of mental illnesses. Aimed at healthcare professionals, academics, service users/providers and the general public. Available on www.stigma.org, and on CD-Rom from booksales@rcpsych.ac.uk (price £11.75).

Printed campaign materials and multi-media resources

(i) For children and young people

Reading Lights. Colourful books for Primary School children (aged 4–7), addressing what it is like to be different, and providing a framework for parents, social workers, teachers etc, to support children. Available from Book Sales, Royal College of Psychiatrists (£12 per set of 4 books). E-mail booksales@rcpsych.ac.uk.

Changing Minds. A multi-media CD-Rom on mental health, for young people aged 13–17 years. For use by teachers as part of the PSHE curriculum (key stages 3 and 4). Contains interviews, articles, video and audio clips, cartoons, music and quizzes, as well as practical information on where to go for help. Available from Book Sales, Royal College of Psychiatrists (price £14.99). E-mail booksales@rcpsych.ac.uk.

HEADstuff. A colourful leaflet for 14- to 17-year-olds, to increase their understanding of mental health problems. For a free copy e-mail to leaflets@rcpsych.ac.uk. Details of bulk orders on request.

Caring around the Clock. A colourful 16-page booklet to help young carers cope with the pressures they face. Available free of charge from leaflets@rcpsych.ac.uk.

(ii) For the general public

Changing Minds: our lives and mental illness. An illustrated book, with personal stories and commentaries from people who have experienced mental health problems. The book describes the impact of mental health problems on individuals and their families, and how they can learn to get on with their lives. Available from Book Sales, Royal College of Psychiatrists (price £10). E-mail booksales@rcpsych.ac.uk.

(iii) For medical professionals

Mental illnesses: stigmatisation and discrimination within the medical profession.
Joint report between the Royal College of Psychiatrists, the BMA and the Royal
College of Physicians, on the stigmatisation of people with mental illnesses by
doctors. Available from Book Sales, Royal College of Psychiatrists (Council Report
CR91, price £7.50). E-mail booksales@rcpsych.ac.uk.

Leaflets for GPs. "Time wasters... does it ring a bell?" Published in conjunction
with the Campaign Roadshows for GPs and primary healthcare workers, held
throughout the UK. For further information about the leaflets or the Roadshow, e-mail
stigma@rcpsych.ac.uk.

(iv) Relating to the media

Guide for Journalists and Broadcasters Reporting on Schizophrenia. Booklet with
facts about schizophrenia, including its diagnosis, treatment, the risk of violence and
correct terminology. Produced in association with the National Union of Journalists.
Available from The Lilly Neuroscience Bureau, c/o Huguenot House, 35–38 St
Stephen's Green, Dublin 2, Republic of Ireland.

Practical guidance on responding to the media. Fact-sheet providing information on
how to complain about inaccurate representation of mental illness in the media. For
use by College members and the general public. Available from External Affairs
Department, Royal College of Psychiatrists. E-mail stigma@rcpsych.ac.uk.

(v) Bookmarks

Laminated bookmarks, with the Campaign website address and the wording "Stop.
Think. Understand. Campaign to reduce the stigma of mental disorders". Available
free of charge. E-mail stigma@rcpsych.ac.uk.

Posters

For the general public

Posters created to advertise the campaign on London Underground (30 cm × 64 cm;
also in A4 versions). Colourful posters with the wording "STOP. THINK.
UNDERSTAND. 1 in 4 of us will suffer from a mental illness in our lifetime. But many
will also face isolation, prejudice & rejection as a result of stigmatisation. Mental
illness affects all of us." Promotes the campaign website www.changingminds. co.uk.
For copies e-mail leaflets@rcpsych.ac.uk.

A3-size posters. Colour posters with the wording "STOP. THINK. UNDERSTAND.
Every family in the land can be affected by mental health problems. Increase your
understanding of mental health problems and reduce stigma and discrimination". For
copies e-mail leaflets@rcpsych.ac.uk.

For further information about the Changing Minds Campaign and its toolkit, please contact:

Head, Department of External Affairs, Royal College of Psychiatrists, 17 Belgrave
Square, London SW1X 8PG.
Tel: 0207 235 2351 ext 127,   e-mail: dhart@rcpsych.ac.uk.

65 Getting our own house in order – The Doctors' Project: Background

Tom Arie

It was brave of our College to open up the uncomfortable topic of our own prejudices, and to invite others to join us in looking at them. Rather than previewing our report, what follows is a short personal essay.

Doctors don't like every patient they see. Many don't like chronic or recurrent illness. On the whole, we prefer cures, and grateful patients. But that simply means we are human – a precious attribute! What really matters is that we should know our prejudices. Worst of all is to be influenced by prejudices which we don't realise we have. We psychiatrists know that insight doesn't come easily – insight is, after all, our métier! God protect us from doctors who are sure they have no prejudices.

The literature on our topic is not large. A *BMJ* headline in 2000 read "Discrimination 'rife' against mental health patients". The study reported there (Mental Health Foundation 2000) found that once a patient acquires the label "psychiatric", some doctors' minds will snap shut: in such patients, symptoms of physical illness were often not taken seriously, being instead attributed to mental causes – frustrating to the sufferer, and occasionally disastrous. But prejudice is more pervasive than that.

Multiple jeopardy

As a psychogeriatrician, I know the double stigma of old age and mental illness. But some patients face multiple discrimination – on account of mental illness, certainly, but often also because of race, age, sex, or sexual orientation; or because of the nature of their illness, as when the patient may be perceived as blameworthy, or as dangerous; and, as we have realised since Hollingshead and Redlich's work in the fifties (1958), because of social class. To such a list we might add features such as homelessness, or personal appearance – mode of dress, say, or hairstyle, or tattoos or body piercing. When there is social distance between doctor and patient, prejudice very easily slips in.

Optimism

Our group never forgot how much has changed for the better. Perceptions and understanding of mental illness and of psychiatry, and education, staffing, location and fabric of facilities – all have been transformed in our time. Read Kathleen Jones or Roy Porter, or *A Century of Psychiatry* (Freeman 1999).

The arts and the serious media, at their best, have had great influence for good, though little is more awful than the populist media at their worst. The roots of prejudice go deep; at times they lie undisturbed, at others they erupt in unexpected places. Thus, there is food for thought in the recent case of Pinochet. Alas, his career is not unique, but he probably is unique in modern times in that when his mental state in relation to "fitness to plead" was officially examined by an appointed team of specialists, it was not considered necessary to include a psychiatrist.

Yet psychiatry is part of mainstream medicine now, in the curriculum, in the general hospital, and in corridors of medical power. Anthony Clare and Raj Persaud are media celebrities. We have had psychiatrist deans, vice-chancellors, a psychiatrist Chief Medical Officer; psychiatrist professors are everywhere. Who knows, the day may come when there is a titular "Royal Psychiatrist".

But if all were well, there would be no need for our working party. So here is a "map" (Table 1) of some of our concerns. There isn't time to say much more about them.

Table 1. A project "map"

Prejudice
- by doctors in general
- by psychiatrists
- by doctors towards doctors with mental illness
- by doctors against psychiatry and psychaitrists

Combating prejudice in doctors
- selection of students
- education of students
- postgraduate and continuing education of:
  - all doctors
  - psychiatrists

Action/publicity
- What to do?
- Whom to target?
- How?
- The media

Aptitudes and attitudes

Student selection has high priority – a vexed question, and it is to our profession's credit that we worry so much about it. (For my generation a main asset for entry to medicine was to be from a medical family – one was actually asked about family connections, though alas I had none to declare.)

Two points must suffice here: most doctors encounter mental illness, whether or not they take a special interest in it. So the ability to accept it and to respond appropriately must surely be among the required attributes of all doctors. It is not enough to measure just intelligence, as Arthur Crisp long ago pointed out (Crisp 1984). In this context no studies are more significant than those of Henry Walton's group (e.g. Walton 1966). I found it valuable to revisit that work, and I commend it to anyone who may not know it.

Walton defined a "typology" of students and doctors – the "physically minded", who have little tolerance of uncertainty and who yearn for "closure", and the "affective" or "psychologically minded", who are able to accept and who even warm to the uncertainties and subjectivities inherent in "human" problems. Clearly, there is little place for the former anywhere in medicine, and certainly not in psychiatry.

Students and doctors with mental illness

A word about students and practitioners who have been or who become mentally ill. We found no evidence that medical schools discriminate against prospective students who are known to have a history of mental illness, though we should be surprised if that did not sometimes happen. Nor did we hear of students being made arbitrarily to discontinue their course on grounds of mental illness per se. And we noted the growing acceptance of support services for doctors in difficulty. But one principle, obvious as it is to us, can do with being spelled out, as a lynchpin of our campaign.

It is that "mental illness" is a portmanteau of disorders as various in their nature and significance as all other illnesses or disabilities. In the context of suitability for a job, what matters is how the illness or disability might bear on the needs of the job. Mental problems are no different in this from physical; they must be appraised sympathetically, confidentially and realistically, simply in relation to how they might affect ability to do the job safely and effectively. Happily, there is now protection in law against discrimination in the workplace.

Finally: Education. The General Medical Council (1987) now requires that all doctors should have good communication skills, awareness of ethical issues, insight into their own personality and values, and compassion and concern for the patient.

To identify and foster such essential and precious attributes, at all points from selection for medicine to the life-long learning of doctors – *that* remains, as it long has been, our target. It is time we stopped just aiming, and actually hit the bull's-eye.

References

Crisp A (1984) Selection of medical students – Is intelligence enough? *Journal of the Royal Society of Medicine* **77**: 35–9.

Freeman H (ed.) (1999) *A Century of Psychiatry*. London: Mosby-Wolfe.

General Medical Council (1987) *Recommendations on the Training of Specialists*. London: GMC.

Hollingshead AB & Redlich FC (1958) *Social Class and Mental Illness*. New York: Wiley.

Mental Health Foundation (2000) Pull Yourself Together. (Quoted in *British Medical Journal* 2000; 1163.)

Walton HJ (1966) Differences between physically-minded and psychologically-minded medical practitioners. *British Journal of Psychiatry* **112**: 1097–102.

66 Getting our own house in order – The Doctors' Project: The report

Arthur Crisp

In Chapter 65 Tom Arie has mapped out the issues to be addressed by this working party. The Management Committee was emphatic that it would ill behove psychiatrists exclusively to aspire to scold the rest of the medical profession on these matters. Such behaviour would be likely to be counterproductive! Moreover, psychiatrists can be as stigmatising and negatively discriminatory as other doctors in respect of people with mental illness. The working party included users and was otherwise constituted so as to be as representative of the medical profession as possible. We were fortunate to secure full participation of the British Medical Association and the Royal College of Physicians. In addition the Royal College of General Practitioners agreed to a collaborative role, and representatives of the Department of Health and Royal College of Nursing attended as observers. My task, briefly, is to summarise the consequent report and indicate how it can be accessed.

The document is labelled CR91 (College Report No. 91). It comprises five sections and an executive summary. The first two sections address the background to the matter. The subsequent three sections respectively focus on details of expected (statutorily determined) medical practice, evidence concerning current recruitment patterns, education and ongoing training of doctors, and, finally, Recommendations. The background to these Recommendations and the Recommendations themselves, five in number, are as follows:

Recommendations (Reproduced with permission from the Royal College of Psychiatrists)

Background

The task is huge – but that must not be an excuse for not beginning. Dealing with prejudice on the part of doctors against patients, medical students, juniors, and colleagues with a history of mental illness is a challenging task. Changing prejudiced attitudes is not easy and requires concerted action by the profession as a whole. In some cases, clear statements and recommendations concerning these matters have already been made by the bodies involved. However, in other areas clear guidance is lacking, and in some there is a need to ensure the implementation of existing guidance.

We present here a list of recommendations that, if implemented, we believe would enable considerable progress to be made. These recommendations aim to combat prejudice by changing minds through the process of selection and education of doctors. They also seek to promote procedures that will militate against prejudice by auditing and identifying prejudicial decisions and attitudes and preventing decision-making directed by prejudice. The working group has given some thought to the means by which these recommendations could be put into practice and some illustrations are contained in Appendix 4 of the report.

1. Creation of an "anti-prejudice" climate

Unequivocal statements, procedures and action by:

(a) Government

- Anti-discrimination and disability legislation potentially includes mental illness as a category (the Disability Discrimination Act 1995 and the setting up of the Disability Rights Commission). This provision must be seen to operate effectively for those disabled by mental illnesses.
- The Department for Education and Employment's Disability Awareness Campaign is most welcome and can usefully feature people with mental illnesses, including doctors and other health care professionals. Clear guidance to managers for addressing the professional problems of doctors with mental illnesses should be developed.
- In March 2001 the Department of Health launched a major new campaign, "MIND OUT for mental health" to stop the stigma and discrimination surrounding mental health.

(b) National Health Service Executive

- The National Service Framework for Mental Health should help in tackling the stigma associated with mental illness. In particular, Standard One requires health and social services to promote mental health for all, working with individuals and communities and to combat discrimination against individuals and groups with mental health problems and to promote their social inclusion.

(c) National Health Service trusts

- Should treat mental illness as they presently treat race, gender, age etc. in all policy and procedures.

(d) General Medical Council

- Should include mental illness as a category that should not prejudice treatment in Section 12 of Good Medical Practice in "Duties of a Doctor".
- Should publicly declare that promulgating or acting on stigmatising attitudes will be regarded as a form of professional misconduct.

(e) Medical Royal Colleges

- Should formally adopt anti-discriminatory policies and awareness campaigns.
- Should publicly state to their members that this is an issue they take seriously.

(f) British Medical Association

- Should formally adopt anti-discriminatory policies and awareness campaigns.

2. Teaching and learning

Organisations with responsibility for training and accreditation should develop clear guidance concerning the need for all doctors to acquire knowledge and skills related to recognition and management of mental illnesses, comparable to those required in respect of all other illnesses.

(a) General Medical Council

- The GMC has statutory responsibility to coordinate all stages of medical education and should ensure that this is achieved in respect of people with mental illnesses. Specifically:

(b) Medical schools

Should ensure:

- That communication skills, including the ability to listen, are taught effectively – these will be especially tested when the doctor and patient come from different ethnic groups or cultures.
- Competence in examining an individual's mental state, which should be comparable to competence in examining an individual's physical state.
- That respect for the uniqueness of the individual is sustained and that he or she is not regarded only as diagnostic label – the doctor should be able to recognise the person suffering from an illness at all times, and register and relate to that person.
- Corresponding recognition that the clinical encounter between a person with mental illness and a doctor can itself sometimes be a powerful instrument for favourable or unfavourable change in the patient's condition, and that it is the doctor's responsibility to maximise the potential for benefit. To accomplish this, student doctors need to develop insight into their temperaments such that they can guard against any tendency to reinforce patients' fears of personal disclosures and experience of stigmatisation.
- The ability to carry out mental state examination as part of pre-registration house officer appraisal.

Should:

- Use input from people with mental illnesses.

(c) Medical Royal Colleges

Should ensure that all doctors, as part of specialist training and as part of continuing professional development:

- Remain able to examine the mental state, recognise mental health problems where they exist and either institute appropriate treatment or refer to the appropriate specialist, and to this end, participate in cross-speciality and multi-professional learning within training schemes (e.g. case conferences/ patient reviews and liaison psychiatry practice).
- Retain respect for the uniqueness of the individual as distinct from the diagnostic label.
- Recognise the importance, in the clinical situation, of their own attitudes to mental illnesses and, if necessary, control these in the interests of patients with such illnesses,

Should:

- Ensure that people with a background of mental illness are not discriminated against in their recruitment or employment procedures.
- Link with mental health groups to help inform relevant policies and develop related educational strategies and audit.

(d) Postgraduate deaneries
Should ensure:

- That all professional education within their remit pays similar, appropriate attention to the problem of stigmatisation of people with mental illnesses.

(e) The medical press
Should:

- Challenge stigmatising material.
- Run series' of articles on the extent and effects of prejudice against mental illness.
- Publish first-hand accounts by people with mental illnesses.
- Provide appropriate training and audit journalistic activity.
- Avoid using stigmatising language.

(f) Medical journals
Should publish:

- Research, reviews and personal views relevant to stigma.
- Educational packages relevant to stigma.
- First-hand accounts by people with mental illnesses.

3. Selection of doctors

Good practice with regard to selection of students and of junior and senior doctors should include avoidance of prejudice on grounds of mental health problems, past or present. It should be based on a realistic assessment of the applicant's health and of any likely effect on their patients.

This initiative should be targeted at medical schools, NHS trusts, medical Royal Colleges and postgraduate deaneries, health authorities/boards, etc. and general practices.

4. Identifying doctors with mental health problems

Systems should continue to be developed for identifying and dealing sensitively with medical students and junior and senior doctors with mental health problems. An occupational health service for all doctors, including general practitioners, is needed.

This initiative should be targeted at medical schools, NHS trusts, postgraduate deaneries, health authorities/boards etc. and general practices as part of the clinical governance agenda.

5. Governance of such a campaign as "Changing Minds: Every Family in the Land"

A campaign of this kind needs an agreed central organisation and structure in order to take forward these recommendations. Its tasks include ongoing communication with the involved institutions; coordination of development and provision of more detailed professional and educational guidelines; and monitoring of progress.

During 2001–02 the report was sent to all undergraduate and postgraduate medical education and vocational training bodies in the UK. It was welcomed and guidance sought as to how its educational recommendations might realistically be implemented. These guidelines are currently being drawn up. Meanwhile, the precis of the Report has been prepared and printed through the offices of the Department of Health, who are about to send it to all doctors practising in the National Health Service in England. The health departments responsible for the other parts of the UK will have it drawn to their attention in case they should choose to do likewise.

The report can be accessed through a link within the Campaign website (www.changingminds.co.uk).

67 Changing Minds: The Workplace Project

Nicholas Glozier

One of the fundamental ways we define ourselves is by our occupation. Working plays a major role in access to social contacts, learning and resources. For many with mental illness this is denied. Of those with "serious mental illness" such as schizophrenia the levels of employment range from 4% to 16%, yet up to nine out of ten of users of psychiatric services wish to return to the workplace (Grove 1999). For those with illnesses such as depression only around 50% are employed (Meltzer et al. 1995). Whilst these illnesses may affect some of the functions required for work, such as concentration, most psychiatric illness is relapsing and remitting. Merely having had a history of a psychiatric illness is enough for employers to be wary (Glozier 1998). Of all barriers to employment, those with mental illness often cite the attitudes of employers. Conversely, few employers understand mental illness. Only large employers can afford occupational health services: less than half of employees have access (CBI 2002). Small and medium businesses in particular have problems: mental illness only being on their agenda when someone goes off sick.

The Workplace Project was initially a collaboration between the Royal College of Psychiatrists and the Faculty of Occupational Medicine and was joined by representatives from Mind, other service users and academic groups. However, the area is beset with difficulties, particularly during an economic downturn. Many of the projects relied upon private interest, and in a world of dwindling training and charity budgets this proved unsustainable. A project assessing stigma amongst NHS staff is ongoing. However, the Workplace Project and its members were able to collaborate with a number of other initiatives designed to tackle workplace stigma.

The Royal College of Psychiatrists have produced a report *Employment Opportunities for People with Psychiatric Disability* aimed at improving employment and vocational schemes across the public and private sectors (Boardman et al. 2003).

The book *Work and Mental Health* (Miller et al. 2002) contains useful information on the effect of psychiatric disorders in the workplace. There are case studies and initiatives designed to help human resource managers and occupational health staff in developing mental health policies and practices aimed at reducing stigma and retaining employees.

Mentality, the mental health promotion charity, was commissioned by the NHS Executive to produce "Making it Happen" and provide a framework for a mental health promotion strategy within the National Service Framework. The key elements are challenging stigma and discrimination. The toolkit, trialled in the Trent region, supporting this is available at http://www.mentality.org.uk/services/resources/toolkit.htm.

The Department of Health launched the Working Minds programme, part of Mind Out for Mental Health in June 2001. Research by the Industrial Society highlighted the damaging lack of awareness of mental ill health that reinforces a negative cycle of ignorance, fear and discrimination. Further, few employers realised the Disability Discrimination Act (DDA) covered people with mental ill health. The Mind Out campaign has become a focus for anti-stigma lobbying and has a collection of useful case studies, policies and information available at http://www.mindout.net/wm/w01_working_minds_home.asp.

Other initiatives supported by this working party include Investors in Health, an evidence based programme of good practice standards for mental health promotion, and Carlton's "Mind Your Head", which provides easily digested information on mental illness, much of it in a work context at http://www.carlton.com/mindyourhead/info.jhtml.

Local programmes aimed at employing people with mental health problems are expanding. A frontrunner was that at St George's coordinated by Ben Davidson.

A useful site with materials about disability associated with mental illness is that of the employers forum on disability: http://www.employers-forum.co.uk.

References

Boardman J, Grove B, Perkins R, Shepherd G (2003) Work and employment for people with psychiatric disabilities. *British Journal of Psychiatry* **182**: 467–8.

CBI (2002) *Their Health in Your Hands: Focus on Occupational Health Partnerships.* London: CBI Publications.

Glozier N (1998) Workplace effects of the stigmatisation of depression. *Journal of Occupational and Environmental Medicine* **40**: 793–800.

Grove B (1999) Mental health and employment. Shaping a new agenda. *Journal of Mental Health* **8**: 131–40.

Meltzer H, Gill B, Petticrew M & Hinds K (1995) *OPCS Surveys of Psychiatric Morbidity in Great Britain. Report 3: Economic Activity and Social Functioning of Adults with Psychiatric Disorders.* London: HMSO.

Miller D, Lipsedge M & Litchfield P (2002) *Work and Mental Health.* London: Gaskell.

68 Changing Minds – The Children's Project

Susan Bailey and Deborah Hart

The Health Education Authority, in the summary of findings from a national survey, *Mental Health Awareness in Young People* (October 1996), concluded that young people at all ages could provide a description for the terms "mental health" and "mental illness". Mental health was described as something positive whereas perceptions of mental illness were largely negative. Language used to answer "what it means to be mentally ill" was negative in tone, indicating mental deficit, disability associated with the brain. Terms like "sick," "disorders" and "ill" were used. The younger respondents were significantly more likely to associate mental illness with physical illness or physical disabilities than the older respondents. In children, negative attitudes have been seen to persist over nearly a decade (Weiss 1994). Medical student share these prejudices to some degree, but those students who reject the stereotype are more likely to choose psychiatry as a career. The more students know about psychopathology, the less likely they are to stigmatise (Byrne 1997).

Attitudes of young people in terms of discrimination and stigma towards minority groups or people with a mental illness are fairly fixed by the age of eight. It is difficult to engage young people with mental health issues in relation to themselves, their peer group, their families and in the wider community (RAMH Education 1996; Weiss 1994).

For the past 10 years the Royal College of Psychiatrists has held a Christmas lecture for young people. In 1996, following Dr Michael Shooter's delivery of a thought-provoking and well-received address "Is it dangerous to be different?" (13 December 1996) to 200 schoolchildren (age range 11–17), 106 children completed a questionnaire asking basic questions of their understanding of and attitudes towards the mentally ill, their own concerns, and their own views of appropriate intervention and help for those experiencing mental health problems, including wanting to understand more and stigmatise less (Bailey 1999).

Being asked to Chair and be part of the Children's Project, Cycles of Understanding, as part of the Changing Minds Campaign has proved to be both a challenge and an education for us both. The key to any project setting out to increase cycles of understanding about the impact of stigmatisation of and discrimination against individuals suffering from an episode of mental illness is:

- learning from what is already known;
- working with the voluntary sector and, most importantly, users;
- working with educationalists;
- harnessing the expertise within our own College, in particular the Faculty of Child and Adolescent Psychiatry;
- developing the personal characteristics to ask others without embarrassment or shame for funding to take the project forward;
- establishing a research and developmental underpinning to all projects.

Children and teenagers make up a quarter of the total population of the UK, approximately similar to that of other European countries. There are approximately 3 million children aged under 5, 6.4 million aged 5–14 and 3.1 million young people aged between 15 and 19. Children and young people from ethnic minority backgrounds make up about one fifth of the total population aged under 20. Of 12 million children there are:

- 400,000 children in need
- 59,700 looked after children
- 320,000 disabled children
- 600,000 live births a year
- approximately 1 million with mental health disorders

In an increasingly stressful world, the mental health of schoolchildren is a growing cause for concern. The middle school years (6–10) and early adolescence (11–14) are characterised by high rates of conduct and emotional disorders. Between 10% and 15% of the population are at risk – with adult-type depressive disorders at 1–2%. Most depression in this period is mixed with other problems such as anxiety or, equally commonly, conduct disorders. Attempted suicide begins as early as 11 years.

These problems can be the result of family difficulties, a chaotic home lifestyle, complicated relationships at school, bullying and social exclusion. This can also lead to stress, eating disorders, depression, self-harm and, in extreme cases, suicide. Conduct disorders often continue into adulthood, with a number of children subsequently showing antisocial personality disorders. Depression in childhood often recurs in adult life. If these problems can be addressed at an early stage, at primary school level, it is more likely that they can be alleviated or even resolved.

A small multidisciplinary group of psychiatrists, psychologists, teachers, service users and representatives from the voluntary sector have been meeting since the beginning of the campaign, under the general heading of Cycles of Understanding. Within that framework, the group has developed initiatives, which go some way towards helping children and young people to understand the origins of intolerance towards mental disorders and the nature of these illnesses.

The group has worked towards recognising and identifying difficulties that can arise for children and young people with mental disorders and those in contact with them. Reading Lights is a series of comic books for 4- to 7-year-olds to talk about what it can feel like for a young child to be different. Being "different" is difficult to accept at any time in your life, but for a young child, it is particularly challenging.

The four books have animals as their central character (Little Raja, the elephant with the troublesome trunk; Streaky, the annoying little piglet; Peaches, the puppy that screeches; and Quackeline, the duck who wanted to be a swan) and are intended to provide a framework for people who wish to support children and develop their strengths and confidence.

Identifying what influences children and young people's understanding of, and attitudes towards, mental disorder has been an important issue for the campaign. HEADstuff is a leaflet for 14- to 17-year-olds developed jointly by the campaign and Mentality, a national charity dedicated to the promotion of mental health. The leaflet challenges perception of mental illness through "facts" and "fictions".

While piloting this leaflet with young people, the researchers found that nearly all the interviewees knew of someone who had self-harmed. Girls were keener to understand a mental health problem and solve it, whilst boys felt uncomfortable talking about it. They were ignorant of the language to use when talking about mental health problems. Schizophrenia was mistakenly seen as split personality and was associated with violent behaviour, mental health difficulties were acceptable only if associated with stress or family problems.

Building on these perceptions, our campaign recently launched a multi-media CD-Rom for 13- to 17-year-olds. This initiative is intended for teachers to use as part of the personal and social health education curriculum and suggests creative teaching ideas for lessons. The CD-Rom includes the voices of young people's experience of mental illness through interviews, writing, video and audio clips and music. It looks at the six main areas of concern for young people themselves: addictions, stress, eating disorders, depression, schizophrenia and self-harm.

Our projects are now an integral part of research evidence based projects now being used in secondary schools.

Our latest projects will evaluate the impact and usefulness of the CD-Rom by means of user views of young offenders, who in turn will help us develop a further CD-Rom that will bridge the divide of mental health, physical health and substance misuse.

The work of Cycles of Understanding (Bailey 2002), we hope, will carry on into a new College campaign looking at the role of, challenges to, and life of carers whilst taking forward new projects about understanding mental health and young people in the context of education, care, juvenile justice and the community.

With the publication of a National Service Framework for children (DOH 2003), the Government is committed to improving the life and health of children and young people. It sets out a challenging agenda, with three key objectives, to put children and their families at the centre of care, to develop effective partnership working so that the needs of the child are always considered and to deliver needs-led services. Part of this journey from childhood into adolescence and on into young adulthood must include reducing the stigma and discrimination against people suffering from mental health problems and helping young people to better understand themselves, each other and then be part of the process of Changing Minds.

However, times are changing. Discriminating against people on the grounds of race, gender or beliefs is now unacceptable to society, and often against the law. It is essential to encourage everyone to stop and think about their own attitudes and behaviour in relation to mental disorders. If we do stop and think, we will almost certainly understand more and more, and, as a result, become more tolerant of people with mental health problems.

References

Bailey S (1999) Young people, mental illness and stigmatisation. *Psychiatric Bulletin* **23**: 107–10.

Bailey S (2002) Let's be mindful of stigma. *Community Care* **1450**: 34–5

Byrne P (1997) Psychiatric stigma, the past, passing and to come. *Journal of the Royal Society of Medicine* **90**: 618–21.

DOH (2003) *Getting the Right Start: National Service Framework for Children Emerging Findings*. DOH, April 2003.

RAMH Education (1996) *The Renfrewshire Experience: School Mental Health Promotion*. Paisley: Renfrewshire Association for Mental Health.

Weiss M (1994) Children's attitudes towards the mentally ill, an eight-year longitudinal follow-up. *Psychological Reports* **74**: 51–6.

69 Changing Minds – The Schizophrenia Project

Deborah Hart

Of the six mental disorders being tackled by the Changing Minds Campaign, schizophrenia, with alcohol and drug misuse, is most difficult to address. In the public attitude survey conducted by the Office of National Statistics (ONS) for the campaign in 1998, schizophrenia was rated the highest in terms of "dangerousness" (71%) and "unpredictability" (77%). With dementia, schizophrenia also scored high on "difficult to communicate with" (59%) and "would never recover" (51%). It will be interesting to see whether there has been any significant change in attitude following a second survey conducted by the ONS this summer.

Although not covered in the survey, there are still many other popular misconceptions about schizophrenia. These include the colloquial use of the term "schizophrenic" as meaning "split personality" and the belief that schizophrenia turns people into knife-wielding maniacs who should be feared and shunned. The word "schizo" continues to be commonly used as an abusive term. These stereotypes are often reinforced by films and media generally.

Set of principles

The first project of the Schizophrenia Working Party was to agree that the campaign should look at the life-style of people with chronic schizophrenia and question the public's notion that once a "schizophrenic", always a "schizophrenic". The following set of principles was agreed about the need to respect and understand the nature of this illness and how it affects people's lives:

Schizophrenia is an extraordinary experience that affects ordinary people

It changes how people see and understand the world around them, often making it a frightening and bewildering place. Not everybody experiences schizophrenia in the same way. It can affect how a person thinks, concentrates and consequently talks with other people. The person having such an experience is struggling desperately to try and make sense of it, in the same way that anybody else would do.

All people are more or less vulnerable to the symptoms of schizophrenia

Under certain circumstances, such as sleep deprivation, different forms of drugs, bereavement or other stresses, we may all have hallucinations (seeing people who are no longer there, hearing people talking to us) or believe that people are against us. For the person with schizophrenia, this lasts a long time and does not go away even when the person is reassured that the events are not taking place. Many of those affected appear to have forms of brain abnormality. In some, the condition seems to run in the family, and in others life circumstances often seem to play a role.

397

There are many people who have experienced schizophrenia who are working, married and living happy and fulfilled lives

Unfortunately for many of those who are affected more seriously, they may live increasingly isolated and poverty-stricken lives through no fault of their own. People with the condition are more likely to harm themselves than harm others.

Once it is recognised, it is possible to treat schizophrenia in a number of ways

There is a range of effective treatments such as medication, talking treatments and learning new skills. The overall aim should be to let the person take charge of themselves and their lives, taking responsible decisions in relation to their family and friends, just the same as the rest of us.

Survey

Little research has been done in terms of addressing psychiatrists' attitudes towards severe mental illness, and schizophrenia in particular. The Working Party obtained the funding to support a survey to investigate psychiatrists' attitudes towards people with severe mental illness. Each member of the College in the UK was sent a questionnaire based on previous research in this area, supplemented with relevant questions on management. There was a 43% response rate.

Psychiatrists' attitudes compared favourably with those of the general population. Amongst other findings, they believed that the risk of dangerousness was over-emphasised, that misdiagnosis of schizophrenia in black people was common and that polypharmacy and the use of antipsychotic medication above the British National Formulary levels occurs too often.

Employment

The Working Party supported the South West London and St George's Mental Health NHS Trust "User Employment Programme" which aims to increase access to employment within Mental Health Services for people who have experienced mental health problems. The Working Party was very impressed by the success of this project, which demonstrated very low sickness rates among employees with a history of mental illness, with only 3% absenteeism. The Working Party felt that, in line with the Disability Discrimination Act (1995), the "Charter for the employment of people who have experienced mental health problems" should be widely adopted by other Trusts throughout the NHS. This proposal is particularly important in view of the fact that 83% of people with long-term mental health problems are unemployed. For people with schizophrenia, however, it is even more difficult to find a job, mainly because of the stigma associated with severe mental illness, but also in view of the unwillingness and existing preconceptions of employers to employ anyone with a psychiatric history.

World Psychiatric Association programme

The Working Party has been monitoring with some interest the work of the World Psychiatric Association (WPA) global programme against stigma and discrimination because of schizophrenia. (www.openthedoors.com). This campaign had been piloting a number of projects throughout the world aimed at different target groups, including emergency room staff, medical students, health policy makers, teenagers, clergy and congregations, business leaders, journalists, and the general public. The Working Party was interested to learn that public attitudes through the media campaign had demonstrated little change, whilst the campaign which had focused on schools had been shown to be successful in changing attitudes.

The WPA programme has also produced an important statement addressing the stereotype that people with schizophrenia are more likely to be violent. In fact, people with mental illness are no more dangerous than the general population and are more likely to injure themselves.

Index of suspicion: strange or unusual behaviour – could it be early psychosis?

The Working Party developed a very simple screening tool for GPs which aims to facilitate the early detection of psychosis in young people. GPs can miss schizophrenia in young people, believing it to be adolescent angst. A delay of several years in the diagnosis of psychosis can impact severely on the young person's prospects for the future. This screening tool has been incorporated in the PriMHE Resource Pack (and CD-Rom) on mental health promotion and managing mental health problems in primary care, linked into the National Service Framework for Mental Health.

Other areas of concern to the Working Party

Polypharmacy: the Working Party had serious concerns in relation to polypharmacy and the side-effects of this practice, which are often stigmatising in themselves.

Physical health and severe mental illness: the Working Party agreed that this is a neglected area which needs to be pushed up the healthcare agenda.

Information giving: the Working Party supported the need to disseminate good information on severe mental illness to patients and their relatives, particularly during a person's first episode. Information giving, however, should be a continual process. The diagnosis of and term "schizophrenia" can in its own right be viewed as stigmatising. The Working Party would welcome a wider debate as to whether the term "schizophrenia" should be abandoned.

Medical students: Professor Steven Hirsch continues to work on producing materials for medical schools to address students stereotypical attitudes toward people with mental illness. It is hoped to target medical students sooner rather than later.

Chairs

Dr Tom Harrison, Dr Tonmoy Sharma, Professor Steven Hirsch

Membership of the Working Party

Dr Bid Allison-Bolger, Janey Antoniou, Claire Brockman, Paul Farmer (Rethink: Severe Mental Illness), Professor David Kingdom, Professor Julian Leff, Dr Chris Manning (PriMHE), Dr Rachel Perkins, Professor Tom Barnes

70 Getting the show on the road

Brice Pitt

The Road Show sub-committee of the Changing Minds Campaign has had the task of going out into the mission field and spreading the word: *challenge stigma!*

The pilot Road Shows

The committee first met on 12 April 1999, with representatives from the College and from Priory Healthcare, who supported the campaign and its literature and sponsored the two pilot Road Shows. The agreeable fantasy of a "travelling circus", or "whistle stop tour", arriving at Town Halls or market-places and setting up a rostrum and preaching the gospel, was modified in favour of an afternoon or evening meeting with lectures, refreshment and generous opportunity for discussion. Although live shows could only reach a minute population, the feedback might be instructive for the campaign.

Two audiences were identified:

- general practitioners (GPs)
- employers

General practitioners

Almost everyone has a general practitioner. GPs provide most psychiatric assessment and treatment and are the gatekeepers of specialist psychiatric services. Their knowledge, enlightenment, compassion and expertise on the one hand, or prejudice, ignorance, disregard, resentment or frank hostility on the other, can hugely affect patients' perceptions of themselves, their disorders and their prospects of being helped.

Key findings from the First National GP Survey of Mental Health in Primary Care by the Mental After Care Association (MACA) 1999 were that:

- GPs spent on average 30% of their time on mental health problems: 1.5 days a week.
- 15% of their time was spent on anxiety and depression. Drugs and alcohol consumed more of the time of urban GPs, while psychosomatic and elderly problems were a bigger concern for rural GPs.
- a third wanted to spend more time on such problems, but felt constrained by the physical element of their workload or daunted by the extensive time required to deal with mental health consultations.
- a quarter wanted to spend less time on such problems, concerned at the knock-on effect on their physical workload, or having no strong interest in mental health or feeling that they lacked the necessary skills and training.

Buchanan and Bhugra (1992) reported that 28% of medical students found psychiatric patients not easy to like. After qualification antipathy doubles to 56%! One study suggested that GPs stigmatised psychiatric patients even more than did the general public (Lawrie et al. 1996).

It seemed, therefore, appropriate to address the alleged antagonism of some GPs to their psychiatric patients with a Road Show entitled "Time Wasters and No-Hopers?" (interestingly, the "?" had disappeared from the title on the day, suggesting that the topic was less about changing attitudes than "What on earth can we do about this heart-sink clientele?").

A psychiatrist on the Road Show committee introduced the Changing Minds Campaign, emphasising the slogans "Every Family in the Land" (including GPs, employers – and psychiatrists), and "Stop–Think–Understand" from the Campaign's booklets (RCPsych 1998a,b).

Stigma is defined as "an attribute, trait or disorder marking one as unacceptably different, eliciting some form of community sanction (discrimination, ostracism, persecution, neglect, deprivation, incarceration)". The stigma of mental disorder induces shame, denial of the disorder and avoidance of help. It is compounded by compulsory admission, chronicity, unemployment, the side-effects of neuroleptics, race, poor hygiene, "Cinderella" mental health services, sensational media coverage, the use of derisory terms like "nutter", "psycho" and "loony" and, among doctors, discomfort over a lack of clear aetiology and organic pathology. Four major stigmatising attitudes to mentally ill people are that they are dangerous, bring it on themselves, are rarely helpable and are hard to communicate with.

The campaign's objectives of raising awareness, changing attitudes, explaining the genesis of mental disorder and the range of treatments, demystifying psychiatry, and encouraging alliances between the wide range of providers and users were described (RCPsych, 1998a,b). On the specific topic of "heartsink" patients it was suggested that disorders like fatigue, insomnia, backache, dizziness, atypical pain, refractory depression, psychosis, personality disorder, substance dependence, agoraphobia and eating disorder may be especially daunting. There may be feelings of being insufficiently trained, of having too little time, or of being assailed by self-pitying, demanding, manipulative, attention-seeking, time-wasting patients unlikely to comply properly with whatever is suggested. While referral may seem a tempting way of getting someone else to see the patient, 82% (according to Buchanan and Bhugra 1992) refuse or the psychiatric services might be perceived as under-manned, under-funded, unresponsive, uninformed or unintelligible!

The GP speaker then took over. His insights as a fellow GP won him crediblity, enhanced by his experiences from time to time as a user of psychiatric services. A highly interactive discussion was largely attributable to his adroit touching of nerve-spots.

The last speaker was also a "user" and a worker for Mind. His wearing a suit for the occasion diminished his "otherness", as did his earnest, plausible manner, though he had a horrifying tale to tell of recurrent psychosis, removal of a brain tumour (acoustic neuroma) and the summoning of octets of policemen by panicking GPs when he showed his perhaps troubled, certainly troubling face at the surgery. The contrast between his composure (though he had had to increase the dose of his antipsychotic for the occasion) and his harrowing story won the audience's respect, though no one seems prepared to admit a prejudice against psychosis.

The discussion about frequently somatising patients who bring other agendas to the surgery, leaving the GP frustrated and feeling inadequate and unsure to what extent psychiatric services could and would help, was animated and generally constructive, though so engrossing that the central issue of stigma in general practice had to be dragged back into the arena. There may be a dilemma in keeping this in the forefront while linking it to a topic that commands the GPs' interest.

Psychiatrists themselves, though often the object of stigma, are not immune from prejudice (Allison-Bolger 1999). Though a Road Show at the Joint Annual Meeting of the Faculty of General and Community Psychiatry and the Collegiate Trainees' Committee in Manchester in April 2001 did not confirm this, the *1 in 4* trailer was unexpectedly unpopular!

Employers

Employers are an important target because so many people's mental health problems are worsened by unemployment (Hayward and Bright 1997). The first Employers' Road Show, however, was aimed rather at the retention of staff in difficulties than the recruitment of those with mental disorder. Of the various disorders highlighted by the campaign it seemed that substance abuse, in particular alcoholism, might be the most pertinent. Alcohol is "our favourite drug", and most people occasionally imbibe. Drinking under stress is well recognised and understood, even if frowned upon. Alcohol dependency affects attendance at and quality of work, among many other aspects of life, and leads to withdrawal or removal from the work force. Hence the title: "Pressure, Panic and Productivity: It Drives You to Drink!".

The Group Marketing Manager of Priory Healthcare Ltd was able to invite a number of employers from London and the Home Counties to an early evening meeting in the Society of Chemical Industry building, Belgrave Square, and there were about 60 acceptances. The particular hope that there would be at least as many Human Resource Managers – the hirers and firers – as Occupational Health personnel was not fulfilled, nor was it possible to find a Human Resource person to speak at the meeting.

Instead there was an introduction, again from a Road Show psychiatrist, pointing out that unrecognised or ill-understood mental disorder in the workplace threatens morale and productivity. Workers may be afraid to admit their problems even to themselves, but "soldiering on" can be stressful and inefficient. Alcohol and drug abuse are common consequences and causes of stress. At work they mean poor time-keeping, strained relationships and impaired productivity. While it is easy to feel hopeless and angry about "drunks and junkies", much can be done to help, which is good for them and good for business.

This theme was developed in presentations on alcoholism by an occupational health physician from Glaxo-Wellcome ("Winning the Battle"), the psychiatrist chair of UK Alcohol Forum ("Alcoholism in the Workplace") and finally, and most effectively, an urbane, disarming, teetotal alcoholic in a talk about his abuse of alcohol and how he had been rehabilitated ("Getting a Life").

It is often alleged that Insurance Companies discriminate unfairly against mentally disordered people. If so, this would be a particularly appropriate target for an Employers' Roadshow. At a meeting with the Communications Manager and the Chief Underwriter of Lincoln Life Assurance it emerged that there are guidelines for every form of mental illness, with indications about whether or not the sufferer be given a policy and what extra premium may be payable for how long. The principal source of information is Lipsedge (1997). It appears that decisions about whether to insure for life or possible disability are based not only upon diagnosis but also upon the individual's psychiatric history, with particular reference to the work record and hospital admissions. At present the actual *mortality* for mental illness is greater than expected by insurance companies, i.e. it appears to be underestimated.

There has been a four-fold increase in disability claims in recent years, a quarter being for psychiatric disorders. A previous history of, say, severe neurosis would carry more weight for *disability* than for life insurance.

While certain people would be unlikely not to have to pay a prohibitive premium (e.g. a person suffering from schizophrenia who was suicidal), sales forces are usually unlikely to turn down people with a history of mental illness, because they are eager for customers and market forces operate. It has thus not been established that the insurance profession's approach to death and disability from mental illness is prejudiced rather than informed.

The "wish list"

The intention to run both of the two shows, for GPs and employers, in different locations and develop templates which might be used locally by Regions and individual members of the College, led to the inclusion of two bids in the "wish list" of 16 presented at a meeting for possible sponsors held by Saatchi and Saatchi in October 2000. Happily, one of these bids "To raise awareness of doctors of the stigma associated with mental illness and how this impedes good practice", was successful, being taken up by Janssen-Cilag. The proposal was:

- Production of a PowerPoint presentation to form the basis of a Road Show for GPs and other doctors around the UK.
- To produce leaflets specially written for GPs.
- To make additional copies of the campaign videotape with new covers acknowledging the sponsorship.
- Training sessions for members of the Royal College of Psychiatrists to enable them to present the Road Shows.
- Campaign videos and leaflets to be delivered to GPs' surgeries with invitations when there was to be a Road Show in that area.
- Road Shows to be integrated with existing training programmes for GPs and hospital doctors.

The estimated cost was £32,500, but in the event the company contributed rather more than that.

"Stigma Alert!"

The plan, then, was to have the PowerPoint package and doctors' leaflets available by June 2001, to have training sessions for psychiatrists and "user" representatives at Road Shows at the Royal College of Psychiatrists in the early autumn (the cost of bringing GPs to such a meeting, which would have had to include paying for their locums, was unfortunately prohibitive) and to have approximately 60 GP Road Shows nationwide within a year, with the title "Stigma Alert!".

The doctors' leaflet, *Time Wasters – Does It Ring a Bell?*, contained a vignette of 32-year-old Jim who complained of tiredness and kept returning to the surgery with the same complaint. The suggestion was that doctor and patient could be wasting each other's time, the doctor by stereotyping his patient as a "'layabout" and not asking questions about recent life-events, Jim by failing to disclose these events and his feeling depressed, perhaps fearing stigma. However, the Changing Minds Management Committee required several revisions of this leaflet in the light of practitioners' likely sensitivity to feeling accused or patronised by psychiatrists! Nevertheless, in 2001 it was distributed to every GP in the UK.

The PowerPoint package included a CD with a wealth of material for use at the lecturer's discretion – slides, animations, the *1 in 4* cinema trailer, the *Stigma* videos, and many clips of users talking about their experience with their illness and with doctors.

The Road Shows were to last up to three hours. They would be open to GPs and local mental health workers and representative users. A local GP would be asked to chair, then a psychiatrist, a GP and a "user" (e.g. from Mind, Depression Alliance or The National Schizophrenia Fellowship (now Rethink)) would speak for 20 minutes each, leaving half an hour for questions and discussion. Refreshments would be accompanied by showings of the *1 in 4* trailer and Dr Mark Salter's *Stigma* video, cases illustrating stigma might then be presented and discussed, and the chair would summarise. The aims were:

- To open debate about and increase awareness of stigma.
- To give information about local resources.
- To provide opportunities for networking and making contacts.
- To enable GPs to get to know local people in the team.
- To help GPs to feel more comfortable about working with people with mental health problems.

The first venues included Aberdeen, Glasgow, Edinburgh, Belfast, Londonderry, Cardiff, Swansea, Birmingham, Manchester, Newcastle, Sheffield and London. Janssen-Cilag representatives set up the meetings and wherever possible arranged for the three speakers to meet before the occasion. Campaign literature was made available to those attending.

Psychiatrists were to introduce the Changing Minds Campaign and what stigma means to those stigmatised and how it affects their daily lives and were to suggest the components of an ideal anti-stigma campaign and at whom it might be directed.

GPs were invited to use a slide based on one GP's experience of mental health problems during a morning in general practice, or to replace this with their own comparable experience, aiming to highlight the frequency of mental illness. There followed a series of slides entitled "Tackling Stigma Head-On". The goal was that delegates should leave the meeting more aware of stigma and how to combat it and influence and enthuse others.

"Users" (notably Stewart Stanil and later Janey Antonionou) produced valuable notes of guidance for other users, listing topics which might provide ideas for their presentation, such as medical training, psychiatric culture, GP attitudes, confidentiality, the Mental Health Act, police and the courts, and mental health, and aspects of treatment including informed consent and forced treatment.

On 4 October 2001 psychiatrists and users (and one highly articulate GP!) attended the College for a mutually appreciated briefing, separately and together, and subsequently 12 (of 20 planned) Road Shows took place in November (eight were cancelled because of low response to invitations). As a result of feedback it was decided that shorter, lunch-time meetings with more discussion time might attract more people and that the overt aim should be to find how GPs and psychiatrists could work together to diminish the stigma of mental illness. The presentation materials were perceived as good and the content of the meetings relevant.

In June 2002 the opportunity arose to present the Road Show programme to a World Health Organization Meeting for south and south-east Europe on Mental Health and Man-Made Disasters, held in Athens, where the response was extremely positive and the materials seized eagerly. "A prophet is not without honour save in his own country"?

Postgraduate training

Ultimately the best place for addressing stigma may not be in sporadic Road Shows, especially as the Changing Minds Campaign draws to its close, but as an integral part of doctors' training.

There are 27 Directors of Postgraduate GP Education in the UK, each responsible for about 20 GP tutors. These directors all received a letter in July 2002 including:

"Psychiatrists are well aware that the bulk of mental disorder is dealt with by GPs. With the radical changes currently under way in general practice and NSF requirements it would be timely to introduce a discussion of stigma – its prevalence, manifestations and how to reduce it – into GPs' Postgraduate Education programmes, and I wonder if I could have your views on whether, and if so how, to achieve this?

We have quite an impressive 'toolkit' (list enclosed, together with some of the materials used in the Road Shows so far). We also have a number of psychiatrists available to participate in lectures, seminars or workshops if called upon. We can also find articulate users of mental health services.

If you agree that this is worth pursuing I'd be most grateful if you would indicate what 'slots' there may be for a 'Stigma Alert!' presentation in the education programmes in your domain and what tutors would be involved."

In the previous month a satellite breakfast meeting at the Royal College of Psychiatrists' Annual General Meeting in Cardiff raised the number of College members willing to speak at road shows to 39. At least one is thus available to every one of the Directors of Postgraduate GP Education, all of whom know who and where they are.

The response has been slow and sporadic, but since a reminder letter in December 2002 it has been growing, and it is hoped that "the show will go on", for hospital doctors as well as GPs, in the highly appropriate setting of postgraduate training.

References

Allison-Bolger V (1999) The original sin of madness – or how psychiatrists can stigmatise their patients. *International Journal of Clinical Practice* **53**: 627–30.

Buchanan A & Bhugra D (1992) Attitude of the medical profession to psychiatry. *Acta Psychiatrica Scandinavica* **85**: 1–5.

Hayward P & Bright JA (1997) Stigma and mental illness. *Journal of Mental Health* **6**: 345–54.

Lawrie SM, Parsons C, Patrick J et al (1996) A controlled trial of general practitioners' attitudes to patients with schizophrenia. *Health Bulletin* **54**: 201–3.

Lipsedge M (1997) Psychiatric disorders. In: Brackenridge RDC & Elder WJ (eds). *Medical Selection of Life Risks*. London: Nature Publishing Group.

MACA (1999) *First National GP Survey of Mental Health in Primary Care*. London: Mental After Care Association.

RCPsych (1998a) *Mental Disorders: Challenging Prejudice*. London: Royal College of Psychiatrists.

RCPsych (1998b) *Changing Minds Campaign "Every Family in the Land"*. London: Royal College of Psychiatrists.

71 Mental illness and the media

Mark Salter

The years since 1945 have seen a remarkable growth in our ability to produce and transmit images. This is not due to technological progress alone; humans have a powerful appetite for images in words, pictures and sounds. The relationship between our desire for images and our gain from them is highly complex. Nowhere is this complexity better illustrated than in regard to mental disorder.

The influence of the media upon our thinking about mental disorder is hard to overstate. The "psycho killer" remains a staple element of Hollywood's output, and garish stories of the latest "care in the community" scandal retain their ability to sell newspapers and boost ratings, regardless of their repetitive nature. Indeed, the predominance of lurid coverage, in print or broadcast media, seems to reflect deeply held cultural assumptions about mental disorder and illustrates a crucial point about the industry: those who work in it are not driven by a need to inform, but rather by a need to sell a product. The need to provide accurate, reliable information is, whether we like it or not, only a secondary or even tertiary consideration. Media output is not simply a commodity to be consumed for education or entertainment. It also has a reflexive quality which is often overlooked; the media choose to tell the story we choose to hear. The media coverage of a story can even become a story in itself.

If exploited, the media can act as a powerful tool for response to – and thereby influence of – events. At the simplest level, this requires tactful complaint, but if more skilfully harnessed, the media can also be used to stimulate and create powerful new – and often unanticipated – domains for informed debate. The incorporation of story lines about mental disorders into soap operas and movies has probably provoked more useful debate about mental illness than most of the public education output of the mental health charities over the past decade.

Such a claim is, of course, very difficult to prove or disprove, but only the most churlish observer would deny the possibility of a causal connection between what we watch, read and hear and the ways in which we think about mental illness. This interaction is highly complex; our own personalities and experiences play a pivotal role in the often uncertain way that we interpret and react to portrayals of mental illness. What is certain, however, is that anyone wishing to promote understanding of people with mental illness requires a basic knowledge of the motives and methods of the various media professions.

The media project

The Royal College of Psychiatrists launched its Changing Minds anti-stigma campaign in October 1998. All of its projects, of course, rely on symbols to some extent, but the media project has made explicit use of the media the central objective of its work. It has sought to harness the power of the image, attaching it to an informational content, on the assumption that greater understanding of mental illness is a prerequisite to a change in belief and behaviour. Five years on, over forty pieces of work have been carried out, ranging from formal conferences, seminars and media training workshops with varying degrees of technical support (for details visit www.rcpsych.ac.uk) through to printed media mail-outs, poster advertising, video films and cinema trailers. Four of these projects are described in this chapter. These descriptions are intentionally brief, and have been chosen because of the general principles of media working that they illustrate, rather than as detailed descriptions of the project itself.

Stigma campaign video

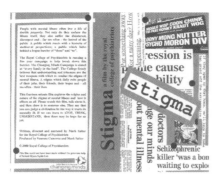

Figure 1. Cover illustration for *Stigma* film.

This 14-minute long "succinct and humane little film" briefly explores the historical, cultural and psychological origins of the stigmatisation of mental illness. It describes how a simple typology of stigma and improved understanding of mental illness may help to combat stigma. It uses entirely static imagery arranged in a rapidly shifting "picture montage" style, laid over a simple soundtrack. This format was chosen to keep down costs and to allow flexibility late into the editing stage, whilst copyright for images and sounds was still being sought. Wherever possible, this was sought free of charge, as was editing and post production, all of which were requested on a charitable basis. The entire film was made within a budget of £3,400, including the first print run of 1,000 copies. The film has received mixed reviews. Those reviewing it as users or care workers were favourable, whilst others regarded its theme of scientific optimism as unduly simplistic. Those with direct experience of producing campaign publicity criticised its attempt to achieve incompatible goals of campaign promotion and education.

1 in 4 cinema trailer

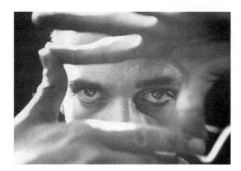

Figure 2. Still from *1 in 4*.

This film of approximately two minutes duration was released with considerable publicity in the autumn of 2000. It has since received favourable critical review and has been adopted by the WHO for screening in 52 countries. The creative input to the project was carried out by a leading London advertising company, WCRS, who have an established reputation for producing powerful television advertisements. Creative input, casting, filming, editing, post production and distribution were all negotiated and carried *pro bono*, each of the contributing professionals being content to be associated with the publicity and humanitarian impact of the project. It was shown as a trailer before every 15+ rated film in all Warner Brothers cinemas during the month of October 2000. It makes use of stark, powerfully emotive imagery that seeks to confront the viewer with the consequences of their own assumed preconceptions. Exit interviews and reviews revealed a wide range of responses, illustrating an interesting paradox of many attempts to harness powerful imagery to the end of challenging stigma: the use of powerful images of despair and loss of control that many associate with mental illness lays producers open to the charge of perpetuating the very misconceptions that the film seeks to challenge. Interestingly, this view appeared to correlate with age, younger viewers instead praising the film for the way in which its imagery personalised the issue of mental illness.

"Stigma" pill box

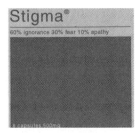 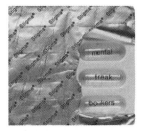

Figure 3. "Stigma" pill box: front and inside detail.

This device was produced as a mail-shot printed item that was sent to every member of the Upper and Lower Houses of Parliament and to editors and health journalists of newspapers and broadcasting companies in May 2000. This coincided with the publication of an opinion poll evaluating the impact of attitudes to mental illness in the workplace, highlighting the way in which those suffering vary degrees of mental disorder continued to experience discrimination at work.

The project was commissioned jointly by the Royal College of Psychiatrists and the Co-Operative Bank, who underwrote the project as part of their humanitarian "customers who care" policy. The original creative idea was produced by commissioning an award for the 1999 British Design and Art Direction Student awards. The winner, Anne McCormack, went on to win the Student of the Year award. The device consists of an ironically printed packet of "Stigma Pills" whose active ingredients comprise "ignorance, fear and apathy". Each of the pills inside the blister pack, designed to resemble a leading antidepressant, contained a pejorative label printed around the circumference. The product information leaflet, accompanying the packet, satirised the language of pharmaceutical products, providing further information about stigma and the campaign in general (see Figures 3 and 4).

Patient Information Leaflet

Stigma™

60% ignorance 30% fear 10% apathy

Why should you read this leaflet?
You are in a position to change the way people think and behave. This leaflet contains essential information to consider before encouraging people to take Stigma™. If you are unsure, please consult your physician.

What is Stigma™?
Stigma™ is derived from prejudice. It is a powerful set of beliefs that we use to deceive ourselves. It is made from three active ingredients: fear, apathy and ignorance.

How does Stigma™ work?
Mental illness reminds us that we are not as rational and civilised as we like to think we are. It is difficult to explain mental illness. What we fail to understand, we fear. Stigma™ reduces this fear, by encouraging the false belief that mental illness only happens to "other" people. These beliefs are often encouraged by the media and others in influential positions.

What are the effects of Stigma™?
Stigma™ helps to ensure that people with mental illness are separated from the rest of society. Stigma™ is an effective, tested method of depriving these people of privileges normally taken for granted. People taking Stigma™ can display disturbance of vision, poor judgement, antisocial behaviour and cruelty. Long term, widespread use of Stigma™ can lead to an entire culture becoming brutalised and intolerant.

What are the possible side effects of Stigma™?
Individuals affected by people who have taken Stigma™ may experience difficulty with any of the following: finding work, making friends, finding somewhere to live, obtaining life insurance, laughing, obtaining legal advice, housing benefit, unemployment benefit, voting, forming sexual relationships, feeling optimistic, travelling abroad, getting married, inheriting money, abstaining from alcohol and other drugs, feeling happy, gaining respect, refraining from suicide.

What should I do if I have taken Stigma™?
Acknowledge it. Knowledge is a powerful antidote to Stigma™. Fear of mental illness is reduced by compassion and understanding. You are in a powerful position to pass understanding on to many other people. Please stop and think how you can achieve this.

Where can I go for help?
Help is at hand. The Co-operative Bank together with the Royal College of Psychiatrists are working to tackle Stigma™. This is part of the five year Changing Minds, Every Family in the Land campaign.

If you require further help, information or ideas please contact The Royal College of Psychiatrists on 0207 235 2351 ext.122

Date of preparation 1/05/00

Figure 4. "Stigma" pill box product information leaflet.

This project received a disappointing response from the target population. Its release led to only three articles in the national press, one in the medical press, nine in local publications, two TV and radio items, and one letter of complaint from a member of the House of Lords. Analysis after the event revealed that the difficulty lay not with the ambition of the idea or the complexity of the device, but in finding a way to attach it to "an angle" which could be readily associated with a simple message relating to the Stigma Campaign.

London Underground poster advertising

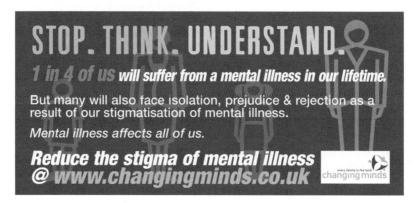

Figure 5. Tube train poster.

In the summer of 2002, Mr Stelios Haji-Iannou of the Easy Group of companies kindly underwrote the design and funding for a simple poster stating the central message of the Royal College of Psychiatrists' anti-stigma campaign. This appeared on the London Tube trains for one month. Measurement of the number of visits to the campaign web site provided an indication of the impact of the device. This increased six-fold during the month of display, settling to twice the pre-display level in the months thereafter.

Lessons learned from the project

The media exploit everyday mental behaviour

The human mind instinctively uses a strategy of stereotyping to reach swift, often inaccurate, judgements about stimuli. Resort to this strategy appears greater for novel or unexpected stimuli, where the subject has little available knowledge of the perceived, or where the stimuli carry strong emotional significance. This concurs with our knowledge of media portrayals of mental disorder. Analysis of media output reveals that a small number of stereotypes are consistently made available to us, among which the themes of danger and unpredictability are by far the most common. Furthermore, people tend to make fewer stereotype-based judgements – i.e. stigmatise – individuals with mental disorders when they possess more information about the subject. Individuals with knowledge of mental disorder appear to make less negative judgements.

The power of the stereotyping instinct is not lost upon the media professions, who treat images of danger and loss of control as stock-in-trade. Fear and uncertainty have always boosted ratings and sold newspapers and, given the deeply ingrained nature of our cognitive styles, seem set to do so for the foreseeable future. People usually make sense of fresh stories and images of mental disorder in terms of ideas already available to them, thus reinforcing previously held beliefs. This accounts for the repetition of a small number of themes in most depictions of mental disorder.

Trojan horses may be the best way forward

These observations have implications for anyone wishing to use the media to challenge the stigmatisation of mental disorders. Protest alone is unlikely to alter a way of thinking that has formed over thousands of years. It follows that to be truly effective, media-based efforts to challenge stigma should first gain access to people's mind via established conventions and thereafter enrich the range of stereotypes actually available so as to include relatively more positive ideas and images. The argument that the Royal College of Psychiatrists' film, *1 in 4*, ultimately reinforced stigmatisation is, from this perspective, a narrow and conservative view that overlooks the way in which its blend of form and content actually enriched the perspective of the viewer. To take another example, the Academy Award winning film *A Beautiful Mind* may have been replete with imagery of despair and loss of control, but it was ultimately a film about schizophrenia with a happy ending. Nevertheless, as the media professions well know, conflict is always welcome, as it is a proven way of drawing attention to a debate. Future forays into the minefield of mental health imagery would do well to heed Wilde's dictum that there is only one thing in the world worse than being talked about.

The media is actually on our side

Another, perhaps more surprising, finding of the media project is that there is an enormous fund of goodwill among the various media professions towards those who work in the field of mental health. This chapter alone describes four projects where creatives, producers, publicists, technicians and many others have donated their talents for little or no material reward, instead happy to be associated with the goodwill generated by the product. Mental health professionals, with their own expertise and their distribution across the land, are well positioned to harness both this goodwill and talent in future. To do this, we need to establish greater dialogue with the media professions at every level, from local press and radio throughout to the largest internet companies. Inevitably, much of this will, at first, need to be set in the media's terms – as we have seen, media workers will *always* place a story or idea in their own context. Knowledge of the motives and methods of the various professions, and a clear understanding of the way these necessarily differ from our own (see Byrne 2003; Salter 2003), are an essential foundation for future mental health/media collaborations.

Mental health professionals long ago passed the point where they could regard media portrayals of mental disorder as an irrelevant or unhelpful distraction. As a new century begins, the media and new technologies seem certain to exert an increasing influence in our culture in general and upon our perceptions of mental disorders in particular. It is an influence that we disregard at our peril, for, as one philosopher has put it: "the image will always have the last word".

References

Byrne P (2003) Psychiatry and the media. *Advances in Psychiatric Treatment.* 2003, **9**: 135–43.
Salter M (2003) Psychiatry and the media: from pitfalls to possibilities. *Psychiatric Bulletin* **27**: 123–5.

72 The nature of stigmatisation

Arthur Crisp

"Doctors came to see her singly and in consultation, talked much in French, German and Latin, blamed one another, and prescribed a great variety of medicines for all the diseases known to them, but the simple idea never occurred to any of them that they could not know the disease Natasha was suffering from, as no disease suffered by a live man can be known, for every living person has his own peculiarities and always has his own peculiar, personal, novel, complicated disease, unknown to medicine."

(Tolstoy, *War and Peace*)

The origins of stigmatisation remain enigmatic. What is the nature of this mechanism, which is so often unfair and deeply damaging to others in contemporary society? In his review of the literature on the stigmatisation of people with mental illnesses, Kelly (1999) concludes "... certainly the experience of reviewing recent research findings related to public attitudes to mental illness *does not bring a strong sense of understanding* [as to why we stigmatise], but rather of acknowledgement that we do think of those with mental health problems in this discriminatory fashion ..." He goes on to state "... the stigma inputed to mental illness appears to be extremely deeply felt in our society and possibly to be growing, despite an increase in awareness of the 'normality' or, at least, the ubiquity of mental illness. The media both fosters and promotes negative images of those with mental health problems, *but* it cannot be said to have created them; the origins of *fear and dislike of those with mental health problems may well from a deeper spring in society ...*" With such an empty canvas it may prove useful to bring the gamut of biological, social and experiential perspectives speculatively to bear on the subject, drawing especially upon many of the preceding texts in this book, and a Campaign working party originally set up to consider the matter. Figure 1 portrays such a schema. It highlights

- an inherent biological mechanism (1),
- other aspects of the human condition (2),
- the interactions between people with and without a "mental illness" (2 and 3),
- the handicaps that the person with mental illness also brings to the encounter (3), and
- the stigmatising and discriminatory consequences of this for the "ill" individual (1, 4, 5 and 6).

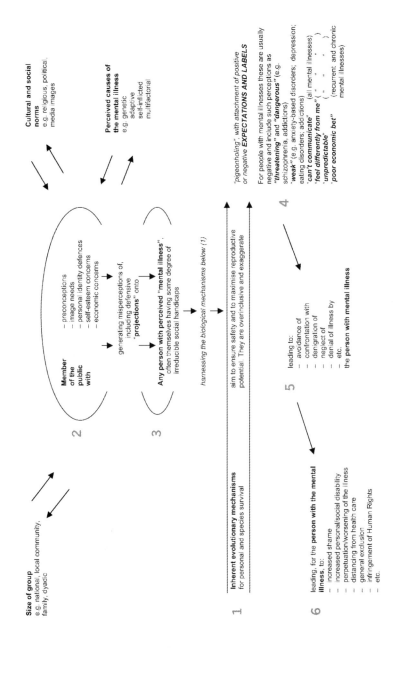

Size of group
e.g. national, local community, family, dyadic

Cultural and social norms
e.g. religious, political, media images

Perceived causes of the mental illness
e.g. genetic
adaptive
self-inflicted
multifactorial

2 **Member of the public with**
– preconceptions
– image needs
– personal identity defences
– self-esteem concerns
– economic concerns

generating misperceptions of, including defensive **"projections"** onto

3 **Any person with perceived "mental illness"**, often themselves having some degree of irreducible social handicaps

harnessing the biological mechanisms below (1)

"pigeonholing", with attachment of positive or negative EXPECTATIONS AND LABELS

For people with mental illnesses these are usually negative and include such perceptions as *"threatening"* and *"dangerous"* (e.g. schizophrenia, addictions)
"weak" (e.g. anxiety-based disorders; depression; eating disorders; addictions)   (all mental illnesses)
"can't communicate"
"feel differently from me" (" " ")
"unpredictable"
"poor economic bet" (recurrent and chronic mental illnesses)

1 **Inherent evolutionary mechanisms** for personal and species survival

aim to ensure safety and to maximise reproductive potential. They are overinclusive and exaggerate

5 leading to:
– avoidance of
– confrontation with
– denigration of
– neglect of
– denial of illness by
– etc.
the **person with mental illness**

6 leading, for the **person with the mental illness**, to:
– increased shame
– increased personal/social disability
– perpetuation/worsening of the illness
– distancing from health care
– general exclusion
– infringement of Human Rights
– etc.

Figure 1. A speculative schema for the stigmatising and discriminatory processes (1)–(6) employed by one person in respect of another with perceived mental illness.

1. Biological

Anatomy is destiny (Freud 1925)

There is a natural tendency, probably rooted in evolutionary biology, for animals, individually or in a herd, to be cautious when confronted by novel circumstances that may threaten survival. Distancing reactions, e.g. flight, to perceptions of predators are over-inclusive in the interests of species and hence usually personal survival. The human brain would seem to be no exception, and Haghighat (2001) has recently reviewed relevant experimental literature.

It would seem then that this basic biological/ancestral mechanism exists in man and can be associated with exaggerated responses in terms of both expansion of the category of perceived threat and the extent of the response. As Bertrand Russell put it, *"what people want is not knowledge but certainty"*. Such pigeonholing into "us" and "not us", erring on the side of personal safety, reduces insecurity/maximises survival. It subserves long term evolutionary interests through the efficient preservation of immediate individual self-interest.

Meanwhile, Gilbert (see Chapter 30) has argued that there are also reproductive evolutionary forces at work that generate social discriminations in humans (and which he claims are especially operative in respect of people with mental illnesses). Thus, evolutionary theory has it that the tasks of survival and ever-greater effective development in the face of competition build into the organism the advantage of discrimination against others who seem biologically and hence perhaps genetically disadvantaged. For instance, they are perceived as "poor reproductive bets". Thus, survival at this primitive biological level may be enhanced by avoiding/rejecting (socially and reproductively), destroying or dominating others seen as territorially weak, inactive, unresponsive, unable to collaborate and strengthen the existing social system, positively burdensome, inappropriately impulsive, ungroomed, physically impaired or uncoordinated, etc.

Such evolutionary "threats" to personal survival and reproductive potential, it is argued, are also capable of being re-framed within mankind's economic and cultural perspectives, but still activate instinctual responses of rejection etc. within us. For instance the evolutionary drive to identify and avoid "poor reproductive bets" and related "territorial weakness" would be re-framed into the stigma of being a "poor economic bet" in terms of ability to generate financial income required for establishing and maintaining a household.

A contrary protective (often maternal) instinct towards biologically weaker and bonded members of the group – usually offspring – is also natural, under particular circumstances. Such altruism can again be seen to have biological purpose that can also be prompted by appropriate social encounters, e.g. by "imprinting".

Indeed, whilst biological mechanisms are popularly seen as enduring and immutable, it is recognised that they are modifiable interactively, e.g. sexual behaviour modified by nutritional status. They can also be environmentally, including culturally, modifiable (e.g. the curbing of "antisocial" instinctually driven behaviour such as violence to others, sexual promiscuity) by legislation, cultural beliefs and customs.

The culture of ignoring or denying the existence of biological mechanisms in human nature, or demanding that they be transcended totally, is more likely to enable their unbridled or distorted expression. Pinker (2002) and Churchill (2002) have recently and cogently addressed this debate and their conclusions – that there can best be a fruitful interaction between nature and nurture born of recognition and understanding of the importance of both these strands of human development – sustain this presentation. But why are these ancestral mechanisms, allowing over-inclusive and distorted negative labelling, so often harnessed and applied powerfully to people with mental illnesses?

2. Personal

Belief systems

> *"Stereotypes and stigma aid people in simplifying their mental categories, justify hostility and serve as projection screens for personal conflicts."*
>
> (Allport 1954)

People's preconceptions of mental illnesses and their attitudes and behaviour towards those so labelled are shaped by a number of factors.

(a) *Their personal experience of such illness in themselves* (and whether or not it has been "concealed" from others), and in those known to them ("Every Family in the Land" and "1 in 4", implying that most of us will have had first hand experience of such illnesses in others).

(b) *The impact of the media.* The media are taken to mean the channels through which information (e.g. fact, opinion, fantasy) is circulated within the population through printed material, the cinema, television and the Internet for example. The term is not usually taken to include the main educational systems such as schools and universities, but the media can itself have primarily educational functions (e.g. the Open University and the more general element of public education inherent in the BBC's charter).

However, the media are also necessarily responsive to the more general needs of the population to be entertained or reassured. This may require that they are sensitive to the fantasies and prejudices of the majority of people and resonate with them. In the process they can confirm and consolidate such prejudices and fantasies. If they fail to attract the public's attention, they lose revenue. Thus, *the commercially based media exist at our will and pleasure and depend upon our patronage.*

Both Clare (Chapter 26) and Byrne (Chapter 27) have drawn attention to the predominantly negative images of people with mental illnesses portrayed over the years in movies. Sensational and often very inaccurate portrayals of people with mental illnesses appear in the daily press, especially some of the popular tabloids. Words like "madman", "psycho", "nutter", are coined to command attention and serve to reinforce negative images; surely again distant from the concept that mental illnesses afflict *every family in the land*. Indeed, Philo (1996) reported that about two thirds of news and current affairs coverage was making a link between mental ill health and violence.

It is this extreme antisocial image, so often portrayed though so rare in reality, and then often linked primarily to substance misuse (drugs and/or alcohol) and/or "personality disorder", that has contributed to the reluctance of some psychiatrists to consider such disorders as part of their practice. This is despite their clinical importance within many areas of medical practice.

The media, whilst they cannot be seen as the prime movers in the processes of stigmatisation of people with mental illnesses, carry a huge public responsibility in this respect because of their invasiveness. Meanwhile, O'Neil, in the fifth of her 2002 Reith Lectures, reminds us not only of their power and unaccountability, but also of their potential untrustworthiness.

(c) *Beliefs as to causation of mental illnesses*, e.g. genetic, adaptive, self-inflicted, socially manipulative (see Part 4 of this book).

(d) *Other aspects of the sociocultural background.* Within anthropological studies, the possible culture-bound nature of stigmatisation and discrimination within human society becomes a little clearer, but not much! Littlewood (Chapter 2) draws attention to the great difficulties, reflected in contradictory findings inherent in cross-cultural studies and in searching for meaningful cultural links to stigmatisations given the multivariate nature of the data and the limitations of languages. He draws some tentative conclusions. Societies (e.g. the Western world) that emphasise individuality can also thereby accentuate the role of personal responsibility for illnesses and their outcome. Competitive societies disadvantage the vulnerable. Loss of employment and poverty reinforce the stigmatised role. Ideas about aetiology underpin attitudes to people with such illnesses. Tolerance of deviance correlates with greater empathy. People who report their beliefs within surveys do not always translate them into actions. Such declarations can be driven by their perceived "social desirability". However, public *behaviour* within the actual setting has to be the marker for such claims.

A recently proposed sociological perspective (Kurzban and Leary 2001) posits that there are two distinct stigmatising mind sets governed by the size of the stigmatising group, i.e. whether it is large or else small to the point of being dyadic – and variously evoking anxiety and anger. Certain threats can also become construed as "parasitic" and evoke disgust. These authors insist that a biological or genetic basis for this is not implied. However, one can readily enough imagine similar relationships between group size and behaviour operating within biological systems. Their theory, so far as perception and reaction to ill people is concerned, has thus far mainly been applied to those with "physical" illnesses such as obesity, cancer, psoriasis, etc.

Meanwhile, the sociological concept of "deviance" has been established as a social label generated by tendencies to differentiate and classify so as to distinguish "us" from "not us". It can be within the economic, physical or behavioural realms. The social categorisation of deviant behaviour is akin to the medical diagnostic process. It has some similar strengths and weaknesses and potential for damaging as well as useful consequences. It may consolidate secondary deviance in the alleged deviant (i.e. influence that person to adopt more fully the given role). Once again, labelling comes into play, e.g. "delinquent", "itinerant" or "madman". A powerful new and negative social role is thus conferred which may overwhelm previously perceived social roles such as "worker", "parent", "student".

Defining social deviance helps to secure comforting social "normality", with an increase of internal social cohesion. Stigmatisation especially arises when such deviance invokes fear, insecurity or self-doubt. Discrimination arises as a *personally* or *socially hostile* or *avoidant* act against the stigmatised person. It can operate throughout personal and social relationships, and within the home, the local community, healthcare and social welfare systems, the workplace, commerce etc.

Experiential

"The lady doeth protest too much, methinks." (Shakespeare, *Hamlet*)

Is the threat posed by mental illness to us as individuals particularly great or unique? Is it greater, for instance, than other groups such as gay/lesbians and ethnic minorities have posed not only in biological or socio-cultural terms, but also in personal terms?

Is it so great as to justify the powerful negative opinions it often attracts?

On the one hand some mental illnesses invoke our commitment to our belief in "free will". Our belief that we can exercise "choice" is embedded in our Western culture. The belief in "choice", despite an undercurrent of respect for and belief in the inevitability of a degree of psychic determinism governing human experience and behaviour, supports our perceptions of "good" and "bad", especially relevant in consideration of "personality disorder" (see Part 5 of this book). It relates to our concepts of "blame" and "responsibility". It supports our social system and its legal underpinning and is a cornerstone of our "moral" judgements.

On the one hand it has been said (Hamilton 1973 personal communication) that free will is a property we each believe we possess, whilst at the same time we often believe that we can predict the behaviour of others. Thus, this latter logic of "determinism", both at a genetic level and within our personal developments, also underwrites the importance that "psychiatry" and society in general also attach to the historical background when either judging or seeking a greater understanding of the present condition of a patient or a situation.

Moreover, so far as mental illnesses are concerned, people with schizophrenia are sometimes judged to have damaged willpower as part of their "organic" illness and may come to be cared for within the social/medical system accordingly, whilst the person abusing alcohol was often construed as having chosen and as being responsible for the initiation and maintenance of his/her lifestyle.

The debate on free will/determinism remains one for philosophers (e.g. see Stout 2002). Meanwhile, it is reasonable to claim that the prospect of personal "choice" can be rendered more realistic by acquisition of available and relevant knowledge and skills concerning one's behaviour and its consequences, amounting thereby to us having "a degree of choice". We are also often comfortable with the idea that processes such as "empowerment" can enable people to behave in new ways for which they have inherent potential. As a consequence of our socialising experiences as humans, most of us learn to curb unbridled impulsivity and strive for a sense of self-control and a perception by others of our social and inter-personal competence. Apparent confidence of this kind might mask inner degrees of fear (e.g. of losing impulse control), self-doubt and fragile self-esteem that resonate variously with the different kinds of "mental illness".

Anxieties about these matters might be heightened by exposure to the mentally ill, who more often exhibit derailment of these functions in a variety of ways and who challenge our interpersonal skills in communication and empathy. Further fears concerning contamination may stem from the popular concept of the person with mental illness having had a "nervous breakdown". This breakdown may be perceived as a breaching of the individual's psychological defence mechanisms, e.g. their erstwhile capacity to deny strain as well as cope with it. This may be experienced as a threat to our own similar defence mechanisms.

Our anxiety may then become relieved through mobilisation of our own mental defence mechanism of *denial* and the related mental mechanism of *projection* (see Hughes, Chapter 31). We deny the strain in ourselves and project its origins – such as poor impulse control, dangerousness and potential "irresponsibility" – more emphatically and judgementally on to the mentally ill person. Indeed it might seem a tribute to the power of the mental defence mechanism of "projection" that, in respect of some mental illnesses, we abandon our notion that others are a product of their genetic and personal developmental past and that their behaviour is correspondingly pre-determined and predictable. Instead we now conclude that, potentially like us, they are to blame for their state and could choose to behave otherwise.

Having attributed such character and behavioural flaws to others, we then wish to distance ourselves from them on the basis of "out of sight, out of mind" (the banishment of others with such "flaws" serves to consolidate our capacity to deny them in ourselves). This accords with the "just world" hypothesis of Lerner (1980). He proposed that we need to believe in a just world so that we can trust that we shall not be damaged. Others, who are damaged, have "chosen" to be so. Once again, as Porter (2002) puts it, *"Setting the sick apart sustains the fantasy that we are whole."* It maintains our self-esteem and sense of personal identity. Haghighat (2001) has framed these matters in terms of "self-interest". In his view, this is not so much concerned with reinforcing one's own mental defences, thereby shoring up one's own mental stability, as with economic self-interest. The mentally ill, often defenceless and with low self-esteem, already besieged and condemned by us, are there to be economically exploited. Economic exploitation, underwritten by economic self-interest, brings us, full circle, back to the issue of interaction between experiential and biological processes.

Additionally, our defences against our mortality may become threatened by those people with mental illness who may manifest personal decay or indifference to survival. To the extent that some of the mental illnesses under scrutiny also seem to have an adaptive/coping purpose, with the individual concerned reluctant to accept any well-intentioned help, we may also become both exasperated and envious.

We may also be trying to cope with specific emotional distress, doubt, despair or occult mental illness within ourselves (e.g. "1 in 4" of us), denying it to ourselves and/or to others. Under such circumstances we may be especially prone to condemn those with explicit mental illness. A parallel might be the extremely negative attitude to, or the persecution of, the gay community by someone with suppressed homosexual tendencies. We are likely also to be especially resistant or hostile to having such a defence pointed out to us.

Finally, mental illnesses are more likely to be seen as synonymous with the individual as a person rather than as an affliction imposed upon them. Mental illnesses by definition reflect and are usually expressed as disturbances of cognition, feelings and/or behaviour – the very stuff of personality itself. The individual may therefore be seen as no more than his or her illness. In addition, mental illnesses are more often attributed to a breakdown in coping abilities in the face of stressful life events. Some mental illnesses are seen as "self-inflicted", others as adaptive. Thus, to the extent that mental illnesses are perceived negatively, so will be the afflicted individual – with little regard for any other aspect of his or her individuality. "She is a neurotic", "he is a depressive", "she is a schizophrenic", "he is an Alzheimer", "she is an anorectic", "he is an addict" are readily taken to be complete statements about an individual.

Such human experiential forces then are likely – sometimes powerfully – to further inflame and sustain our ancestral propensities to categorise and then negatively label those amongst us with mental illnesses. We especially avoid those whose illnesses are severe and condemn those who are perceived as having "brought the illness upon themselves". This parallels attitudes to those with "physical" illnesses (Crandall and Moriarty 1995).

3. The person with the "mental illness"

Labels

The person with the "mental illness" has had this label attached to him or her, usually by a doctor. Illness labels stem from the medical need to seek out diagnostic categories that will enable doctors to (a) recognise the next similar disorder that comes their way,

(b) predict its course from background knowledge concerning it and related risk factors, and (c) select and recommend treatment that is known to improve outcome. This "medical model" approach has often proved effective and indeed essential to good practice. However, it carries the hazards of over-inclusiveness, incompetent application, ineffectual treatments and the generation of a potentially harmful label. Moreover, by its very nature, it often excludes recognition of the uniqueness and individuality of the person so labelled. Of its several possible meanings, the term "shrink" best describes and represents this process! In a busy practice, or if professional indifference or burnout prevail, then the ancestral mechanism that has been outlined earlier as underlying the stigmatisation processes can now be even more specifically activated. The label now provides further reinforcement and a focus for stigmatisation of the mentally ill person.

With "bodily" disease, the diagnosed illness is more often perceived as an infliction upon the person concerned, whose autonomy and individuality remains respected. The diagnosis of mental illness, by contrast, carries a further potential for losing sight of the person as a unique individual. This may be partly due to the fact that mental illness is sometimes perceived in a reductionist way as "brain" disease, despite, in some cases, more apparently than is the case with physical illness, being related to personality, relationships and life events. Mental illness labels are thus often especially feared. They can render the individual a victim unless they lead to effective treatments.

Social handicaps that can arise as products of mental illnesses

Many illnesses and related disabilities, acute and chronic, generate definite and unavoidable social handicaps. Infectious diseases may demand or invoke social distancing because of risks of transmission. In the process they can provoke a variety of attitudes within others, dependent upon perceptions of the disorders (e.g. resistant staphylococcal infection, tuberculosis, sexually transmitted diseases or the common cold). Illnesses associated with offensive smells (e.g. those causing putrefaction, faecal incontinence) have similar potential impact. Recurrent epilepsy may make social interaction difficult and lead to social avoidance. Physical disfigurements, with and without restricted mobility, blindness, deafness and other sensory losses, all compel some social disadvantage. The list of such other disabling bodily disorders is extensive. Many people with such "physical" illnesses strive to minimise their associated social handicaps.

Some few medical disorders carry a cachet, usually either by immediate association or because of presumed or apparent aetiology. Obesity, now often perceived as reflecting self-indulgence, has been revered in the past as evidence of health, strength and wealth. In some cultures this attitude still prevails. Gout has been called "the patrician malady" (Porter 2000), again because, in the past, its aetiology was associated with wealth and good living. Bipolar affective disorder and, sometimes, forms of personality disorder, may be perceived as related to the creative arts in particular (see Part 7 of this book) and afflicted individuals correspondingly respected, muting the social disadvantages (Schildkraut and Ottero 1996).

But mental illnesses can sometimes generate a variety of unavoidable social disadvantages for those so afflicted. Impairment within mental illnesses is in such realms as cognition, affect and behaviour. Such processes are fundamental to many social interactions. Moreover, sometimes the related disorder has specific links with and is sensitive to social settings and interpersonal relationships (see below).

Mental illness in individuals is not always recognised by others. It may be concealed successfully from others or personally denied. It has been said that no more than half of people with acute or chronic mental illness have obvious social handicaps. Even then the mental illness may go undetected. Some mental illnesses are accompanied by evident physical disabilities (e.g. movement disorders as unwanted effects of medication for schizophrenia) or abnormalities (e.g. stunted growth in anorexia nervosa) that generate additional social problems. The stigmatisations of people with mental illnesses not only fuel their low self-esteem (self-stigmatisation) but generate secrecy and denial, further hampering abilities to communicate.

Mental illnesses are sometimes also linked to personality. The latter can also generate social handicaps for the individual, especially within the realm of so-called personality disorders (see Part 5 of this book), e.g. related to antisocial behaviour or drug/alcohol dependency. Co-morbidity is quite common. For example, anxiety may accompany severe depression; anxiety and/or severe depression may co-exist with alcohol or drug misuse. So may schizophrenia. Eating disorders can co-exist with severe depression and addictions. Early dementia and depression may occur together.

Social handicaps associated with mental illnesses can provide a major basis for the stigmatising processes. The six groups of disorders that we are concerned with here (see e.g. Parts 2 and 4 of this book) are addressed separately from the standpoint of illustrative, sometimes irreducible, social handicaps/disabilities that can accompany each of them. Such handicaps are not exclusive to those with mental illnesses. They can also exist in others as aspects of personality.

Anxiety disorders

Nineteen percent of females and 14% of males at any one time have an anxiety disorder (including mild depression) (data drawn from ONS (2001) – this does not include patients in hospitals or other caring institutions).

Phobic anxiety

The person with a specific phobia will not experience panic so long as the phobic object/situation can be avoided. Others may then be unaware of its existence. However, if it limits mobility and freedom, the individual may come to be experienced by others as either a social burden or, if the phobia is concealed/denied, then bafflingly tyrannical and manipulative as they strive desperately to protect themselves from exposure to the dreaded object or experience.

Phobic individuals will go to great lengths to avoid exposure to the phobic object/situation, but if this fails (e.g. a person with a flying phobia is compelled to fly, a socially restricted house-bound person with agoraphobia is compelled to travel, a person with a thunder phobia is unavoidably exposed to thunder etc.), panic erupts, and flight and/or somatic symptoms (e.g. hyperventilation, sweating, palpitations) occur. Such panic may invoke some support but may also be experienced as threateningly contagious. Others may then prefer to distance themselves or at the least may feel uncomfortable and disempowered.

Phobias are common. They may be unitary or multiple and may be linked to more generalised anxiety. The latter may be associated with reduced appetites, including reduced libido. Difficulty in sleeping may also have social repercussions. All such factors can have adverse effects on personal relationships.

Obsessive compulsive disorder (OCD)

Obsessional fears and ideas and/or compulsive and ritualistic thoughts and behaviour preoccupy the individual who has OCD. He/she may well become uneasy and irritable if distracted. Obsessional fears and ideas may focus on dirt (leading to excessive and intrusive cleaning) or sexuality (impairing intimate relationships) and also generate other unexpected behaviour. Such fear and ideas, sometimes not acknowledged, can also leave the individual severely socially restricted in other ways, e.g. unable to mix with the public or use public services. Attention to personal hygiene may be excessive or reduced.

Severe depression

There is a 10% lifetime expectancy for severe depression. A person with severe depression has reduced energy and spontaneity and has difficulty with eye contact and conversation. Appetite and libido are usually reduced. Self-neglect may arise. Personal relationships become impoverished. The feelings of defeat, hopelessness and worthlessness may be communicated. The capacity to work is reduced and the individual becomes unproductive. Agitation and complaints about sleeplessness can be major features and socially intrusive. As with the anxiety disorders above, the individual may resort to alcohol consumption as an attempt at self-medication. Other self-destructive feelings and thoughts may be detected by others, invoking a variety of reactions ranging from the protective to the defensive.

Schizophrenia

Schizophrenia (with a lifetime expectancy of 1%) can confer severe social handicaps, especially if the psychotic symptoms are acute or severe. For example, if hallucinations are active, the afflicted person may act as if they are hearing something that others cannot. They may respond to their hallucinations in ways that are startling to others. False beliefs may lead them to be puzzlingly suspicious or threatening. They may say bizarre or inappropriate things in conversation. Their speech and manner may seem odd. They may also show side effects of medication, such as obesity, odd movements, restlessness, strange facial expressions. In general, those unused to being with such a person may find them very odd, unpredictable and unsettling to interact with.

Violence, sometimes amounting to homicide, is a much publicised alleged attribute. In reality such violence is slightly more common than arises generally, *but* it is rare. It is more likely if the individual is intoxicated with street drugs or alcohol, although this is more a characteristic of such intoxication and is not specific to those afflicted with schizophrenia. Over the last several decades the proportion of homicides in the population attributable to people with schizophrenia has steadily fallen.

People with chronic schizophrenia may seem "burnt-out", i.e. emotionally unresponsive, without purpose and energy and uninterested in personal hygiene. People affected in this way are only a proportion of those with schizophrenia, which is itself a rare condition. Nevertheless, care in the community has resulted in the public becoming more familiar with the condition, which then is sometimes perceived as indicative of all mental illness.

Because schizophrenia can take this publicly identifiable form, it is often not realised that some people with schizophrenia can have a single short illness, or long periods of remission with and without treatment.

Dementia

This condition, which affects 20% of those aged over 80, is a process of progressive deterioration/disintegration of intellect, memory and personality, due to physical changes in the brain. It becomes commoner with age and is common in the eighth and later decades of life.

Often recent memory becomes most impaired. Good judgement and well-being can fail at the same time, and previous intellectual interests wither. Personality can change. Some traits disappear; others come to the fore. Ability to relate in a friendly manner may be lost, and evil intent by others may be imagined and acted upon.

Wandering, driven by fragments of such beliefs and residual memories and related distress, may become a feature and then incontinence arises. Fleeting insight into what is happening and emotional outbursts can occur. Depression may be an early symptom. Such deterioration in a loved one can be especially difficult to bear. Not being recognised or being positively misidentified, watching a parent becoming a caricature of their old self and thus confronting one's own possible outcome, can lead powerfully to denial and rejection as well as feelings of helplessness and depression.

Eating disorders

These affect 2% of people, but arise mainly in young adult females (EDA 2000).

Anorexia nervosa

The person with anorexia nervosa is as she/he needs to be and will defend this position to the exclusion of all else. This may require her/him to be totally in control of food intake and deceitful as needs be, solitary and otherwise tyrannical. Preoccupation with food and avoidance of its ingestion because of its weight-gain consequences often totally absorbs the individual's attention and concentration. If weight gain occurs or is threatened by social pressures, then panic erupts. Obvious despair or tantrums may also occur. This pattern of behaviour, often coupled with concealment of its origins from others, though psychologically protective, is socially seriously damaging and handicapping.

Until health is seriously undermined by severe starvation, the person with anorexia nervosa, who is often basically conscientious, can sometimes remain industrious and achieve relative success educationally or in the workplace. The person with established anorexia nervosa is infertile and asexual, as well as emaciated and physically unattractive to most others. All this resonates with her/his desire to be left alone but is obviously a serious barrier to social interaction and development. People who attempt to help, simplistically encouraging the person with anorexia nervosa to eat, quickly become disempowered and usually give up. The same can happen in relation to the other relentlessly self-destructive components of anorexia nervosa such as suicide itself.

Ironically enough, such underlying severe social pathology may be further overlooked by others, especially when the disorder is not associated with severe emaciation. They only (enviously) perceive instead what they construe to be admirable "self-control", rather than the reality of the panic-driven avoidance behaviour.

Bulimia nervosa

The extreme avoidant component which can stigmatise those with anorexia nervosa is absent in bulimia nervosa. Outwardly the individual may be highly sociable for much of the time. She/he is more impulsive and this may be condensed exclusively into the domain of eating/bingeing. Since obesity is feared after bingeing, vomiting and purgation are necessary defences. Such behaviour can be remarkably well concealed, but usually declares itself socially sooner or later.

Excessive cigarette smoking can arise as a defence against the impulse to eat. Behaviours can take on the force of a compulsion and addiction so that indifference and insensitivity to surroundings creates an additional social barrier for the individual.

Other impulse-ridden behaviours can erupt, taking such forms as sexual promiscuity, shop-lifting, and drug and alcohol dependence, all with the potential for invoking major disapproval by others. Other major co-morbidity includes depression.

Alcohol use, misuse and dependence

Thirty-eight percent of males and 15% of females are identified with "hazardous drinking", including 7% of us assessed as alcohol-addicted (ONS 2001). Denial of addiction to/consumption of alcohol and the craving consequent upon addiction can handicap normal social interactions in many ways. The addict's single-mindedness and desperation can disempower people who are close to them. Communication can wither. Intoxication can produce varying degrees of personality change and lead to the expression of strong emotions. There may be little lasting memory for behaviour and events during the period of intoxication, leaving others feeling imposed upon, angry and helpless, especially when the addiction and intoxication have arisen partly as a product of close but conflict-laden relationships with the afflicted person. The disorder often comes to impair sexual function and can become associated with morbid jealousy and violence, including a much higher than usual risk of physical abuse of others, homicide and suicide. Severe intoxication can lead to stupor, coma and delirium, with accompanying social embarrassments.

Recurrent intoxication can lead to permanent tissue damage throughout much of the body, including the brain. Memory and personality then become permanently damaged. Alcohol dependence amounting to addiction is common and many afflicted people manage to survive socially for a long time and may recover, especially with help. In other instances the syndrome declares itself in the workplace to the social and economic disadvantage of the individual concerned. Pursuit of alcohol can impoverish the individual and his dependents and come to involve criminal activities. Alcohol dependence can co-exist with high levels of social anxiety, low self-esteem and other formal mental illnesses, especially depressive illnesses, personality disorders and addiction to other substances. In such instances the social handicaps caused by those disabilities compound the problem.

Alcohol is "used" by the majority of people in our society for recreational purposes and in ways that fall short of it being a fully addictive process. It is commonly used in social settings to reduce handicaps such as shyness, social anxiety and low self-esteem, through its disinhibiting and anxiety-reducing effects. There is a spectrum from using alcohol in this way through to socially handicapping and damaging addictive and intoxicated behaviour, such as that referred to above. The term "misuse" is often applied to its excessive and "deliberate" consumption to produce intoxication and consequent antisocial behaviour. Some societies and cultures prohibit or generally disapprove of alcohol consumption. In our own society there are those, including health care professionals (e.g. Johns, Chapter 35), who suggest that it, but not the individual, should be formally "stigmatised".

Drug use, misuse and dependence

This occurs in 20% of males and 9% of females aged 20–24. The overall prevalence is 4% (ONS 2001). As with alcohol, social handicaps can arise both from the egosyntonic need to secure the drug and from its intoxicating effect. Such behaviours, especially when buttressed by denial, or secretiveness, can especially baffle and dismay others and have a distancing effect. The handicaps, to an extent, depend upon the particular drug. The need to secure it, especially if the individual is addicted, dominate and generate violent and/or criminal activity. As with alcohol, drug usage significantly often overlaps and interacts with one or other mental illness, or with personality traits that further hamper normal communication. Single-minded drug dependence can also lead to personal neglect and destitution, and impoverish communication with others.

4. More specific public perceptions of the person already labelled as "mentally ill"

In 1998 the Management Committee decided to survey the reported perceptions of the adult British public concerning people with mental illnesses before the start of the Campaign. We invited such consideration in respect of each of six diagnostic categories of mental illness: anxiety disorders, depressive disorders, schizophrenia, dementia, eating disorders, drug and alcohol misuse/addiction. The more detailed outcome of this survey is described by Gelder in Chapter 3 and in Crisp et al. (2000). Briefly, people with drug and alcohol misuse/addiction and with schizophrenia were reported as being especially *dangerous* to others; those with eating disorders or drug or alcohol misuse/addiction were commonly perceived as having "only themselves to blame" and as being capable of "pulling themselves together". Major problems with "communication" and "empathy" were perceived as common across the board, as was the (consequent) perceived characteristic of "unpredictability". It is these additional descriptive labels, again over-inclusive and often exaggerated, that further define the negative and stigmatised status of people with mental illnesses.

5 and 6. The personal and social impacts of such stigmatisation

These are profound and have been movingly described by people with mental illnesses in Part 2 of this book in particular. Some such effects are briefly listed in Figure 1 and are dealt with extensively in this book and in the literature (e.g. Dunn 1999; Sayce 2000). They take us beyond the realm of stigmatisation per se, the subject of this chapter. Both psychological and social in their nature, they add hugely to the burden and distress of the person with the illness.

Interventions

The schema in Figure 1 invites interventions at all six levels. Corrigan and Watson (2002) have recently proposed again that interventions to curb stigmatisation can properly be construed as falling into three categories, namely Education, Contact, and Protest. These correspond comfortably with well-established vocational educational programmes, e.g. for medicine, that are framed in terms of Knowledge, Skills and Attitudes.

Some approaches to attempts at destigmatisation are described elsewhere in this Part. The Campaign Toolkit (www.changingminds.co.uk) also reflects an attempt to inform and empower us in this respect (see the appendix to Chapter 64).

It may be equally important to understand and respect our human biology. Personal growth, facilitated from childhood, that maximises self-understanding, openness, good communication skills, respect for diversity, wariness of the media, are goals to aim for. We might also aspire to develop a "new look" declaration of human obligations to match our current concerns with human rights.

References

Allport GW (1954) *The Nature of Prejudice.* New York: Addison-Wesley.
Churchill C (2002) *A Number.* London: Nick Hern Books.

Corrigan PW & Watson AC (2002) Understanding the impact of stigma on people with mental illness. *Journal of World Psychiatry* 1: 6–19.

Crandall CS & Moriarty D (1995) Physical illness: Stigma and rejection. *British Journal of Social Psychology* 34: 67–83.

Crisp AH, Gelder MG, Rix S, Meltzer HI & Rowlands OJ (2000) Stigmatisation of people with mental illnesses. *British Journal of Psychiatry* 177: 4–7.

Dunn S (1999) Creating accepting communities. In: *Report of the Mind Enquiry into Social Exclusion and Mental Health Problems*. London: Mind. 21: 21–42.

EDA (2000) *The Need for Action in 2000 and Beyond*. Eating Disorders Association (www.edauk.com).

Freud S (1925) *Some Psychical Consequences of the Anatomical Distinctions Between the Sexes. Standard Edition of the Complete Psychological Works of Sigmund Freud*, Vol 19. London: Hogarth Press.

Haghighat R (2001) A unitary theory of stigmatisation. *British Journal of Psychiatry* 178: 207–15.

Kelly JM (1999) *General Public Attitude to Mental Health/Illness. A Summary of Existing Research Prepared for the Central Office of Information on Behalf of the DoH*. COI Ref RS 4206. London: The Stationery Office.

Kurzban R & Leary M (2001) Evolutionary origins of stigmatisation: the functions of social exclusion. *Psychological Bulletin* 127: 187–208.

Lerner MJ (1980) *The Belief in a Just World: A Fundamental Delusion*. New York : Plenum Press.

O'Neil O (2002), *Reith Lectures*. London: BBC.

ONS (2001) *Psychiatric Morbidity Among Adults Living in Private Households*. Office of National Statistics.

Philo G (1996) *Media and Mental Distress*. London: Addison-Wesley.

Pinker S (2002) *The Blank Slate: the Modern Denial of Human Nature*. London: Allen Lane, Penguin Press.

Porter R (2000) *Gout: The Patrician Malady*. London: Yale University Press.

Porter R (2002) *Madness*. Oxford: Oxford University Press.

Sayce EL (2000) *From Psychiatric Patient to Citizen. Overcoming Social Discrimination and Exclusion*. Basingstoke: Palgrave.

Schildkraut JJ & Ottero A (1996) *Depression and the Spiritual in Modern Art*. Chichester: Wiley.

Stout R (2002) Review of "Living Without Free Will" by Derk Pereboom. *Times Literary Supplement*. December issue: 28.

Epilogue

Concluding message from the Royal College of Psychiatrists

John Cox

The College is embarked upon the second public education campaign in its 30-year history, and perhaps its most ambitious to date. "Defeat Depression" was the slogan of our campaign initiated in 1992 – a war analogy, initially perhaps a more audible clarion call than Changing Minds. Yet as this campaign has shown the possibility to reduce stigma and change minds can indeed occur.

The College much values the contribution of the Royal Society of Medicine and the Sir Robert Mond Memorial Trust for their support of the campaign and their production of this important book, edited by Professor Crisp. I am sure members of the College who read it will be changed in their own attitudes a little.

Stigma has been shown to be a multi-faceted public and private attitude; the marking out, the branding and distancing of the person; the reassuring belief that only others are irrational and that only others can have a mental disorder. "Every Family in the Land" has encouraged us to "come out" with regard to our own family's experience of mental disorder, and to appreciate more fully as the *1 in 4* film concludes, "it could be your aunt, your son, your mother, your spouse, it could be you – it could be me".

The campaign slogan takes time to leave *its* mark. Yet the survey evidence showed that despite changing family structures, and in many instances their replacement by non-familial supports, we still do have a sense of family and can recognise that mental health problems may occur not only in other families but also in our own.

Most of us can identify a family member with a mental illness; when my father for example was offered a necessary and substantial loan by his more affluent elder brother which never materialised, was this an act of brotherly generosity or a symptom of a manic illness – or was it both? Why was it that his treatment in a mental hospital was never really talked about?

Many of us may have experienced a mood disorder or realised that a hallucination is not restricted to those with frank mental illness. Some may have seen a close relative suffer from a brain/mind disorder and welcomed the anonymity of a consultation with a psychiatrist arranged by a familiar general practitioner. Some have recognised that stigmatised attitudes towards mental disorder are more conspicuous in the carer than in the service user.

As this book makes clear, these mental disorders are widespread. Some are very conspicuous and obvious to a passer-by; others more internal and recognised only by the individual or by those in the close family.

Why *do* we feel the need to preserve our own false sense of rationality by marking out others? After all, next time the stigmatised could be one of us and this could restrict our access to thorough investigation and appropriate treatment critical to our future well-being and quality of life.

Mental disorders are "brain disorders". Our brains, like other parts of our body, can become disordered when the external stressors are extensive, or when adverse memories of the past intrude into the present. There are *no* pure mental illnesses without a physical basis, as the emphasis of this campaign correctly points out. All mental disorders are partly explicable by changes in brain function – though not necessarily by observable structural abnormalities.

Psychiatrists are in a holistic sense brain doctors who specialise in disturbances of a person's behaviour, mood and cognition and are to some degree stigmatised by proxy.

This campaign rightly therefore challenges first the medical profession. If stigmatising attitudes are not replaced by a more realistic understanding of the need for consultant psychiatrists and for other mental health professionals, then the public (including doctors) will not have available help when it is needed because of recruitment and retention problems. Doctors do indeed need to put our house in order and eliminate stigmatised attitudes towards those with psychiatric disorders and those who specifically care for them (mental health nurses, psychiatrists, psychologists).

Yet let us also understand that experience of a mental disorder can be a characteristic of an artist, and hence a risk factor for some of the most creative people in society. Doctors are also at risk, not only because they work in stressful environments, but also because they often carry the burdens and fears of others. I remember reading a book called *Wounded Healers* (Altschul 1985), which consisted of accounts of mental illnesses experienced by health professionals, and the way this affected their professional lives, and increased their sensitivities to others' difficulties. Is a mental health professional, who has never experienced a mood disorder, likely to be less empathic with a patient and therefore less therapeutic in the daily task?

We need therefore to *stop stigma* before stigma stops us from accessing help when it is needed or from carrying on working when there should be a period of sick leave. There is no them and us; no doctor who could not be a patient.

The aims of the Royal College of Psychiatrists – an independent international and democratic organisation – are to maintain standards of education and training as well as to enhance understanding of the causes and management of mental disorder. Psychiatry is not "fringe medicine" as my Oxford physiology tutor once advised me. On the contrary, the present day advocates for integrative medicine, in which brain and mind, body and soul come together, could change attitudes towards psychiatry and reduce the stigma towards the so-called mental illnesses and also towards those who have the specific training to provide therapy for those with mental disorder.

If the false divide between mental and physical illness can be demolished, if it can be realised fully that anyone can develop mental illness – and that all require unimpeded access to help if this should occur – then this campaign could yet be very successful indeed. For this to happen leaders of public opinion, and not just show business personalities, need to feel more free to talk about their own mental health difficulties and episodes of mental illness, and for employers for example to realise that a past history of mental disorder, far from being a liability, could be a substantial asset.

Furthermore, great art, whether music, poetry or painting, has gained its dramatic force and aesthetic beauty from externalising and hence healing some of the inner experiences of the creative artist and hence those of the onlooker. These artists have out of their own sufferings helped us, and in so doing have reduced the negative stereotypes which can so often characterise our perception of an individual with mental disorder.

Through this campaign the Royal College of Psychiatrists is indeed endeavouring to put its own house in order. From its commitment to research and high standards of training it aims to ensure that a future generation of doctors are more likely to have worked through their own stigmatising attitudes, and hence are freer to describe their own difficulties and listen to the discrimination experienced by their patients. In this way they will become stronger advocates for change.

Reference

Altschul A (1985) There won't be a next time. In: Rippere V & Williams R (eds). *Wounded Healers: Mental Health Workers' Experience of Depression.* Chichester: Wiley: 167–75.

Appendix

Notes on the Illustrations and Artists

The illustrations

The paintings and sculptures illustrated in this book are all held by the Bethlem Royal Hospital Archives and Museum.

The Bethlem Royal Archives and Museum were first opened to the public in 1970, and house art and historical collections spanning many centuries, which are of great interest and importance in the field of mental health. The historical collections included the archives of Bethlem Hospital (the original 'bedlam', founded in 1247) and the Maudsley Hospital (founded as a mental hospital early last century), as well as other historical material relating to the history of these two hospitals. An outstanding exhibit in the tiny museum is the pair of statues known as *Raving Madness* and *Melancholy* from the gates of 17th century Bethlem.

The art collection has come together from many different sources, not only from these two hospitals. It consists mainly of paintings and drawings by trained or practising artists who have suffered from mental illness, but also includes works produced under the influence of abnormal mental experiences of other kinds. It is particularly famous for the exquisite watercolours of the Victorian artist Richard Dadd, who painted throughout his 42 years of confinement in Bethlem and Broadmoor, but contains many powerful, disturbing and often deeply moving images, including works by contemporary artists.

The collections are owned and managed by a charitable trust - the Bethlem Art and History Collections Trust. The current objectives of the Trust are to enlarge the building in order to provide better access to the collections and encourage their use for educational purposes, and to develop the resources of the archives and museum to inform and educate the public about mental illness and mental health issues, and to contribute towards the destigmatisation of mental illness.

The artists

The following text is based on biographical material from the Bethlem Museum and on material from Robert Howard's series, 'Mind Odyssey – Psychiatry in Pictures', published each month in the *British Journal of Psychiatry* since July 2001.

Anon (A 'Fisk' out of Aqua)

Presumably an oblique and distorted expression of the artist's experience of his or her situation, *A 'Fisk' out of Aqua* is an imaginative and witty "psychotic realist" painting. The picture is one of the most popular with both staff and visitors to the Bethlem Royal Hospital Art Collection. We know only that it was painted at Bexley Hospital in the 1950s and that the artist was somewhat dismissively described as a "chronic paraphrenic".

Anon (Let Me Be)

The artist, a person with anorexia nervosa who wishes to remain anonymous, painted herself and her circumstances – "me as I am" - within art therapy. She conveyed her aborted existence within the illness and thereby provided a personally relevant building block for the psychotherapy.

Bryan Charnley 1949-1991

Of all Bryan Charnley's paintings, it is his final sequence of pictures that is most famous. They were painted whilst he took himself off medication in order to experience his schizophrenia in an unadulterated form, which culminated in his suicide. *Broach Schizophrene* formed part of his portrayal of his personal experience of his illness. In an "Artist's statement" to accompany his pictures, he wrote in 1988: "Sigmund Freud, commenting on his work on the mind, said that wherever he had been, an artist or poet had been there before him. I hope, to some extent, my work might exist in a similar way. I try to avoid being too direct about the privations suffered as a schizophrene and try instead for more oblique poetic metaphors as I feel the truth can be more nearly approached this way. My work is also a much needed form of exorcism. Apart from my pictures, I regard my illness as completely negative, involving the sufferer in a vicious downward spiral. Current medical practice attempts to suppress both the patient and his symptoms, convenient but evasive. My paintings stand as an attempt to penetrate this wall of silence and I hope they can throw some light on a condition which has largely eluded medical science."

Caius Gabriel Cibber 1630-1700

A Danish-born sculptor who worked mainly in England, Cibber came to this country at the beginning of the Restoration period. He was appointed "Carver to the King's Closet" for his services to William III. Cibber worked for a time for Sir Christopher Wren and produced the reliefs on the square pedestal on which the Monument in the City of London stands. He is best known for his statues *Melancholy* and *Raving Madness* at the Bethlem Museum in London. His son Colley was Poet Laureate to George II.

Richard Dadd 1817-1886

An English-born artist who began exhibiting his work in 1837, Dadd gained a reputation as a promising young artist. However, when he was 25, whilst travelling around Europe and the Middle East, he developed symptoms of severe mental disturbance and was suffering paranoid delusions by the time he returned home. These were so severe that he stabbed his father to death believing him to be the devil in disguise. Dadd fled to France but was arrested. He was extradited after 10 months and committed to the asylum attached to Bethlem Hospital. He continued to paint throughout his 42 years of confinement. It was here that he painted his *Sketches to Illustrate the Passions*. About 30 have survived; they each take the form of a scene dominated by figures from literature or history. Dadd was always unpredictable, occasionally violent and never completely lost his delusions. He died of consumption in 1886.

Olivia Gillow b.1972

Trained at art schools in Brighton, Glasgow and Munich, Olivia Gillow is a professional artist whose current work focuses on paintings of landscapes and the experience of mental illness. Over the past 10 years, despite initial compliance with mood-stabilising drugs, she has had several in-patient admissions for bipolar disorder and maintains regular contact with the Manic Depression Fellowship. During one of her admissions she shared a room with a woman with obsessive-compulsive disorder who had distressing hand-washing rituals. This disorder has been the theme of other works by Gillow, in particular an installation involving a door. When turned, the door handle goes round and round without any other action. Carved around the doorframe are the words: "If you were suffering from obsessive compulsive disorder you would have to turn the door handle again... and again... and again... and again before you could enter the room."

Dorothy H. 1899-1980

Dorothy H. spent most of her life as a patient in St Augustine's Hospital in Canterbury. Diagnosed with schizophrenia, she believed that she was married to the Chinese Emperor. She embroidered pictures all of which featured stories about him. Her description of *The Story of a Chinese Emperor* is as follows: "Three bridges are the theme of this picture. A green Dragon, mighty in winged splenders, climbs the top bridge of rope ladder connecting roof to roof. A lady opens a window and hands him a nice pot of thea. The young Empress plays Ma-Hong on the roof with her baby boy, sable winged. Only dead Converse with Caste, in mauve descaced walks up arm out off over green shrub angels soon forecasting the failure, guillotine and cross and thorne crown ere God his tiny people will hear on the Sun platform the legless Emperor Jesus wears real crown forget me not on guise Tron. Nor Man a woman huddles her bade to breast, rearing, charging steads plunge forward in man's arms and slumbers two more. Second bridge connecting door of stone houses stone constructed. My own family in left two bays in red below a tame peacock feeding out of bogs best basket bonnet. The stone work is covered with blossoms. Right boy naked climb from sailing vessel to rope ladder. A marble woman holds air up in glass slaps water bark in blue ball stands on ash sand ridge cosmos square. Centre piece charging bull Hercules follows stone shield held high. Cage holds corpre in spikes slowly ground for ammunition. The stone bridge is divided by monument holding gigantic ball over-roofed. Passing in mauve holy man swings Owl lamps, to light Una Dea - Confisscius Pallas on bridge with scarlet banner sometimes raising ded. Two Hearse bearer carry first war victim. A general my fathers uniform cock helmet look of Roman Dynamite in ton one child brings to explode the other babe stands on head kicks its wells to fire. Mother looks on her door is Alp violet under Glass Fish Roof. Three princes under clef and procede past drinking tea, veiled nurses hold bamboo sticks. Two pairs of men women dancers hold between them, to the beat of the bango the ladies gracefully rotate holding sword in sun shade their arrival and death burning under fish signal war and child's protection. The base is a cross bridge swung on invisible golden boxes. In the distance 1600 bridges pines snow laden are seen towers of execution, pagodas like front. On the other side a floss carrying a fisherman under his red flag beseeching his son to hand him baby down. A nice kind second dragon hides all a bit from enemy. I forget on right over Pagoda a one eyes tortured cat myself the Zar H. Romanoff Christ Next to her cross staffed red bearing Nepomak on sandstone block, the signpost to my hill castle holds. In middle the Imperial Rickshaw is open a ring of bamboo alone draws attention to the royalty, a kakadu in cage and bells ring admirably in. The Empror wears shell pink of the ocean wife plays mondoline to beguile her fair sposer back from the journey he never starts, overhead a foul murderess stabs his pulsating heart."

Bibi Herrera b.1956

Bibi Herrera was the daughter of a prominent communist activist, and in 1973, on the day of the coup that brought General Pinochet to power, she was arrested and held for over three years, enduring interrogation, torture and rape. She arrived in Britain as a political refugee in 1977, but soon felt isolated and unable to face the brutality of her past and this resulted in her first suicide attempt. In 1993, after receiving news that a close friend in Chile had been killed in an accident, she cut her wrists, damaging nerves and tendons so severely that she has permanently lost the use of her left hand. During her subsequent admission to the Bethlem Hospital she was encouraged to talk about her experiences in Chile. She recalls that at this point she was "extremely unhappy, angry to be alive and reluctant to do anything". It was here that she was offered occupational therapy in the form of pottery. Her pots and their decorative designs draw heavily on her memories of Chilean Indian art and traditional symbols. "My pots remind me of my people and I like the colours. I think the reason is, when you've been through so much, everything is black and white. I think it's that I want to see that life is not only black and white." Herrera believes that without pottery she would almost certainly have not been able to come to terms with her traumatic and degrading experiences and would have made further serious attempts to end her life. "My life has been quite black but I want to show that there is still much beauty in the World and we can all find something better. Pottery has given me a reason to carry on living. I can make something instead of destroying it, especially my life."

William Kurelek 1927-1977

Born into a Ukrainian immigrant community in Alberta, Canada, Kurelek grew up terrified of his father and suffered psychological problems throughout his youth, which he attributed to this relationship. He briefly attended the Ontario College of Art but left and hitchhiked to Mexico, spending five months at an art school there. He then went to seek psychiatric treatment in London, where he was admitted to the Maudsley hospital. While he was there, he painted *The Maze,* which he described as follows: "The subject, seen as a whole, is of a man (representing me) lying on a barren plain before a wheatfield, with his head split open. The point of view is from the top of his head. The subject is then roughly divided into the left hand side of the picture, with the thoughts made in his head represented as a maze; and the right hand side, the view of the rest of his body. The hands and feet are seen through the eyes, nose and mouth, tapering off into the distance and the outside world. The Maze. An exitless one, it occupies and divides the inside of the cranium into groups of thoughts, the passageways being calculated to do the grouping. The white rat curled up in the central cavity represents my Spirit (I suppose). He is curled up with frustration from having run the passages so long without hope of escaping out of this maze of unhappy thoughts. Outside World. Grasshoppers and drought (sun before the clouds) represent the mercilessness of Nature, which bankrupted my father, a farmer, and brought out of him the cornered beast. The thorny, stony ground is a kind of T.S. Eliot Wasteland - spiritual and cultural barrenness: the pile of excrement with flies on it represents my view of the world and the people that live on it. The loosened red ribbon bound together the head of a T.S. Eliot Hollow Man, and was united by psychotherapy (Dr Cormier), but since the outside world is still unappealing, the rat remains inert. Before the head was opened, burrs (bitter experiences) choked the throat and pricked the sensitive underside of the tongue, and when it was opened the sawdust and shavings (tasteless education) spilled out from on top the tongue: mixed with the sawdust are symbols of (to me) equally tasteless Art, painting, literature and music. The burrs also represent, in the eye socket, the successive evaluations of my character by any friend during the process of acquaintance, all repellant but hopeful till the last, when the heart is discovered to be a grub. On the tongue and in the throat, the Kurelek family (big burrs produce little burrs), representing my father as the hard domineering blue burr opening up the mushy yellow burr, my mother, to release a common lot of burrs, my brothers and sisters, and one unique orange one - myself. The last burr, spearing culture, is I at the university. The inverted one is I as a child, trapped painfully between two aspects of my father, the one I hated and the one I worshipped." He became a Catholic in 1957, and he attributed his full recovery to this rather than his treatment. He returned to Toronto in 1959 where he married and spent the rest of his life painting and writing, dying of cancer aged 50.

Stanley Lench 1934-2000

Episodes of manic-depressive illness punctuated Lench's life from his childhood and he was first a patient of the Maudsley Children's Department. Self-taught as an artist, he had a West End exhibition when he was only 21 and from this he gained a place at the Royal College of Art. His pictures record his obsession with appearances and the very different reality that may underlie them. He called this theme "the illusion of illusions". He worked as an attendant at the Tate Gallery and took perverse pleasure in the fact that many visitors who were eminent in the arts world failed to recognise the true artist in their midst. On one occasion, Lord Clark came by with a small entourage, satisfactorily ignoring Lench and triggering off a series of stylish and mocking paintings.

Jonathan Martin 1782-1838

The son of a tanner, Martin was born in Northumberland. One of his brothers, John, was a popular history painter; another, William, was an inventor and pamphleteer. After a period in the Navy, Martin followed in his father's footsteps, becoming a tanner. He then became inspired by prophetic dreams and converted to Methodism. Several times, his religious fervour brought him before magistrates for disrupting church services. He was sent to the asylum before escaping and settling down to work in Darlington, but he continued to believe that he had a personal mission to expose the corrupt state of the established church. His conviction led to a failed attempt to burn down York Minster. He was sent to gaol and then the asylum at Bethlem. Martin's paintings depict his prophetic visions and are filled with rich imagery, high drama and extravagant fantasy.

Vaslav Nijinsky 1890-1950

Born in Kiev, Nijinsky was the son of Polish parents who were both dancers. He entered the Imperial Ballet School at the age of ten and had achieved success as a soloist, even before graduation. World fame and iconic status was attained when he joined the Russian ballet company *Ballet Russes* to choreograph and perform. During 1918, while living in Switzerland to await the end of the war, he began to suffer a mental breakdown that was eventually diagnosed as schizophrenia. It was during this period that he made most of his paintings. They are all based on the circle, which not surprisingly for a dancer, he regarded as the perfect line. *A Mask* seems to be related to a group of less figurative drawings which he was making as his mental state approached a crisis, described by his wife in her biography of him: "His study and rooms were literally covered with designs; no longer portraits or scenic or decorative subjects, but strange faces, eyes peering from every corner, red and black, like a bloodstained mortuary cover, They made me shudder. 'What are those masks' 'Soldiers' faces. It is the war'."

Elise Pacquette (née Warriner) b.1968

Elise Pacquette suffered from severe and at times life-threatening anorexia nervosa between 1986 and 1997, and painted *The Anger Within* during her final year at art school. "The real element of the painting is the incredible contrast between the somewhat passive outside image of the person and its contrast with the inside which holds all the emotion." As the title suggests, the picture is an expression of her anger during the illness, hidden within a formless bubble of a body without arms or legs and with only a line for a mouth. "This is all of the outside or peripheral bits of me that could express emotion and which are shut down. Inside is turmoil. Everything is happening here. Emotions are bubbling up. My anger was important. It gave me energy and allowed me to do things and masked my fear, frustration and loneliness. It allowed me to express the way I was feeling in a way that I could use as a tool against other people. If I showed how lonely I was, people would come to try and get close to me, to try to change me. I didn't want that." The anger is a hidden monstrous presence of which only the artist has awareness. "It is all inside. Nothing of that can be seen on the outside. It is as if all the senses are on the inside". Elise Pacquette is now completely well and working in the theatre and with the deaf.

Marion Patrick 1940-1993

Marion Patrick was born and brought up in Lancashire. She suffered from a severe bipolar illness and was first admitted to hospital at the age of 15. After training at the Burnley School of Art, she painted and exhibited her work until the 1970s, when she gave up, distressed by the mess it made in her home, now in Gravesend, which she kept obsessively clean. She specialised in painting disturbingly sad and isolated young children - perhaps because she was told when she was young that she should not have children because of her psychiatric condition. Her pictures are always unsentimental and capture the awe-inspiring solemnity of small children. In 1969, she said, "My work is an attempt to communicate beyond the isolation of the individual."

Charles Sims RA 1873-1928

Born in London, Sims trained at art schools in London and Paris and quickly became a critical and academic success. His eldest son was killed during the First World War and, in 1918, Sims himself was sent to France as an official artist. These experiences, together with the move from his home in the country, seem to have marked the beginning of a change in his personality, which became more reserved and aloof. Two years before he committed suicide, he worked on the series *Spiritual Ideas*. During this period he was undergoing treatment by a "nerve specialist". He was experiencing severe insomnia and dreading the approach of old age. The paintings are unlike his usual style: he used abstract form and colour, with the background of all the paintings suggesting a torn curtain through which some mystical experience is glimpsed.

Louis Wain 1860-1939

A graduate of the West London School of Art, Wain began his career as an art journalist but became famous for his humorous drawings of cats - the 'Louis Wain cat' was much in demand from the 1880s to the First World War. However, after the war there was less call for his work and he experienced great poverty. Always known to be an eccentric, he now began to develop signs of serious mental disorder, becoming increasingly suspicious, abusive and occasionally violent. He was certified insane in 1924 and was admitted to Bethlem Hospital the following year. He then moved to

Napsbury Hospital, dying there nine years later. Although he grew increasingly disordered, he continued to paint and draw with his old skill. Thus his work is of great interest because comparisons can be made between works from before his illness to those after, such as *Ginger Cat*, which is quite revealing of his psychotic condition: the cat's eyes are fixed, almost hostile, perhaps because he thought that the world was looking at him in a menacing way.

Cynthia Weldon (née Pell) 1933-1977

Cynthia Weldon, a graduate of Camberwell College of Art, developed a devastating bipolar illness at 16 and was first admitted to St Bernard's Hospital, Southall, in 1961. During the next decade of her life she made several suicide attempts and had frequent admissions to St Bernard's, where she was treated with antipsychotics and electroconvulsive therapy. In 1973 she was admitted to Bexley Hospital and while she was there produced some of her most haunting images. Britta von Zweigbergk, Cynthia's art therapist, became the unofficial "keeper" of her drawings and paintings. She said that she began to see Cynthia as being like a war correspondent reporting from the war-torn battlefield of her experience of severe mental illness: "Her drawings and paintings were her dispatches often sent in a hurry with scant regard for personal safety, the Art Therapy Department acting as a base from which her materials were supplied". In her pictures, Cynthia portrayed with great simplicity and feeling scenes from the daily life of the hospital, of her own suffering and that of other patients. In July 1977 she killed herself by cutting her throat while von Zweigbergk was on holiday.

Index